Youth and Internet Addiction in China

A form of "electronic opium" is how some people have characterized young people's internet use in China. The problem of "internet addiction" (*wangyin*) is seen by some parents as so severe that they have sought psychiatric help for their children. This book, which is based on extensive original research, including discussions with psychiatrists, parents, and "internet-addicted" young people, explores the conflicting attitudes which this issue reveals. It contrasts the views of young people who see internet use, especially gaming, as a welcome escape from the dehumanizing pressures of contemporary Chinese life, with the approach of those such as their parents, who medicalize internet overuse and insist that working hard for good school grades is the correct way to progress. The author shows that these contrasting attitudes lead to battles which are often fierce and violent, and argues that the greater problem may in fact lie with parents and other authority figures, who misguidedly apply high pressure to force young people to conform to the empty values of a modern, dehumanized, consumer-oriented society.

Trent Bax is in the Department of Sociology at Ewha Womans University, South Korea.

Routledge culture, society, business in East Asia series

How and what are we to examine if we wish to understand the commonalities across East Asia without falling into the powerful fictions or homogeneities that dress its many constituencies? By the same measure, can East Asian homogeneities make sense in any way outside the biases of East-West personation?

For anthropologists familiar with the societies of East Asia, there is a rich diversity of work that can potentially be applied to address these questions within a comparative tradition grounded in the region as opposed the singularizing outward encounter. This requires us to broaden our scope of investigation to include all aspects of intra-regional life, trade, ideology, culture, and governance, while at the same time dedicating ourselves to a complete and holistic understanding of the exchange of identities that describe each community under investigation. An original and wide ranging analysis will be the result, one that draws on the methods and theory of anthropology as it deepens our understanding of the interconnections, dependencies, and discordances within and among East Asia.

The book series includes three broad strands within and between which to critically examine the various insides and outsides of the region. The first is about the globalization of Japanese popular culture in East Asia, especially in greater China. The second strand presents comparative studies of major social institutions in Japan and China, such as family, community and other major concepts in Japanese and Chinese societies. The final strand puts forward cross-cultural studies of business in East Asia.

1 Youth and Internet Addiction in China
Trent Bax

Youth and Internet Addiction in China

Trent Bax

Routledge
Taylor & Francis Group

LONDON AND NEW YORK

First published 2014
by Routledge
2 Park Square, Milton Park, Abingdon, Oxfordshire OX14 4RN

Simultaneously published in the USA and Canada
by Routledge
711 Third Avenue, New York, NY 10017

Routledge is an imprint of the Taylor and Francis Group, an informa business

First issued in paperback 2015

British Library Cataloguing in Publication Data
A catalogue record for this book is available from the British Library

Library of Congress Cataloging in Publication Data
Bax, Trent.
Youth and internet addiction in China/Trent Bax.
pages cm.—(Routledge culture, society, business in East Asia series; 1)
Includes bibliographical references and index.
1. Internet and youth—China. 2. Internet addiction—China. 3. Families—China. I. Title.
HQ799.9.I58B39 2013
004.67'80835—dc23
2013004276

ISBN 978-0-415-65691-7 (hbk)
ISBN 978-1-138-64356-7 (pbk)
ISBN 978-0-203-79689-4 (ebk)

Typeset in Times New Roman
by Book Now Ltd, London

Contents

	Introduction: turn on	1
1	Log in	12
2	The Internet Addiction Disorder	23
3	Critiques of the Internet Addiction Disorder model	46
4	The humanistic intensive internet use model	69
5	The family war-machine and the search for freedom	95
6	Push and pull factors	123
7	*DSM-IV* – Internet Addiction Disorder	165
	Conclusion: log off	180
	Notes	186
	References	210
	Index	220

Introduction: turn on

In a groggy and confused existential state Huang He ("Yellow River") walks clumsily along the enclosed hallway of the "Cure Internet Addiction Centre" inside the Linyi No.4 People's Hospital, Shandong Province.[1] His groggy and confused demeanor stems not from his parent's belief that young Huang He is "addicted" to the internet, but rather from the 12 sleeping pills they had secretly fed him so they could transport him from home to hospital. With Dr. Yang Yongxin's hands firmly grasping his shoulders, Huang He looks around the enclosed space between the corridor and the now infamous room no.13 where he is about to be unknowingly subjected to electric-shock treatment and asks:

"What's this all about then?"

His father tells him he has been brought here (against his will and under forced sedation) to cure his internet addiction. Huang He replies: "Cure internet addiction, cure what internet addiction?"

Dr. Yang Yongxin, again holding him from behind, asks rhetorically: "So you don't get online then?" "I get online," he replies, adding: "At present how many young people don't get online?" In the dark as to why he is there, Huang He then turns to his father and enquires: "What are you doing bringing me here? Not once have you told me. You are deceiving me, what's the meaning of all this? I will tell you, I won't accept any medical checkup. Forget it." The father, in a search for justification, then informs Dr. Yang, who is holding the son firmly by the arm, "He breaks things."

Dr. Yang then asks Huang He, "You get online and break things, don't you?"

"I am 18 yrs old, I am an adult. Have you sought my permission for this?" protests Huang He. Sensing trouble, one of Dr. Yang's big burly "assistants" now encircling Huang He chimes in with a not-so-veiled threat: "You cannot leave, don't even bother trying to leave."

"Are you really saying that I can't leave?" an increasingly anxious Huang He retorts. Dr. Yang confidently replies, "Well go and leave then. Don't block him, let's watch him leave." Yang Yongxin, his half-dozen henchmen, and his father, all follow him as he attempts to exit the hospital. Not finding a way out after walking around in circles through the confinement of the enclosed hospital ward, he says to Dr. Yang, "You really think I can't leave?" While encircled by Dr. Yang and his "security" personnal, Dr. Yang replies without a hint of irony,

"Well, no one is blocking you from leaving." Therefore, Huang He rolls up his sleeves and attempts to smash a window with his fist in order to flee. The window – and fortunately his hand – fails to break. Defeated, he is lead away to be "treated" with electro-shock therapy. This little episode we should see as the dark-side of China's *battle with the internet demon*.

While Huang He's battle highlights briefly the extreme lengths parents and mental health professionals in China are willing to go to in order to "rectify" the behavior of youth they see as extreme, the following letter by Xiao Chuan allows us to enter the pre-treatment lifeworld of this young person labeled an internet addict (*wangyin*) by Chinese society's authoritative figures (parents, medical and psychiatric professionals, government officials, and media representatives). This very personal letter, written by 16-year-old Xiao Chuan to his parents, provides us with a window into observing not only the "internet addict"'s' *intra*personal life-world and *inter*personal relations within the family and his peers, but also the *extra*personal structural conditions that all go into constituting his social existence.[2] It is this interrelation between the intrapersonal and interpersonal lifeworld, alongside the intimate interconnection between the real world and virtual world of this person seen as an internet addict, that essentially differentiates the humanistic-based model presented here (what I call the *Intensive Internet Use Model*) from the biomedical-based *Internet Addiction Disorder* concept (what I call the *Young-Tao Model*) this book holds up to the light of critical analysis. The Internet Addiction Disorder concept is given center stage simply because it is this biomedical model that currently dominates both the professional and popular discourse of what should more appropriately be called "socially problematic internet use." This letter is presented in order that, from the outset, we begin to take seriously the most important question we can ask in order to unravel the mystery of an internet addiction phenomenon that has seemingly been sweeping through Chinese society like some neo-SARS virus: *What is the nature of the relation between the "internet addict" and his or her social existence?* In order to answer this question, new concepts and a new approach to this phenomenon are required, most of which are briefly introduced in this chapter. All these concepts will, in turn and in good time, be dealt with – both theoretically and empirically – throughout the book where and when appropriate. And so to Xiao Chuan's *thwarted lifeworld*, as experienced by him:

Dear Mum & Dad,

My exam grade was really bad this time, but I tried my hardest. On Saturday and Sunday I revised for two days, but I could not get my mind to concentrate. Even though you did not let me get online, you still don't understand where I am coming from. All I wanted was a little distraction from study so as to walk into time's gap, for doing so allows me to have a small taste of extreme happiness. But as soon as I return back to reality from being online, I begin to suffer again. You didn't allow me to get online, and so I didn't get online again. You made me study, so I studied. Therefore, you should not get angry again. I have lost too much for you, and done too much for you, but still you want to give me a telling me off. I am not willing to let you.

My best friends are on the internet, and I am able to reveal to them my true intentions and am able to laugh with them. They are extremely important to me, even to the extent that they are more important to me than you are. My family is inside the game, and we never argue, rather we always mutually help each other. I have already lost too much for you, and have paid out too much, so don't force me again. I do not have a broad mind set and I have no thoughts or plans for the future.

The questions in the math exam were quite simple, but because I was careless then I only got a mark of 78. As for the English exam I got 56. I thought that this was an ok grade because I originally thought I was only able to get a mark of 20. History, Geography and Biology I did not remember very firmly. I remembered but then forget it during the exam. As for after the exams, I do not dare to make any guarantees to you, but I will try my best.

From your son, Xiao Chuan[3]

What we should note is that Xiao Chuan, like all the apparent internet addicts presented in this book, is not merely having trouble controlling his internet use, but, much more problematically, he appears to be having trouble with *the normal pattern of living*. As seen through the biomedical lens, however, this person is often presented as living in a kind of social vacuum and so what is overly focused upon is this one-to-one relation between the internet user and the internet – and online games in particular. Once caught in what is often visualized as a kind of dark virtual pit, as though equivalent to the opium addict trapped within an opium den, this "electronic opium" (*dianzi yapian*) is said to have *caused* the now "mentally diseased" internet addict to have cut oneself off from the "true" and "real" world. But what we should note when we glance at Xiao Chuan's letter is this central feature: the "internet addict" is not the only actor in their world.[4]

Yet through the lens of the biomedical-based internet addiction disorder concept this person is often conceptualized as a kind of physical-chemical system or organism, who must first be drained of their interpersonal social existence before they can become an "object of scientific study" so as to be diagnosed with suffering from an *individual pathology* called internet addiction disorder. In order to uncover the underlying mechanisms driving socially problematic internet use, I propose conceptualizing this "internet addict" not as mentally disordered or pathologically sick but principally as a *person related to persons*.[5] As we see with Xiao Chuan, these persons this internet addict is centrally relating to are, first and foremost, his/her parents and then usually his/her "best friends."

Or more precisely, we see that Xiao Chuan is having serious trouble relating on any level to his parents, who he feels do not understand him and the function the internet plays in his life. Moreover, he feels his parents have forced him to "pay out too much" and as a result he feels he has "lost too much" to them. But paid out and lost too much for what exactly? He, like his best friends who he feels – and this is significant – are more important to him than his own parents because they "never argue" and "always help" each other, has devoted his time and energy to school partly *for* his parents and for the normal functioning of society; and in the process paid for it with his happiness. Is this not why he is so attracted to the internet because it offers him both a distraction from this forced "addiction" to schoolwork and school grades and, more importantly, allows him to experience a "small taste of extreme happiness" – happiness which the normal functioning of society too often denies him by making him, as he says, "suffer?" Perhaps what is central to unraveling the mechanisms driving this internet addiction phenomenon is not principally this one-to-one relation between internet user and internet but, rather, their relation to home and school. For it is no coincidence that the vast majority of the entire Chinese population said to have "come down with internet addiction" (*ranshang wangyin*), as though it is somehow an incredibly effective socially selective virus, are adolescents in their mid-to-late teens.

It is also no coincidence that *Xiao Chuan's* letter begins and ends with him highlighting his school grades, for school grades are as important to this internet addiction phenomenon almost as much as the internet itself is. That is, one does not exist without the other. In reality, the internet addiction phenomenon pivots around the competition – between China's education system expressed through the parents and its consumer-based society expressed through the online gaming industry – for the *hearts and minds* of youth. In order to "lock in" the young person to either of the social categories, *student* or *consumer*, we see parents spending vast amounts of personal resources through hard-won gains and sacrifices, while on the other hand, gaming companies spending vast amounts of resources through investment, research, science, development, and advertising, so they can hopefully convince growing and transforming (i.e., individualizing) youths to devote their time, energy, passion, and resources principally to either work or leisure – work in the form of study and leisure in the form of online play.

During this battle for the hearts and minds of individualizing young people who themselves are searching for personal freedom and independence (power), "normal" parents are often chaining their children to schoolwork out of what I call a "chained love" for the child. Yet, at the same time, parents are acting in response to a very real and potent fear that the only-child's successful future may never be realized because they refuse to stop gaming and start studying. By "chaining" I am not merely referring symbolically to the way parents use material rewards in order to buy off the child's devotion to schoolwork – i.e., grades-for-goods – which often results in further deepening the child's already flourishing *love-of-consumption*. But I am also referring to the very concrete way parents use symbolic and physical violence upon a child who loses interest in "boring old school" and, instead, becomes very passionate about the stimulating leisure pursuit of online gaming that provides extreme feelings of happiness, excitement, and satisfaction. For a revealing and symbolic example, we can refer here to the father in Chengdu who literally attached a 14-metre-long metal chain to his 10-year-old son for the whole weekend as a strategy in which to prevent the son from running off to play video games.[6] Not too dissimilar to the actions of the parents presented earlier in this chapter, the son was pulled out of a video game parlor by his mother on a Friday night, after which his father chained the boy to a pillar in their yard, in the hope that he would stay at home and do his homework.

While this son was reportedly watching television while his parents were busy at work, therein forcing us to think about the parent's behavior as a contributing factor in online gaming, later we see more clearly what results when parents beat up or lock up the son as a way in which to prevent him from going to the internet bar so that he can "firmly grasp his studies." In a similar way to which a resistant Xiao Chuan wrote that he "was not willing" to let his parents give him another telling off after he had generally obeyed their orders to "study, study, study," later we observe such parental disciplinary measures produce within the child *fan gan* (a rebellious psychology). The biomedical model, however, argues that this internet addict is very "vulnerable" to the "lure" of online games because he/she possesses "weak self control," as though their own will, volition, and motivation for getting online has somehow been spirited away to the online world. Through *fan gan*, however, we understand that there are very real "push" and "pull" factors – as I call them – driving and motivating young people to seek a social life lived electronically.

We can understand these diverging push and pull factors, and the humanistic model presented in this book, by simply referring to a TV program aired in China on "internet addiction." The chat-style show, one of many aired across China since 2004 discussing "internet addiction," featured a 15-year-old girl sitting beside her mother and sitting next to the show's guest Mr. Tao Hongkai.[7] As will be shown, the Intensive Internet Use Model presented here stems from my participant-observation research with family educator Tao Hongkai. Like "Xiao Wang" in Chapter 2, this 15-year-old girl said that while at school she is "thinking" about getting online, and when she has free time she runs off to the internet bar. As we will see, the biomedical Young-Tao model conceptualizes this process as the user having a "preoccupation" toward the internet and so such thoughts, which is called a "symptom," expresses one of eight *signs* of internet addiction. I will argue, with reference to the American Psychiatric Association's *Diagnostic and Statistical Manual (DSM-IV)*, that such thoughts only make *valid* sense once her entire social existence is factored in.

In fact, this book seeks to demonstrate that the biomedical-based Young-Tao model does not actually adhere to the *DSM-IV*'s definition of a mental disorder. This is important because proponents of the Young-Tao model have been advocating the inclusion of "internet-use disorder" in the next edition of the manual, DSM-V, to be published in 2013. Such advocacy could be said to have partly succeeded, as "internet-use disorder" has been included in the DSM-V as a psychological condition "recommended for further study." This book, however, is precisely this "further study," and the results tell us that "internet-use disorder" is not a legitimate psychological condition of the mind or body.

In any case, the presenter of this particular TV show then asks her to highlight the greatest pleasure she derives from the internet. The girl replies that actually it is just like a kind of "narcotic" (*mazui yao*), as it temporarily gives her a very "cozy feeling" and when she is online she feels very happy. It is this presumed equivalency to narcotics which is central to the biomedical interpretation of "excessive" internet use. The biomedical model argues that online gaming *is just like* smoking opium, with the effect being that this relation between subject and technology "poisons" the mind with what later we see some call "information pollution." This presumed comparability to drugs is then seen to justify the bio-medical model being based upon the same behavioral addiction model that was designed to diagnose drug addicts and compulsive gamblers. However, we know with reference to the famous *pharmakon* concept used by Aristotle and Plato that a substance like a narcotic contains both the poison *and* the remedy.

As Xiao Chuan alludes to, as this girl clearly states, and as the following empirical data and narratives authenticate, rather than simply being a kind of poison poisoning the minds of China's youth, online gaming functions as a kind of "medicine" to existential needs for the survival, maintenance, and even inflation of the self, and thus does not simply result in them "playing the hurt away" as one expert put it. In short, it is through the *creation of tension* while gaming and in the battle with others, which brings "infinite pleasure" as Xiao Kang termed it in his letter, that online gaming can have a liberating, even cathartic, effect for the player because such activities can loosen and even free socially produced stress-tensions. In this sense, online gaming can serve as a kind of antidote or remedy to the stress-tensions being produced within the person by a society like contemporary China going through profound social transformations and disorienting change. For as this girl then says, the biggest effect (*houguo*) of going online is that it allows her to *fa xie* (give vent to) her feelings of frustration, anger, etc. That is, and this comment should be given our full attention, going online allows her to *blow off steam*.

However, their desire to blow off steam through online play only makes sense if we understand the *pressure cooker* that is their so-called "normal" life. Like Xiao Chuan, she adds that "in reality there are too many unfair matters."[8] She adds that pressure, in the "real" world, is sometimes so great that one may not be able to find a good orientation because they feel that real life is too distressing. It is here at the taken-for-granted "normal" functioning of society that the seeds of what is called internet addiction are sown.

The biomedical model holds that the problem of mental health in a society is generally only that of the number of "maladjusted" individuals and not that of a possible maladjustment of the whole social system itself. Turning this problem on its head – using Erich Fromm's *pathology of normalcy* concept – I propose that socially problematic internet use does not principally stem from the maladjusted and pathological individual but, rather, from a maladjusted or "pathological" social system – of which what I call a *culture of excess* or *living out of balance* is ever-present.[9] This pathology of normalcy, as seen through the experience of young people like Xiao Chuan, can be understood to mean a social structure that, in general sense, is adverse to genuine human happiness and self-realization. To be specific, it is because of the *disordered* nature of their lifeworld and the social system they live in that "excessive" internet use has emerged and flourished. And so instead of simply seeing how online games poison both the mind and what is called the "social functioning" of the gamer, perhaps we should focus our attention upon the ways the gamers' whole social existence is itself being "poisoned" by, for example, stress and pressure to achieve within an excessively competitive education system.

It is through the disordered nature of the normal functioning of contemporary Chinese society that the "thirst" for online games is produced, which, in turn, is like a kind of weapon used during the individual's intense confrontation with an often *excessive* and *dehumanizing* modernization process. Central to this dehumanization is, as Xiao Chuan highlights, the immense pressure placed by parents over schoolwork, and school grades in particular. What we see is the child being evaluated not for his *use value*, his humanistic qualities, but, on the contrary, primarily for his *exchange value*, that of school grades, which upon graduation can (hopefully) be exchanged for white-collar employment. We must understand their internet use as partly a response to this set of social and historical conditions. Only by taking this phenomenon into the home by focusing upon the interpersonal relations within the family nexus – relations partly driven by *filiarchy*[10] – does this internet addiction phenomenon begin to make empirical sense. What we discover within the family is not a mentally disordered child, but rather a socially dysfunctional family unit, which can be understood as a kind of *war-machine* because it is composed of two fiercely opposed sides often violently fighting and striving to defend their position and advance their own interests. We can understand the driving forces of this war-machine – when we bring in the work of British psychiatrist R.D. Laing – through the way parents both *engulf* their child by "loving them to (existential) death" and the way they, and the entire education machinery, inadvertently *depersonalize* them through trying to turn them into *grade-making machines*. These factors, among others, basically constitute the push factors driving young people online as a way in which they can *preserve* their (increasing desire for an) autonomous-self. And so far from simply "escaping reality," they are, on the contrary, using the internet *in order to* deal with this [ab]normal pattern of living.

In order to see the other side of this motivational coin – the pull factors drawing them in to the functions of online games because they provide them with *existential trophies* – we can refer to the words of another online gamer on the chat-show mentioned earlier. When asked what pleasure he derived from the internet, this young man said that when playing online games he is able to "obtain great satisfaction," for when his online character is "stronger" and more "impressive" than another's then this makes him feel like "number one." This desire to be *someone* through feeling like a winner by dominating others – what could be called *the laoda effect* – signals not that they have detached themselves from the real world, but, on the contrary, that they are trying to adhere to dominant ethics such as ambition, competition, aggressiveness, and self-assertiveness so central to both contemporary China and online gaming. In effect, powerless individuals living in an authoritarian yet individualizing society, whom are gaining no pleasure from school and home life, are able to feel like a master of their *own* universe and in control while immersed in a social system that constantly reinforces the high social value of individual success and achievement and an individualized life. Again with reference to Fromm, the premise of this process can be conceptualized in the following way: "domination [over others] is the outcome of a thwarted life."[11] Or for our particular purpose: *excessive online gaming is often the outcome of a thwarted life* (and not a disordered mind).

The social and ethical problem for the "internet addict," however, is that he/she is playing the wrong game: the game of *use value* (leisure) and not *exchange value* (work). That is to say, these so-called internet addicts are condemned because they cut themselves off from the normal functioning of society (the society-of-work), and, instead, escape into what is believed to be a world of fantasy. And while "caught" there – like moths to a lamp – they are thought to produce nothing real, and because they are being non-productive they are then said to be "wasting their precious time."[12] But by handing back agency to this person, and through analyzing the functions internet use plays in their lifeworld, we see that what the internet addiction phenomenon amounts to is this: individuals are forced to seek biographical solutions to socially produced problems."[13] This, generally speaking, is because by focusing excessively on economic development the Chinese Party-State has created a system which is, by and large, adverse to producing genuine human happiness and self-realization. That is, it too often does not meet the existential needs of its citizens. And so the actions of these so-called internet addicts glaringly reveal the following structural problem: citizens cannot live on economic reforms alone.

As China-watchers like Duncan Hewett have repeatedly pointed out, China's young generation are caught in the eye of an unprecedented social transformation wherein they are trying – too often without appropriate guidance and the right moral tools – to navigate between a conservative and authoritarian social system and rapidly evolving new lifestyles.[14] In their *search for freedom* from authoritarian structures and their desire to carve out new ways of *being in the world*, these youth labeled as internet addicts reveal the full impact of this social – from Mao-to-market – transformation upon the lives of those straddling the decline of a failed socialist project and the rapid emergence of a technology-driven consumer-based society. And because the internet is at the forefront of this transformation it is having a profound impact upon the development of Chinese society. Tai Zixue, who like many has been writing about the way the internet is contributing (positively) to the emergence of a civil society in China, implores us to "look at how the internet has affected the life of ordinary Chinese citizens to understand the cyber revolution that is taking place in China."[15] This book is designed to do exactly that, but by looking at how the internet is affecting the lives of "ordinary" non-political families this text offers an alternative interpersonal narrative to a more techno-positive discourse centered upon the contributions this cyber revolution is rightfully playing vis-à-vis civil society in China.[16]

The main goal of this book is to critically unpack the dominant discourse around "internet addiction" so as to reveal the contradictions and inconsistencies within the dehumanistic biomedical model, and to then – by way of the empirical social reality of this person wrongly labeled an internet addict – shift the discourse by introducing a humanistic-based theoretical model as a way in which to understand his or her entire social existence. By discarding "internet addiction" in favor of "socially problematic internet use," I am arguing that we are dealing here with a problem of development rather than with a problem of pathology. And because of this, I believe we can better understand this issue if we closely examine people's lives. But this close examination of the lifeworld of those labeled internet addicts, in particular the family nexus, does not then lead us to claim the push and pull forces highlighted later "cause" socially problematic internet use. Of course, some adolescents living in similar social arrangements to those examined later do not have socially problematic relations to online games. This book merely seeks to show the probable, and not definitive, social forces driving this phenomenon. Beyond demonstrating that this phenomenon cannot be reduced to an individual pathology, the broader message is to show those labeled internet addicts are, themselves, living within what we could call an "addict-ogenic culture" wherein "pseudo addiction" (a life of excess) is a general social and historical condition.

Book structure

In order to convince the reader of the need to return back to a modernist humanist tradition as an appropriate way in which to understand the *experience* of living in contemporary Chinese society, I begin in Chapter 1 by describing, in a very straightforward and descriptive manner, my own experience of first entering into and then coming to understand this internet addiction phenomenon. In describing the methodology I am, at the same time, also introducing "the two Taos" – Tao Ran and Tao Hongkai – for they are the central figures both within the internet addiction phenomenon and within this book. The fact is that the humanist perspective presented here was not imposed upon the subject matter simply proactively, but rather grew out of the experience of the field, in particular, the way young people being dehumanized by authority figures such as Tao Ran, during an often dehumanizing modernization process, are themselves responding to this process in ways that could be called *the search for a humanistic life*. In this sense it could be said I am writing on two different narrative levels. On the one hand I am writing on the subject of internet addiction, yet on the other hand I am writing about the thwarted life that resides "underneath" internet addiction. Thus my use of Erich Fromm and R.D. Laing is not simply about imposing them onto a topic or country neither has specifically written on, but rather of bringing to the surface – revealing, with reference to the work of Tao Ran and Tao Hongkai – the *pathology of normalcy* and *culture of excess* that constitutes much of contemporary life in China.

In Chapter 2 I present the (dehumanistic) Internet Addiction Disorder Concept by first presenting the first part of a letter sent by Xiao Wang to Tao Hongkai outlining his relationship to the internet and internet games. I present the first part of this letter as a way in which we can understand both the biomedical visualization and conceptualization of this person they call an internet addict. By only focusing on the *surface* of Xiao Wang's lifeworld, in particular his one-to-one relationship to the internet, I am arguing that the main shortcomings of the biomedical model is its over-emphasis on the *signs* or apparent *symptoms* of internet use and, more importantly, the subsequent negation of the social condition of this person. I also present and critique the two main pillars holding up the Young-Tao model (time spent online and harming social functioning).

Chapter 3 goes to the heart of the Young-Tao model: the eight-point symptom list. This aspect of the model is given extensive attention because the eight-point symptom list is being presented to the academic community, and the American Psychiatric Association in particular, as a valid and reliable model psychiatrists can potentially use as tool to diagnose "internet addiction." By analyzing the literature that relates directly to the eight-point symptom list I am calling into question, even before I use my own empirical data as a critique, both the reliability and validity of the Young-Tao model.

In Chapter 4 I present the theoretical underpinnings of my interpretation of the internet addiction phenomenon, which I call "the Intensive Internet Use model." This model is a "replacement" for the Young-Tao model not in the sense that this model can "diagnose" internet addiction, but rather because internet addiction does not empirically exist, and, therefore, we need new concepts in order to conceptualize and deal with socially problematic internet use among China's youth. The goal is to shift the discourse around internet use by offering a humanistic-based model as a beginning to this discursive shift. In order to differentiate the Intensive Internet Use model from the Young-Tao model I present the second part of Xiao Wang's letter. Part-two of the letter expresses the social condition that Xiao Wang's internet use stems from – phenomenon which must be brought to the surface for analysis if a reliable and valid model is to be authentic. In presenting the Intensive Internet Use model I am also introducing and explaining all the relevant terms and concepts within the model that are later used when, in the main section, the model is applied to the empirical data.

Chapters 5 and 6 constitute the heart of the book, wherein I structure my argument around letters written to Tao Hongkai by the parents of "internet addicts" as a way to understand the entire lifeworld of not simply these so-called internet addicts but, more importantly, their *inter*personal relations with their parents and peers. The letters chosen are referred to as "ideal types" not because they offer ideal or causal examples, but rather because they closely approximate representative examples containing the common themes that consistently emerge from the letters and thus the phenomenon itself. So while I am referring to one letter in particular, in fact this letter is speaking more generally about the common characteristics specific to the parent's narrative. Understanding the social existence of the children contextualizes their behavior and through the parents' narratives we are able to understand certain social conditions that "push" young people to seek a life lived electronically.

But I also move beyond the interpersonal toward the *extra*personal by locating internet use within materialism in general and the consumer-driven society in particular. Doing so allows us to see that far from their behavior simply being "pathological," intensive internet use, on the contrary, drives to the heart of the consumer-driven society and the policies of the reform era. Taking the argument to this more structural and organizational level calls into question the assumed "cause" of problematic internet use, for the Party-State has created the specific conditions for excessive or intensive internet use to exist and flourish. In this way we learn that the "internet addict" is not a product of mental illness but rather a product of their time, for the *intensification of life* is emblematic of China's culture of excess. To complete the main body of the text I focus the analysis upon the *intra*personal factors contributing to increased internet use. Through Xiao Kang's letter we learn about the aspects which "pull" them in to the virtual world. Far from seeing their attraction to online games as a mechanism which allows them to *escape reality*, we learn through Xiao Kang's experience that intensive gamers are, on the contrary, using online games in order to seek and obtain contemporary China's dominant social values. In this way intensive gaming is not remedial in a medicinal sense, but rather life-changing in an existential sense.

Chapter 7 functions as a kind of litmus test for the Young-Tao model while, simultaneously, providing empirical support for the validity of the Intensive Internet Use model. The filter for this litmus test is the American Psychiatric Association's *DSM-IV*, because, as already mentioned, it is this manual the proponents of the Young-Tao model are using to seek legitimacy. But once the entire lifeworld of the "internet addict" is factored into the equation then it is clear that they do not adhere to the *DSM-IV*'s own definition of a mental disorder, and thus the Young-Tao model is not only misguided but illegitimate.

In highlighting the serious shortcomings of the Young-Tao biomedical model the concluding chapter should be read as the end-of-the-beginning, for a new approach to dealing with problematic internet use is proposed. This approach does not simply force individuals to change but rather seeks to uncover the intra-, inter- and extra-personal factors underlining socially problematic internet use. Quite simply, it is not that those labeled internet addicts have unhinged themselves from the "real" world, but rather that the normal functioning of society is not satisfying their existential needs. Only by uncovering their "biopsychosocial" needs are we able to seek real-world solutions to their psychosocial problems.

1 Log in

A walk into the wild frontier with Renfei

Initially, I envisioned becoming an ethnographer by employing the ethnographic method of participant-observation to acquire knowledge of this phenomenon called "internet addiction." By observing, and thus by implication participating in the activities young people engage in while *hanging out* in internet bars, I envisioned understanding the world of those in China whose waking and dreaming lives are dominated by computer technologies. The initial set of probing questions centered upon discovering what is it that attracts them to games such as *World of Warcraft* to such a degree that they are willing to spend in excess of six hours at any one time plugged into it – and then finding themselves labeled as "internet addicts" by their parents and people such as Tao Ran. I was also interested in discovering what is it about the internet bar which attracts China's youth with such intensity and devotion that they are willing – in their tens of millions – to spend large amounts of their waking, eating and sleeping hours in this light-deprived/light-intensive smoked-filled space seemingly isolated from the normal functioning of society, yet at the same time, plugged into a virtual world with both virtual and real characters.

Ever since the production of Malinowski's *Argonauts of the Western Pacific* have ethnographers embedded themselves into a social setting with the desire for understanding, from the ground up, the social reality of social organization. Understanding the social reality of young people labeled "internet addicts" is especially important because, as one of China's leading film makers Jia Zhangke pointed out, when many of China's young speak, nobody listens.[1] As a result they have few opportunities to express their ideas and to assert their opinions about society.[2] By "letting them speak" and by focusing upon the conditions in which their social reality arises we can, as R.W. Connell argued, paint a collective portrait – using language – of a group of people caught up in a certain process of social transformation.[3] Michael Burawoy said real workers should be examined in real productive circumstances, and so should real internet users be examined in real productive circumstances.[4]

Therefore I first sought out a close and trusted friend, called Renfei, to introduce me to the world of online gaming. I decided to hang out with Renfei not only because we already had an established trust-based relationship,[5] but also because for Renfei the internet is not simply part of his life but, as he put it: "The internet *is* my life." Therefore I lived with 26-year-old Renfei in Dalian city, Liaoning Province, for two months at the end of 2008 as a way of observing, at close hand and in a natural intimate setting, the lifeworld of a young Chinese man who could, if subjected to the commonly held criteria for categorizing internet addiction, in theory be labeled as an "internet addict" because he was spending about 12 hours per day online – thus exceeding, by double, the six-hour-per-day threshold currently being advocated (details are provided later). Through Renfei and his family and friends I sought, following Turkle's method for understanding internet-mediated relations, to enquire into a) how netizens and those concerned about internet use perceive the technology, b) what motivates people to use this technology, and c) what users obtain and lose by using it. As Turkle argued, this is to highlight not only what computers do *for* them but also what computers do *to* them.[6] Basically, this required hanging out with Renfei in order to see the dynamic flux of experience as it becomes through, and not outside of, time.[7]

I quickly discovered that surrounding Renfei's apartment one could literally locate an internet bar on every street corner.[8] I was attracted to one internet bar in particular because of its auspicious name: *The Free Space Internet Bar*. As Renfei had informed me beforehand, if I purchased a rechargeable membership card I could acquire 110 hours for 100 yuan, or 50 hours for 50 yuan, which is half the price of the normal rate of 2 yuan per hour. Thus, the more one "invests" in internet time the cheaper it is, which means that the economic model of the internet bar must be seen, from the outset, as playing a part in enticing young people to spend longer and longer periods of time online.

The first thing observed in the internet bar is that which one observes when encountering the Chinese city: atomization. Netizens were intensely focused on the machine in front of them, with many males constantly yelling out – to themselves, their friends or opponents within the game – the harshest possible expressions within the Chinese language. While it is easy to frame their cursing as a sign of moral decay, this strips away the functional component of these expressions as, for example, mantras or slogans "recited" by the frustrated, the angry, the estranged, and the competitive. While many would come to the internet bar with friends, or come to meet friends, socializing was mostly conducted through their separate computers as they were either playing against each other or playing as a team against others. We could say they were together-apart. This is partly an outcome of the physical structure of the internet bar itself, as it is designed – with computers lined up in rows – generally for individual and not group play.

With each user attached to the computer in front of them in a state of intense play, and often wearing headphones, then it was very difficult to make contact with them. In a way the netizen is not in the internet bar itself, but paradoxically, in cyberspace. For the lone user the internet bar is a kind of interface between the real and virtual world. Thus after a number of unsuccessful visits to different internet bars I realized that to understand the online gamer *in action* one needs to go where they existentially are, and that is in cyberspace. Renfei therefore said: "You need to get inside in order to understand the research. You have to get lost in order to be clear."

I very quickly became lost in *Perfect World*. Before playing the Chinese manufactured game *Perfect World* a technician in an internet bar helped to open my account, showed me how to create my avatar and how to begin to play the game. Once left to my own devices, however, I quickly became lost, unable to carry out the basic tasks required to advance within the game. Nevertheless, I have since learnt that *Perfect World* can be visualized as a kind of metaphor for understanding what is so attractive about the internet for China's youth. The game is designed to have your avatar – as the center of a perfect world – meet up with other avatars that will help you while, at the same time, other players come to you asking if you want to play with them. The emphasis is on "warm" social relations based, ideally, on equality, trust, sharing and mutual benefit. Interestingly, one's avatar also has the power to fly, which can be understood as a metaphor symbolizing the *search for freedom* I outline later as an important "pull" factor drawing them in to cyberspace. Or as Renfei's ex-work colleague sang while sitting on a mini-stage in a private karaoke room surrounded by her work colleagues: "Come along with me to a faraway frontier borderland."[9]

Perfect World is a kind of enchanted pastoral world, full of green rolling hills, trees, sparse physical infrastructure, no cars, meandering dirt tracks, and few people. Basically, a world that is in important ways the binary opposite of their "real" life, which is densely urban and bursting with buildings, cars and certain strangers who rather than wanting to help you sometimes want to deceive you or even dismiss you completely. For example, while chatting to "rain" online I asked her what is good about the city of Jingzhou where she lives. "Everything is good," she replied, "but the people." She said they are "bad" because they often steal. Likewise, Renfei himself said one day: "There are so many thieves around it is frustrating." And while hanging out with Renfei's friend Zhaonan in his home-city of Anshan late one evening she received a call from her worried mother. According to Zhaonan there are "lots of bad people around." This fear of the stranger and of becoming a potential victim of crime resulted in Zhaonan ringing her mother once the taxi had arrived at her apartment, wherein the mother came down to the street level to collect her hopefully-safe daughter. Little wonder that young people are so attracted to going to a perfect world. Nevertheless, it teaches us that the virtual world only makes sense if we understand their real world – and, most importantly, the interconnection between the two.

Renfei subsequently taught me how to play the video games *World of Warcraft* and *Counter Strike*. In order to experience, first-hand, what it was like to spend hours in a smoke-filled internet bar playing games with friends we frequented on a number of occasions one of the local internet bars to play *Counter Strike*. Instead of just "killing" each other we instead decided to do what most gamers do, and that was to form a team so that we could then work together to achieve the goals set out within the game. The effect of doing so was to strengthen our friendship, as through working and strategizing together you become a team. As Renfei said, playing online games together cannot only bring friendships closer together but can also turn acquaintances into "true" friends. In a society where making "true" friends is often difficult, we should not be too surprised that online games are seen as so attractive to people searching for a sense of belonging and relatedness.

In addition, he also helped me to open up a QQ address so that I could chat to people.[10] On QQ I discovered a whole range of chatrooms where netizens can go to find a friend or partner, chat about online games, favorite hobbies, music, etc. I used these chatrooms in order to chat freely with people throughout China, wherein I asked them about their lives in general and their feelings toward, and opinions on, online gaming and the internet. Unlike meeting these complete strangers in an internet bar face-to-face, wherein one would be guarded about what one says, I found them to be incredibly open and forthright. In trying to make sense of this phenomenon, Renfei noted that young people in China are generally more open in expressing themselves while messaging online. "They don't care about losing face," he explained, "because online they don't have a face, it is faceless." He also said that while the appearance online can be faked (name, address, gender, age, etc), the feelings and emotions expressed are often very real. They may change the "façade" or outer appearance of their presentation-of-self while online but they tend to not hide their feelings.

While hanging out with Renfei and his family and friends provided me with useful empirical and experiential data, and while the conversations I had on QQ with people scattered across China supplied me with worthwhile auxiliary material, I had yet to encounter my first "internet addict." In order to move from the lives of "normal" young people wherein the internet is deeply embedded into their entire lifeworld, and toward the lives of "abnormal" young people called "internet addicts" where the internet is said to have consumed their life, I decided to make contact with Mr. Tao Hongkai.

The two Taos and the oscillating Keith Bakker

Before outlining my experience with Tao Hongkai it is imperative we first situate not only the work of Tao Hongkai, but also the complicated relationship to his nemesis and the main proponent of the internet addiction disorder, Mr. Tao Ran.

Tao Hongkai is an educator who spent 18 years working in the US and returned to Wuhan in 2003 to retire quietly. One day, however, his attention was drawn to a newspaper article about a girl said to be "addicted" to the internet and her seemingly helpless and distraught mother. Tao Hongkai subsequently called the family and after several hours chatting with them the daughter agreed to give up the internet and return back to focusing on her schoolwork. After this initial success, Mr. Tao encountered unexpected fame and became an idol for parents whose children spent too much time online. Parents from far and wide began seeking out his guidance. Between 2004 and 2011 he spent his days and nights traveling all over China appearing on TV programs, giving interviews, taking courses, and visiting schools and boot camps spreading an education- and communication-based method. By describing his method as "quality education" (*suzhi jiaoyu*), Tao Hongkai was attaching himself to a debate over national education policy and ideology that, since 1985, has focused on using education to improve the "*suzhi*" (quality) of the Chinese population.[11] At the same time he has been involved in a very public battle with military-psychiatrist Tao Ran over the public discourse of problematic internet use. While Tao Ran has been advocating – using the internet addiction concept – a psychiatric-based medicalized discourse for framing the problem, Tao Hongkai has been arguing that what China is facing is a set of societal problems, in particular a problematic education system and counter-productive parenting.

In order to understand the diverging worlds of Tao Ran *the doctor* and Tao Hongkai *the educator*, we can refer to the experience of Mr. Keith Bakker as emblematic of the differences between these two opposing forces. In 2006 Keith Bakker was the first person in Europe to open up a "detox clinic" (in Amsterdam) for game addicts offering in-house treatment using essentially a biomedical model as his guiding method. Echoing the biomedical model outlined later, Bakker initially said: "Video games may look innocent, but they can be as addictive as gambling or drugs and just as hard to kick."[12] At the end of 2008, however, Bakker had a major methodological and theoretical change of heart. "The more we work with these kids the less I believe we can call this addiction," he told the BBC. "What many of these kids need," continued Bakker, "are their parents and their school teachers – this is a social problem." While starting out thinking "game addiction" was an individual pathology, Bakker is now of the view that the gaming problem "is a result of the society we live in today." In particular, Bakker has observed that 80 percent of the young people his clinic has seen have been bullied at school and feel isolated. Therefore, he (like Tao Hongkai) believes many of the symptoms they have can be solved by going back to "good old-fashioned communication."[13] Echoing Bakker's findings, Tao Ran has actually observed the same troubled social existence of his own "patients." In direct contradiction to his diagnostic-based psychiatric model, as we will see, he has said the following crucial statements:

1) Every child in this rehab center has a sad or miserable history, because their parents didn't treat them justly.[14]
2) Of the kids that come to our base, 58 percent have been cursed and beaten by their parents.[15]
3) Parents who are violent toward their children and in families where relationships are not good drive children to seek consolation from the internet.
4) [Of the "internet addiction sufferers" confined to his military hospital] 95 percent are boys who lack the love of a father.[16]

While emphasizing their troubled social existence, Tao Ran does not then base either diagnosis or treatment upon this foundation but rather focuses upon individual pathology, therein washing over the interpersonal dynamics involved. However for Bakker, as it partly is with Tao Hongkai, the root cause of the huge growth in excessive gaming lies not with individual pathology but generally with parents who have failed in their duty of care. "It's a choice," Bakker says. "These kids know exactly what they are doing and they just don't want to change."

Bakker has learnt that feelings of anger, frustration and powerlessness often exist *prior* to their gaming, and that alienated youth bond in the virtual world in order to find a sense of community and belonging. In reflecting upon his methodological and theoretical shift, Bakker says that calling gaming an addiction strips away the element of choice or agency these youth have. Finally, he adds: "In most cases of compulsive gaming, it is not addiction and in that case, the solution lies elsewhere."[17] In short, we could say this: Bakker started out as Tao Ran and ended up as Tao Hongkai. Or we could say that instead of merely focusing upon the overt signs and symptoms stemming from excessive internet use Bakker chose to focus upon the entire social existence of the gamer.

Understanding Tao Hongkai's approach to problematic internet use can be summed up by simply referring to the title of his first book: *Internet addiction is not the child's fault*. Tao Hongkai lays a large portion of the causes of "internet addiction" not simply at the feet of the child, but rather at the feet of the parents and the "unharmonious" interpersonal relations between them brought about by the parents' problematic educational and socialization methods. Because of the one-child policy, the excessively competitive education system, and the rise of materialism and consumerism, Tao Hongkai believes parents – who themselves are under immense pressure to conform – are spoiling and thus smothering their kids.

After observing the actions of thousands of families he says that for the parents the main concern is the child's school grade, and so when the child does well the parents and the grandparents will reward the child by saying that he/she can choose want they want as a reward. This, he says, creates a culture-of-dependence, and so parents, if they want to develop "quality education" within the home, must be much stricter on their own actions if they are to produce a child who has both independence and self control. His criticism of the parent's misguided socialization measures toward the child can be summed up in the famous saying *wang zi cheng long* (wishing the child will become successful).[18] Tao Hongkai counters this wishful thinking by saying parents should not be wishing their child will become successful, but rather should be: *jiao zi cheng long* (educating their child to become successful).[19] Therefore, he attempts to get "engulfing" parents to take a step back from their child's lifeworld so that the child can become a) more independent, b) more able to control their own actions, and, c) able to "love oneself." An independent, autonomous, self-loving and self controlling individual, Tao Hongkai believes, will be less likely to become enthralled in the internet because they possess the existential tools needed to "resist" the pull factors of the internet in general, and online games in particular.

Becoming an "expert" on internet addiction

After contacting Tao Hongkai expressing an interest in meeting with him to learn about both his work and this social phenomenon, I was promptly invited by him to attend a series of events he was involved in, first in Wuhan, then in Jinan, and finally in Beijing. In Wuhan I took part in the filming of a TV show appropriately titled "*Communication*" (*goutong*), wherein Tao Hongkai and a host of families who had sought his guidance discussed internet addiction.

In Wuhan I also took part, as suddenly a "foreign expert on internet addiction," in a seminar Tao Hongkai was giving at Huazhong Normal University with Mr. Jin Rui, an official from the Communist Youth League's Ministry of Culture.[20] In seeking to put forth "suggestions" rather than "explanations,"[21] I suggested to the sixty or so students attending the seminar that perhaps we should think about the linkage between the exponential and simultaneous growth of both "internet addiction" and Christianity in China. I used the example of a friend's cousin whose family labeled him an internet addict as he would spend days at a time in the internet bar. Their method of fixing – or getting rid of – the problem was to send him off to the People's Liberation Army (PLA); which he subsequently escaped from. I focused on the fact that not only had his parents divorced when he was young, but his mother had left for South Korea and his father had basically rejected him therein forcing him to live with his maternal grandparents. Little surprise, I suggested, that he preferred the internet bar over home. I connected this anecdote to the general argument that it is a *search for belonging and relatedness* that is driving the rapid growth of Christianity in China, and so instead of simply accusing the son of being an addict is it not more productive to say he is himself in search of a sense of belonging, and so the internet and the internet bar serve that function?[22]

In Jinan city, we visited a military-style boot camp called "The Shandong Healthy Internet Training Base" where Tao Hongkai acted as a consultant. The owner of the camp, like the majority across China, is an ex-PLA officer who had opened up this very lucrative operation with other ex-PLA personnel after Tao Hongkai had "saved" his son from online gaming.[23] A press conference was given in front of local journalists and a TV crew, while the students at the camp – all dressed in military fatigue uniforms – were ordered to put on a brief military display in the camp's courtyard so as to signify to both the "distinguished guests" and the public their uniform obedience, discipline, goodness, and purity. After a tour of the camp, myself and the two other foreign guests gave speeches to about 30 parents whose children were currently staying in the camp and who themselves had come to receive Tao Hongkai's guidance. I suggested to the parents that we ask why is it that when people engage in acts that are considered abnormal, deviant, and criminal that they are almost automatically said to have a mental illness.[24] I suggested that we think through the reasons why most young people reject the label "internet addiction," as does not this stigmatizes them and label them as "sick." I wanted to put forth the suggestion that the internet addiction concept is maybe not the best tool for creating solutions to their problems.

Besides interacting with parents, sessions were organized so that we could meet and chat with the "internet addicts" themselves, away from both their parents and the camp's authorities. The conversations (and fun) we had with them further solidified the view that they are in no way "mentally ill," but are, using unconventional methods, generally grappling with having to grow up during a time of gigantic and disorienting social transformation. In this sense, the epistemological premise of this book is Marx's famous quote "It is not consciousness that determines life, but life that determines consciousness."[25] Or we can rephrase this by saying "It is not mental illness that determines internet addiction, nor internet addiction that determines mental illness, but life that determines socially problematic internet use." This is to say that thoughts and actions are formed under the pressure of the material and social circumstances in which they live, and thus these thoughts and the actions accompanying them are attempts to make sense of their situation and to guide their everyday actions.[26]

In Jinan we also participated in a TV program on Shandong TV called *Tianxia Fumu*,[27] wherein the title of that particular show was called "*Curing Internet Addiction*" (*Jie Wangyin*). The centerpiece of the show was a family in which the apparently "internet addicted" father, who refused to appear because he considered his playing to be a hobby, was accused by the mother of turning the son into an "internet addict," after playing online games together seemingly "caused" his school grades and interest in school to decline. The son, who himself claimed he began playing online games because all his friends were, said that when he did not get a good school grade he felt terrible and so this would prompt him to want to go and play games. I suggested to Tao Hongkai that his online gaming is a symptom rather than a cause of his (life) problems.

In Beijing I attended a four-day course Tao Hongkai was taking in conjunction with a recently opened treatment center. The course – costing 3,750 yuan per family – was attended by ten families and twenty-five parents and children. To begin the course a seminar was held where I was asked to speak to the families (and a number of educators, lawyers, and non-governmental organization workers). I began by pointing out that the actual origin of the concept internet addiction came from a joke made by Ivan Goldberg in 1996 and, until now, no reputable university or organization had, at that point, accepted it as a scientific definition. I also said that the topic of internet addiction could fit into a quote from Mao Zedong's famous Little Red Book that reads: *xian shengchan, hou shenghuo* (first production, then life).[28] In many ways the problem of playing online games is encapsulated in this quote for there is a value placed upon work and production and a devaluation placed upon leisure – even despite the fact that market reforms have produced a whole consumer-based-culture industry of desire and pleasure in contemporary China. Attending the four-day course gave me an opportunity to spend time with the parents and the children and to observe directly the problems existing between them.

I also visited the "Adolescent Excessive Use of the Internet Intervention Studies Centre" in the suburbs of Beijing. Although there were only four students staying at the center at the time – and one of these was there because his mother thought he was homosexual and so was trying to rectify his "abnormal" thoughts – the very large center can house forty-eight students. Whereas the military-style boot camp places emphasis on military discipline and so separates the child from the family,[29] this school, in contrast, sees the solution to the problem involving factoring in the parents as one important piece of the puzzle. Therefore instead of employing ex-PLA soldiers, this center has employed fresh graduates who have majored in communications, management, and psychology. There is also a dormitory for the parents to stay in. In addition to a number of large glasshouses where local residents grow fruit and vegetables, and a large sports facility, the center also has "therapy dogs" and a host of other animals to help in the therapeutic process. The premise being that adolescents who find human relations cold and loveless can take comfort, and find love, in the warmth of these animals.

The letters

In addition to the empirical data gained by observing and participating in Tao Hongkai's work, I have chosen to place central importance upon a different set of data I came into contact with through him. In addition to thousands of parents attending his lectures, seminars, and courses, around 3000 parents have written to him directly begging him to "rescue" their child from "internet addiction." I was given complete access to all these letters, and so randomly chose fifty to translate and interpret (e.g., Xiao Chuan's). Obviously this collection of letters is not a random sample in the conventional statistical sense. But it is a random sample of a "natural" kind, written by parents across all of China who can be taken as representative of a larger population of parents seeking help for their child's "internet addiction."[30] As it happened, all the letters were written by a parent concerning the behavior of the son. While this fact would prompt many to then look to gender-related factors such as "masculinity" as explanatory tools, I have decided to concentrate upon a deeper humanistic level so that the model can be more inclusive. This is not to deny the importance of gendered factors, rather it is to present an alternative model in thinking about internet use to the dominant biomedical model so that, in future, we can refine this model to include a more nuanced set of tools and concepts.

The importance of the letters stems from the central fact that it is the parents, and not the child, who are attaching labels such as "internet addiction" upon their child's deviant behavior. And so the letters offer us a direct window through which we can view the way the parents (in particular, the mother) regard, and thus evaluate, the behavior of their child. At the same time, and often inadvertently, we are also able to observe the problematic behavior of the parents themselves. Because of the very serious "cry for help" underpinning the letters we understand that parents are not intentionally suppressing facts or trying to be misleading, for they are anxious – dreadfully anxious – to be as helpful as possible for they see Tao Hongkai as literally the last port of call before the family sinks into some kind of permanent and entrenched state of war.[31] What is significant about the letters – which in essence comprise the parent's interpretation of the family – is the way crucially important events within the family are seemingly discounted or denied; or more specifically, the way very serious implications *in* the facts are discounted or denied that call into question, and actually negate, the internet addiction disorder concept.[32] The death, absence, neglect, and/or violence of the father and the divorce of the parents are exemplary examples, as these "acute and chronic stressors," as Horwitz calls such social phenomena,[33] are the primary reasons for the emergence of symptoms of distress within the child, which diagnostic psychiatry sometimes mistakenly classifies as mental disorders, and, as we will see, authority figures misguidedly classify as "internet addiction."

The parents' letters, which we shall see share many common characteristics, can be understood with reference to what Arthur Kleinman calls "the illness narrative." For Kleinman the illness narrative is a story the patient tells, and significant others retell, in order to give coherence and meaning to the distinctive events surrounding their illness and suffering. We can understand the illness narrative, or in our case the "internet addiction narrative," as the story parents tell *on behalf of* the child as a way to provide Tao Hongkai coherence to what the parents believe are distinctive events surrounding the child's descent into internet addiction. Kleinman argues that "plot lines, core metaphors, and rhetorical devices that structure the illness narrative are drawn from cultural and personal models for arranging experiences in meaningful ways and for effectively communicating those meanings."[34]

To simplify, the dominant internet addiction narrative about the child spending all their time at internet bars (or at home) playing games is couched around the core metaphor of "internet addiction," whereby parents, almost as a knee-jerk reaction, frame their child's "excessive" gaming as stemming from internet addiction and so criticize and force them to accept the parent's interpretation of events. The child rejects this interpretation and, through *fan gan* (feelings of rebellion), returns back to the internet bar. Upon returning the child is usually beaten physically, which results in them running back to the internet bar for longer periods. Around this point communication usually breaks down between the child and his/her parents. The narrative then hits a wall of disbelief whereby the parents do not know where to turn next as they have run out of resources and strategies for dealing with a disobedient child; and so the narrative can take a number of different routes. One is to seek the help of family and friends. One is to send the child off to a private school. One is to contact a psychiatrist. One is to send the child off to an Internet Addiction Treatment Clinic/Camp or the military. One is to seek the help of Tao Hongkai. And one is to try some or all of these methods as each step, in turn, fails to adhere to the parent's best wishes.

The parent's internet addiction narrative signifies that these methods are designed not simply to "cure" the child but rather to restore "order," "control," "balance," or "stability" to the wayward child so that, above all else, the child will return back to school. As one 14-year-old girl told me while she was going through treatment at the boot camp in Jinan, one of the major effects of the camp is that it does not allow you to think of the internet as all the talk is centered around getting into a good university.

As Kleinman points out, the web of meanings enmeshed within the narrative only make sense in the context of the lives of *all* concerned. But to understand these lives and the narrative it creates, we must relate life and the distress and suffering it creates to cultural, social, economic, and political context. Thus the letters are employed to illuminate the significant interpersonal relations and the structural conditions of the child labeled an internet addict. More generally, the narratives – which is my interpretation of the Chinese family said to have an internet addict for a child – is filtered through the *DSM-IV*'s definition of a mental disorder. The letters, along with the data stemming from fieldwork with Tao Hongkai, must not be understood as "second-hand" and "first-hand" data, respectively, but should, instead, be understood as a couple, with each informing the other. If distinction exists, then the letters can be visualized as the (private) "back-stage" of the family relations, and my encounters with these families as the (public) "front-stage."

However, there is something significant about the letters that an outsider like myself has difficulty obtaining from face-to-face encounters with parents of so-called internet addicts. The value of the letters resides in the parent's revelation of deeply private, distressing, and intimate thoughts and feelings relating to very serious problems existing within the family nexus. In this way the letters cast an illuminating light upon a central part of their lives that is normally only discussed with family members and close friends.[35] While Tao Hongkai gave permission to freely translate and publish them in their original state, in order to ensure complete confidentiality all names and places have been altered.

2   The Internet Addiction Disorder

Xiao Wang: I am an internet addict, save me

What follows is the first part of an extraordinary letter sent to Tao Hongkai in the hope that he could *save* this young man from the clutches of "internet addiction." This letter is extraordinary because unlike most young people who are sent by their parents, almost always through deception, to military-style and medicalized boot camps and treatment centers, Xiao Wang actually sought out help on his own accord. For example, of the approximately 3000 letters that accompanied this one in Tao Hongkai's office, perhaps 5 percent were written by the "internet addict" him/herself. The other 95 percent or so are written by a parent, usually a mother, imploring educator Tao Hongkai to save their child from the dreaded internet addiction. And so to Xiao Wang's internet use:

> I have already lost confidence in my own life. I am already close to desperation.

> I'm Xiao Wang, I have just turned 18. My home is in Shanmei, Shanxi province. My father works at the county Public Security Bureau, and mum was laid-off from a state-owned enterprise a few years back. From primary school to middle school, you could say that my school grades were not too bad. But in the second semester of the first year of middle school, from within my quiet study life, there emerged "the internet." In the weekends I would meet my classmates and together we would go to the internet bar and hang out. It took quite a long period of time for me to slowly feel that it was good fun. Gradually the number of times I went to play took a bee-line upwards. Basically by the third year of middle school I was going every day, returning home to eat dinner and then using an excuse to say that I had lots of homework to do. At that time my school grades had already taken a bee-line downwards, and so dropped down to the bottom ten in the class. My father caught me at the internet bar during lunchtime and so got me by the collar and took me home and beat me.

> From then on my pocket money said goodbye to me. I didn't go to the internet bar again for a while, but after a period of time, I couldn't restrain myself. But I had to labor under the fact that I didn't have any money, so one night, after

Mum and Dad had gone to sleep, I secretly went into their room, and stole 50 yuan out of mum's clothes' pocket. That evening I prostrated with fear! Thankfully the following day she had not discovered it missing.

Then an old weakness arrived, and I again went to the internet bar. But my parents found out what I was doing and so I was again given a full beating! After some time I went to the internet bar again! But my dad and mum were controlling me more and more severely. But sitting in school my mind was always unable to be calm, as I was always thinking about going to play. I therefore began cutting class. Slowly I began skipping a whole day. The teacher discovered that I was often not in class and so rang my home. After getting home dad and mum locked me in the home, and wouldn't let me out. This carried on for more than half a month until I wrote a guarantee that from now on I wouldn't go to the internet bar again.

During the period after the exam I couldn't resist the lure of the internet bar, and so my time spent there became more and more. The internet addiction was getting bigger and bigger! Since getting online, I slowly discovered that my life and environment had gone through a big change. My eyesight had gotten worse, things that are three meters away became a blur. My character has also changed, for a person who was not originally that open has become even more introverted, and I now also speak less. It is like I have become an individual.

But following the changes in relation to reality, my form within the internet has also started to change! Real-world friends have become less and less, while virtual friends in the virtual world has gotten more and more. It has simply become an inverse ratio!

It would appear, on the *surface* at least, that Xiao Wang offers us a classic case of "internet addiction" – at least as it is commonly conceived. Xiao Wang seemingly presents us with all the *overt signs* of a person addicted to the internet. Like a train leaving the station for a virtual world, he writes of slowly feeling that internet use was fun and then, gradually, this usage speeds up exponentially. This addiction, as he himself defined it, was characterized by him being unable to restrain himself from heading back to the internet bar. As though stuck on a seesaw, his internet use took a bee-line upwards while, conversely, his school grades took a bee-line downwards. This apparent inability to restrain himself from the fun and excitement of the internet became a kind of "old weakness" that would *compulsively* repeat itself. It would appear that he had lost control over his own behavior, or, conversely, that the internet had somehow taken control of him as he was unable to resist its alluring qualities. That is, like the opium addict of the nineteenth century, it looks as though he is hooked on the twenty-first century's *electronic opium*.[1] After all, even while sitting in school, far away from the internet bar, he was unable to maintain a calm mind because he was always thinking about going to play at the internet bar. In order to placate this thirst and eradicate these apparent withdrawal symptoms, Xiao Wang began cutting class. Like a snowball rolling down a snow covered hillside, the more he was sucked into the vortex of this addiction the bigger it all seemed to get.

Thus everything began to change for Xiao Wang, for example, his eyesight worsened, his "relatively introverted" character became more and more introverted, and, like an "inverse ratio" or a world turned on its head, real-world friends decreased while simultaneously virtual-world friends increased. Tao Ran, a psychiatrist, PLA Colonel and Communist Party member, has written the following about these perceived physiological effects of internet addiction Xiao Wang seems to find himself *caught in*:

> Internet addiction causes network autonomic dysfunction, gastrointestinal disorders, eye fatigue and other somatic symptoms. This will result in serious physical discomfort for young people. This discomfort will add to their emotional disorder, leading to further internet use, and thus to reduced social or outdoor activities.[2]

Or as Tao Ran put it much more succinctly and poetically, yet a lot less scientifically, to a journalist: *Their souls are gone to the online world.*[3]

Tao Ran and the war on gaming

The first casualty of war is truth.

Hiram Warren Johnson[4]

War is a game of deception.

Sun Zi[5]

Tao Ran, who is the director of the most well-known internet addiction treatment center in China at Beijing's Military General hospital, had previously worked in the psychiatric profession treating perceived opium addicts and alcoholics before embarking on the very lucrative endeavor of treating those whose souls have seemingly gone to the online world. Due to his professional background as a military psychiatrist treating "addicts,"[6] then we should not be at all surprised to hear him say the following about internet addiction: "If you let someone go online and then he can't go online, you may see a physical reaction, just like someone coming off drugs."[7]

After all, does not this statement gel smoothly with Xiao Wang's own narrative, in that he could not calm his mind because he was thinking about playing online when he should have been thinking of schoolwork? And likewise, it seems to make sense both vis-à-vis Tao Ran's professional history and Xiao Wang's self-analysis, for Tao Ran to say the following about the behavior of the internet addict: "Today you go half an hour, and the next day you need 45 minutes. It's like starting with drinking one glass and then needing half a bottle to feel the same way."[8]

After all, did not Xiao Wang himself say that the number of times he went to play online took a bee-line upwards after he discovered how much fun and alluring online gaming was? For Tao Ran, drug addiction, alcoholism, gambling addiction, and internet addiction are all comparative because, according to him, "the effects are the same." That is: "Some addicts drop out of school, some mug people for money, steal and sell their families' things to keep playing games. Some end up killing themselves because they feel life has no point."[9]

In order to make this dramatic and often tragic connection between the actions of the internet addict and the desperate and down-and-out drug addict, Tao Ran offers examples such as one of his patients who, like a snake hibernating from a cold environment, apparently went into an internet bar in the winter and did not come out until spring, some six months later.[10] Such a comment does make one think, however, about the coal miner who spends most of his working life lodged, and sometimes trapped, down a dark pit far removed from what is called the normal functioning of society. If Tao Ran's young patient was addicted to the internet principally because of the prolonged period of time spent doing an abnormal activity removed from the "real" world, then is it not appropriate to also say the coal miner is "addicted" to mining? Let us return to this important problem of *value judgment* because it is central to the internet addiction phenomenon.

Or during a TV debate on Anhui TV's *Focus Point* program Tao Ran forcefully reminded the other panelists attacking his biomedical model of the 22-year-old who infamously poisoned his parents, allegedly because he was addicted to the online game *Legend*.[11] What Tao Ran did not remind his antagonists of, however, was that because the media had been (falsely) reporting that Tao Ran's definition of internet addiction – which we will get to in a moment – had been accepted as a legitimate mental disorder, then the family was more than willing to label the son an internet addict. They were *attributing* the son's poisoning of the parents to what they (mistakenly) thought was a new mental disorder called internet addiction because doing so was the only way the family would be able to have the son's death sentence reduced. According to Chinese law a person recognized as suffering from a mental disorder can, in certain circumstances, be exempted from full responsibility for his or her actions and thus will not be held criminally liable.[12] Let us return to this important problem of attribution later.

Alongside Tao Ran's own dramatic stories, there are also ample reports in the mainstream media highlighting the extraordinary lengths internet addicts will apparently go to in order to continue their addiction. For example, a teenager in Nanjing was reported to have colluded with his friends to steal and then sell his parent's car to raise money for what the newspaper confusedly called first his *habit* and then his *addiction* to the internet.[13] This comment, however, raises an interesting dilemma that will need to be explored: when is internet use a habit and when is it an addiction? And, perhaps more importantly, what distinguishes the two from each other? This report, like most about internet addiction, offers up more questions than answers. For example, if the son needed a quick injection of cash in order to fuel his addiction then why was it reported that it was his friend, and not himself, who both suggested stealing and selling the car and who then promptly drove away in the car alone never to return? One is left to wonder what role *significant others*, such as friends and peers (let alone parents and teachers), play in this assumed one-to-one correlation between internet user and internet. If we refer to Xiao Wang, we see that in the weekends he would meet his classmates and together they would go to the internet bar and hang out, and that only *after* doing so did his enjoyment and his time playing online games increase. Any conceptualization of the causes or the catalyst of Xiao Wang's internet addiction must surely take into serious consideration the powerful variable and/or contributing factor that is the peer group. This is an issue of importance we will have to address.

Likewise, there was the media report about a 150-kg 26-year-old man in north-east China who died after what the paper described as a "marathon" online gaming session over the Lunar New Year period. Like almost all the reports on the dramatic lifestyle of the internet addict this newspaper report offered little in the way of contextual information as to his obviously problematic physical and psychological health *prior* to this marathon session. Nevertheless, the article did offer one very important piece of contextual information. A local teacher said the "dull life" during the holiday prompted many young people to turn to computer games for entertainment. "There are only two options," the teacher complained of Chinese social life, "TV or computer. What else can I do in the holiday as all markets, KTV and cafeterias are shut down?"[14] This comment prompts us to think of the role both the government and the marketplace play when there is cheap, accessible, and ubiquitous internet available for Chinese youth in the city. One also wonders if this young man had devoted the same amount of time to a marathon session of study or work, and consequently died as a result, whether he would have then been called a study or work addict? In fact, the giant telecoms firm Huawei attracted media attention for its "wolf-like" and quasi-military style corporate culture not only because at least five employees committed suicide there, but also because two employees reportedly dropped dead while working on the computer at their work stations.[15] No one blamed the computer nor did anyone call them computer addicts.

And finally there is 23-year-old Xiao Cai who was said to be so addicted to online games that his mental state of mind had been adversely affected.[16] As a result he wanted to commit suicide, and so when trying to overdose on sleeping pills and pesticides did not bring about the desired result, he eventually, on his third attempt, ate some small steel blades. While recovering in hospital a newspaper reporter visited him, and as though out of a scene from *One Flew Over the Cuckoo's Nest*, the reporter said that Xiao Cai was mouthing phrases from the online games and laughing occasionally while glancing toward the reporter. Somewhat more sober was Xiao Cai's uncle who attributed the internet addiction to his "introverted personality," a psychological condition we will see is important within the lexicon of the internet addiction phenomenon. The other attributed cause leading to Xiao Cai's internet addiction and eventual suicide attempts – all three of which "failed," which is significant in itself – was that after getting online in junior high school he met, and was subsequently betrayed by, a female netizen. This interpersonal and emotional episode was said to have hurt him so much that he then put the majority of his time into playing online games. As noted earlier, this reasoning raises perhaps the most important question of all in relation to internet addiction: *what is the nature of the relation between the "internet addict" and his or her social existence*? Only by tackling this question are we able to say whether their internet use is, for example, an expectable or unexpectable response to their social existence.

If Xiao Cai tried to kill himself because online games adversely affected his mental state, then what are we to make of the ten Foxconn employees in Shenzhen who committed suicide within the factory walls in the first half of 2010?[17] Much has been made of the excessive hours, oppressive work conditions, and military-style dormitory system adversely affecting the workers' mental state of mind as they monotonously and hurriedly manufacture Dell laptops, iPhones, and Play Stations. Therefore, can we conclude that Foxconn is responsible for their deaths in the same way online games are said to be responsible for making Xiao Cai sick and suicidal? Surely Foxconn, at least in the first half of 2010, is a more dangerous place for Chinese youth to be than on the internet.

It is incidents such as workplace accidents which, by contrast, highlight the *disproportionate* attention given to the relation between youth and technology. For example, in 2008 official statistics reported 101,480 people died in workplace and transportation accidents in China.[18] Arguably, if company bosses and management were not so "addicted" to the profit motive, and invested more on work safety, then they would be able to save thousands of lives. Likewise, while a war on gaming has been playing out within public discourse there has been a much more tragic outcome from a different kind of relation between adults and technology. In the first quarter of 2009 15,464 people were reportedly killed in road accidents and 63,102 injured.[19] As we know from the work of Stanley Cohen, one of the defining features of a moral panic is its disproportionality, in that the topic under concern does not accurately or objectively reflect social reality.[20] Tens of thousands are dying on the roads and at work and hundreds of thousands are seriously injured and yet this has recently received less public attention than adolescent internet use.[21] This signals that the internet addiction phenomenon is not simply a public health problem, requiring medical or psychiatric solutions, but is more so a socio-political problem, requiring a sociological analysis.

Moral entrepreneur and medical crusader

It is young people like Xiao Cai (and Xiao Wang) that Tao Ran has been most focused upon because, as he explained on *Focus Point*: "We want to tell adolescents and parents as early as possible that internet addiction, if taken to a certain degree, can transform into a mental illness."[22] Leaving aside for the moment the confusion that stems from trying to comprehend how internet addiction can transform into a mental illness when it is claimed that internet addiction *is itself* a mental illness, we should instead first focus on his visualization of the internet addict.

For Tao Ran the internet addict appears to pivot on a see-saw like axis of differing forms of mental disorder or mental disease as he or she moves further and further away from the perceived normal functioning of society – the real world – and more and more toward the unreal virtual world.[23] The result of which is, as Xiao Wang expressed it, a person who was not originally that open becomes even more introverted, and now speaks even less. And so the more they push and pull on their joysticks and on the computer mouse as they play on the internet, the more new physiological and mental disorders they are said to create for themselves (including, according to Tao Ran, autism, self-contempt, conduct impediment, and personality impediment[24]). And as their momentum accelerates, and as their psychological problems accumulate, then their problems snowball, or grow exponentially, and thus the further they move away from the real and true world the closer they get to their eventual destination: the dark pit of virtuality. Once enveloped in this dark virtual pit the internet addict is said to be cut off from the *true world* and can only exist in this inverse ratio, or world turned on its head, where what was virtual has seemingly become real. Or as Xiao Wang nicely put it: "Real-world friends have become less and less, while virtual friends in the virtual world has gotten more and more." And so the young diseased and addicted person who is brought to Tao Ran's hospital, usually after being deceived by his or her parents and thus often in a resistant, agitated, aggressive, scared, and rebellious state, is diagnosed by Tao Ran in the following clinical way: "We have found that internet addicts will also have combined trace elements in the body and spirit containing abnormal symptoms such as: affective disorder, depression, anxiety symptoms, obsessive-compulsive symptoms, psychomotor retardation, sleep disorders, physical and psychological problems."[25]

Likewise, Tao Ran's contemporaries, psychologists Wu Zengqiang and Zhang Jiangguo, have offered us a less clinical and biomedical conceptualization of the internet addict, but a no less darker visualization, as a way in which to allow us to comprehend the apparent turbulent and afflicted psychology of the internet addict. "Youngsters on the internet," according to Wu and Zhang,

> [R]esemble a small ship floating on the ocean. Although the sun shines bright while this ocean seems to be calm, behind this calmness are turbulent undercurrents. Without experience youngsters cannot find a clear direction, and so they can only drift along with the tide while being pushed and swallowed by this tide ... This is fearful, and you cannot imagine this world constructed by this – or the next – generation who grow up in this unprincipled situation.[26]

Part of the reason Wu and Zhang conceptualize Chinese youth as vulnerable little ships being tossed around by the rising and receding tide of the internet is because they are said to possess *weak self control*. And having this perceived weak self control over their internet use, and their lives more generally (and their schoolwork in particular), then they are said to be wasting their "golden time" and "precious youth" (read: study time) surfing the web. The net result, argue Wu and Zhang, is that all of the abundant online information that youth are being pushed around by and swallowed up in is leading to them suffering from what they call *information pollution*.[27] That is, the internet is said to be polluting or diseasing their mind. With this very polluting lexicon in hand, President Hu Jintao himself declared at the beginning of 2007 that the Chinese Communist Party (CCP) had "vowed to *purify* the internet" in order for them to be able to "master the country's sprawling, unruly online population."[28] Likewise, in 2007, in a TV documentary that was never aired publicly extolling the virtues of his hospital's treatment methods, Tao Ran, following Hu Jintao's lead as both a PLA officer and Communist Party member, said "We need to purify our internet environment of these pornographic, violent and gambling phenomena. We definitely need to take charge [of the internet] and get into a position to properly supervise it."[29] That is, an unprincipled situation needs to be made principled, or the out-of-control needs to be brought back firmly in control. This is an argument beyond the role of a psychiatrist, because he is saying that it is not simply that "sick" youths need to be cured, but that, more importantly, deviant youths need to be controlled.

In order to cleanse their mind of this information pollution, that has caused unprincipled, control-less, unruly, and weak youth to have become disordered, depressed, anxious, obsessive, and even "retarded," Tao Ran offers the following cacophony of traditional Chinese medical theory and modern Western-based treatment:

> Effective drugs during hospitalization are used to correct patients with neuroendocrine disorders and the accumulation of heavy metals in vivo, accompanied by the spirit of improving the symptoms of qi, blood, and adjusting the body's yin and yang balance so that patients return to normal patterns of life.[30]

Quite simply, in order to bring these unruly youths under control, medication is the means, and the return to normal patterns of living is the ends. But as psychiatrist R.D. Laing noted, a psychiatric diagnosis and subsequent medicalized treatment methods such as Tao Ran's is based upon a false epistemology: the illness is diagnosed on the basis of human social behavior and conduct, yet it is treated biologically.[31] As already mentioned, let us focus upon what Tao Ran uncritically refers to as the normal pattern of living, for when we look closely at the life of the assumed internet addict then it is clear that this "normal pattern of life" was never really obtained. On the contrary, it is precisely because of the *disordered* nature of their lifeworld, and the social system which they live in, that excessive internet use has emerged.

For Tao Ran, however, these internet addicts need to go to his hospital in order to have their conduct impediments, mental disorders, and physiological problems rectified or corrected not only because their excessive behavior is considered harmful to a harmonious home environment, but if their behavior continues along this mentally diseased track then they are likely to bring harm to, or pollute, society. But medication, which is meant to "cure" them, does not to any satisfactory degree rectify or correct interpersonal behavior; this is why the boot camps and treatment centers use military-style drills and exercises. In this way a combined medicalized and militarized treatment method seems to force the subject to take on two very different social roles. They are seen as both a deviant in need of rectification, and, at the same time, as a sick patient in need of treatment. That is, they are both "bad" *and* "sick" –and so simultaneously, yet contradictorily, both responsible and not responsible for their actions.

While Tao Ran attempts to attack their diseased and disorder bodies – their *body-out-of-balance* – with drugs, elsewhere around the world video games themselves are actually being used to help develop social and spatial ability skills in children and adolescents with severe learning disabilities or other developmental problems, such as speech problems and children with "autism" and "attention deficit disorders."[32] Thus while Tao Ran argues that video games are the *poison* poisoning youth, others are saying that video games can be understood as part of the *remedy* to psychological and developmental problems.

Nevertheless, another picture has emerged of how, in actual practice, Tao Ran "cures" some of those under his care. A number of Tao Ran's ex-patients told Tao Hongkai that in order to be "released" from a hospital they believe is harming their physical and mental health they are willing – against their will – to say such things as "I don't want to play games anymore, I love my parents." Likewise, the son of the president of a university in Beijing told Tao Hongkai that he was forced to go to Tao Ran's clinic, but like many who see the sign "internet addiction" draped across the entrance, he escaped. He was subsequently found and sent back, wherein they tied him up, first subjecting him to electric-shock treatment and then force-feeding him doses of unknown drugs. He struggled against this initially but came to the conclusion that if he was to have any chance of getting out then he reasoned that he will have to comply with their demands – i.e., be obedient. Tao Ran's clinic then forced him to write five "confession" letters to his parents:

1) In the first letter he had to blame his parents for his present circumstances and say that he will not forgive them for putting him in such a place.
2) In the second letter he had to complain about the clinic by describing it in negative terms.
3) In the third letter he had to express his dislike and disgust of the clinic highlighting how he is sick there and cannot eat the food.
4) In the fourth letter he had to write he is missing home cooking and his comfortable bed.
5) In the fifth letter he had to express that he wants to go home, that he wants to go back to school and study hard, and that he will never play games again as he is now cured.[33]

The clinic is then able to use this confession as "proof" that they have managed to "cure" him of his internet addiction and through renouncing his bad behavior he is now fully rehabilitated and ready to lead a "normal" life. However, when the boy returned home he said to his father: "I am going to devote the rest of my life to making your own life a living hell for putting me through that hell. I am not going to study. I am not going to get a job. I am not going to get married.

I hate you."[34] In short, Tao Ran's clinic, like many across China, far from curing his so-called internet addiction, further fractured the already seriously fractured relations between parents and child.[35] Little wonder, perhaps, that one of Tao Ran's ex-patients would tell me that he thought his methods were "hopeless."[36]

In order to highlight the harm internet addiction is causing to Chinese society Tao Ran likes to say things like the following: "Why in our prisons now do 76 percent of juvenile criminals have internet addiction or *some kind of relation* with the internet?"[37] The underlying assumption being that the content and structure of so-called violent video games "teach" the gamer to fight, steal, and kill, and as a result the gamers' moral system, and moral judgment in particular, dissolves under the constant exposure to, and proficiency toward, virtual violence. In brief, online gamers cannot apparently make a distinction between what is real and what is virtual.

However, the letters show that the so-called internet addict does not encounter real-world violence in the virtual world – because the virtual world is a virtual representation of violence in two-dimensional images – but rather encounters real physical violence first-hand in the family. For example, Xiao Wang tells how he was beaten severely a number of times and then, like one of his father's criminal suspects, locked in the house. What we see through the letters is that *parental violence actually contributes to increased internet use.* In any case, if video games were teaching young people how to fight, then we would expect to see young people clicking on a computer mouse and tapping on a keyboard as a way in which to beat up his/her adversary in a real-world setting, for this is how video games "teach" people to fight. Nevertheless, co-authored research by Britain's leading psychologist on "video game addiction," Mark Griffiths, investigated the assumed correlation between video game addiction and aggression and concluded from a sample of 7069 that, at very best, there was only a very weak "link" between the two.[38] Moreover, a US 2-year $1.5-million multifaceted study involving 1,254 children and 500 parents investigated the assumed (causal) link between video game violence and real-world violence. Not only did the results not support the "big fears" predominant in the media – that violent video games make children significantly more violent in the real world and that children who play video games will engage in illegal, immoral, sexist, and violent acts – but they also encountered one unexpected finding: "Boys who didn't regularly play video games (i.e., not at all, or zero days during a typical week) were more likely than even boys who played M-rated games to get into fights, steal from a store, or have problems at school."[39] That is, since video game play is now the norm for boys in the US (as it is in China) then non-players are by definition considered *abnormal.*

In practice, neither the judicial system nor the prison system is diagnosing juvenile criminals for internet addiction in China, and in any case, no such mental disorder has thus far been classified in the Chinese Classification of Mental Disorders and thus no valid definition exists. But if they were asking juvenile criminals if they have "*some kind of relation* with the internet" then one would suspect a figure closer to 100 percent. Nevertheless, we could ask a counter question in relation to juvenile crime: "Why in Chinese prisons now is it said that 59 percent of juvenile criminals come from broken homes?"[40] Thus youth crime researchers such as Liu Guiming are more inclined to locate the problem of youth crime not at the feet of internet addiction, and so-called violent video games in particular, but rather on "the influence of broken families, the depletion of school education, and incomplete social management."[41] Such complicated realities call into question the approach of Tao Ran the *moral entrepreneur* who is lobbying both the public and the government for the creation of new social rules around youth behavior,[42] and Tao Ran the *medical crusader* who is attempting to influence public morality and behavior by presenting a narrow medicalized picture of socially problematic internet use.[43] The fact is the social context is central for understanding the behavior of the internet addict, for by "diagnosing" young people who are angry, agitated, resistant, and even scared because they were brought to Tao Ran's medical operation through deception and unwillingness then this social context is lost. Or we could say it has been spirited away to Tao Ran's biomedical world during his (lucrative) war on gaming.

By presenting a social problem as principally a psycho-medical problem, people like Tao Ran are able to impose a process of "medicalization" upon problematic internet use. This process of medicalization, which Conrad and Schneider refer to as a process involving the transformation of "bad" people into "sick" people, contains three distinct levels of medicalization.[44] The first step is *conceptual medicalization*, wherein a social problem gets translated using a biomedical lexicon into a medical problem. The second step involves *institutional medicalization*, whereby treatment settings are created to deal with the problem now conceptualized as a medical problem (and legitimated by organizations such as the American Psychiatric Association). The third step is *interactional medicalization*, in which medical personnel directly care for people with the new problem they themselves have created.[45] That is, Tao Ran has conceptualized a social problem (i.e., socially unacceptable forms of internet use) as a medical problem (internet addiction), and in the process has turned "bad" kids (i.e., those who do not conform to social norms) into "sick" kids (i.e., those in need of undergoing his treatment methods). Likewise, he has created treatment settings, out of existing treatment settings, to deal with this newly created problem. And he has created the mechanisms needed for paid interactional medicalization to occur so as to "cure" these newly termed internet addicts.

Yet while Tao Ran presents the internet addict as a potential criminal with a physiologically and psychologically diseased mind whose soul has been lost to the virtual world, he has also said "our kids are all very special and intelligent."[46] And since they are special and intelligent then, according to him, "It's only normal for people to make detours when they're young." Employing the classic discourse of a moral entrepreneur, Tao Ran finally says, "Our mission is to help them get back on track before it is too late."[47] But conflating (moral) badness and (bio-psycho) sickness creates confusion, and not clarity, when attempting to explain the causes underlying socially problematic internet use.

On the one hand we are lead to believe that the internet addict is a very *abnormal* and mentally diseased individual who needs to be cured by medical means, and since his/her behavior is bringing suffering to him/herself and society then this behavior, through militarized disciplinary means, needs rectifying or correcting before it gets out of control. Yet on the other hand we are led to see the internet addict as a *normal* individual who has simply made a detour off the right track (i.e., the normal functioning of society) and so just needs to be guided in the right direction. But to be suffering from a mental disorder and to be socially misguided are two very different conditions. The former is premised upon the assumption that there is something malfunctioning *within* the individual (an internal dysfunction) whose presumed ordered psychological system has somehow been made disordered, while the later posits a kind of disjunction between individual conduct and societal norms and expectations. In short, one is seen as sick while the other is seen as bad – both of which are judgments of a different kind.

Xiao Wang, for example, said that while sitting in school his mind was unable to be calm as he was always thinking about going to play. Is this Xiao Wang suffering from "withdrawal symptoms," and therefore his online gaming had disordered his mind by filling it with unwanted, and turbulent, urges to game? As Wu and Zhang argued, does Xiao Wang not resemble a small ship floating on the ocean whose thoughts are caught in turbulent undercurrents? Alternatively, we could say that while doing what he *should* be doing he cannot help but think about that which he *should not* be doing. In reality, Xiao Wang's thoughts only make empirical sense in relation to the social context his thoughts and his actions take place, which in this case involves him sitting in a classroom we can assume he does not want to sit in. In relation to this non-stimulating work-based environment then we should not be at all surprised – or even expect – that he is thinking about the stimulating and fun internet bar and online games, for this is the center of the battle for the hearts and minds of youth by the education system and the gaming industry. But this visualization only becomes legitimate if we suspend our value judgment toward the classroom as something inherently positive and the internet bar, and "violent" online games in particular, as something inherently negative.

Tao Ran's diagnostic standard for internet addiction disorder: time spent online

For us to determine if Xiao Wang is an internet addict, as seen through Tao Ran's biomedical-based lens, then what criteria does Tao Ran use in order to make the important distinction between the *normal* internet user and the *abnormal* internet addict?

The first part of his two-part standardized diagnostic model, or what he confusedly refers to as the two "large symptoms," relates specifically to time spent on the internet. As he has said: "It is not necessarily about *liking* going online as such, but more about the long period of time spent online every day that is internet addiction."[48] While trying to downplay the personal motivations for getting online he also makes a very clear – subjective and social-value judgment-based – distinction between the kinds of activities underpinning this long period of time spent on the internet:

Firstly, spending above six hours a day online for non-work and non-study related purposes can be considered internet addiction's standard time. If in order to work you spend more than ten hours online then this cannot be regarded as internet addiction. Secondly, if this kind of online state is continued for more than 3 months, only then can this constitute the standard course of the internet addiction disease. During the summer holidays some kids will continuously go online for two months, but if after going back to school they can walk out [of the internet] and put their heart back into their studies, then this cannot be regarded as internet addiction.[49]

To summarize: the person who uses the internet for more than six hours per day for non-work or non-study-related purposes for a period exceeding three months, that happens to fall outside of school holidays, is (if he/she also meets the second criterion) an internet addict. It should be noted, by contrast, that England's leading psychologists working on "online gaming addiction" referred to those who played *EverQuest* for more than 30 hours per week as "dedicated players."[50]

Here Tao Ran attempts to downplay the significance of the distinction between someone liking or wanting to go online for a prolonged period of time and someone who feels compelled by a force stronger than their own will to go online because, for example, "they cannot restrain themselves." This distinction negates, or at least contradicts, his previous statement in that the effect of internet use is the same as the alcoholic who feels compelled, or *needs*, to drink more and more every day in order to "feel the same way." This, I would surmise, is because his focus on making a subjective distinction between internet use for work and internet use for leisure largely cancels out this important part of the control aspect of a legitimate addiction model – i.e., is he controlling his internet use or is his internet use controlling him? This is because most internet users would say they *have to* use the internet at work (have no control over it or "need" to) while they generally *want to* play online for leisure (have control over its use).

This must surely be the first addiction model ever constructed wherein the potential addict is exempted from being labeled an addict when his/her use of the object under question takes place during either working hours or school holidays. Is this not equivalent to saying that the night-club hostess who drinks herself into a stupor at work every evening and while on holiday does not have a drinking problem, or is in fact exempted from having a drinking problem, but whose heavy drinking in her own leisure time classifies her as a problem drinker or alcoholic?

While, on the one hand, Tao Ran focuses his model upon youth as the vulnerable target group, at the same time he presents either the computer as containing a kind of internet addiction virus that could affect anyone at any time, or the Chinese population as all possessing addictive impulses that are triggered when they come in contact with a computer. As he has said: "There is no trend for internet addiction as far as social or economic status, or geography, are concerned. So long as they can get access to a computer, there will be addiction."[51]

If, as he argues, internet addiction knows no social boundaries then how come, according to his standard, no one at work can become addicted to their work computers? How come the worker who has to use the computer every day, sometimes for 12 hours, is somehow miraculously saved from internet addiction? Do the workplace and the workplace computer, which must be causing the same negative physiological consequences, somehow insulate or inoculate people from internet addiction? If the aim is to be objective and scientific then surely a subjective distinction between the internet used for work and the internet used for leisure seriously calls into question the *validity* of this so-called standardized diagnostic criterion. How can it be that too much leisure can make you "addicted," but too much work only seems to make you, say, "exhausted'? Does this not point to the central fact, as Durkheim long ago argued, that the normal/pathological binary is a moral rather than a medical distinction?[52]

Moreover, if he had referred to his own research data he would easily recognize a very distinctive characteristic about the internet addiction phenomenon that highlights a very restricted social boundary demarcating internet addiction. In a paper analyzing the "epidemiology" of 607 of his patients we observe 95.4 percent of the 607 patients are males, while of these males the average age was 17.7 years.[53] Likewise, he has said elsewhere that the majority of the "internet addiction disorder" patients addicted to internet games are mostly young men, while those said to be addicted to online chatting are mostly young females.[54] The central fact is that the vast majority of the entire Chinese population "catching" the internet addiction disorder and/or succumbing to its alluring qualities are in reality adolescent males still in school (or meant to be in school), who are still living at home under parental control and discipline. This central element, wherein internet addiction is mainly affecting 17-year-olds, will need to be properly explained if we are to fully comprehend the internet addiction puzzle.

Nevertheless, Tao Ran's conceptualization of time itself is especially problematic for describing internet use. Paul Virilio, for example, has vividly argued that in the age of the internet there are now two different sets of time. First there is what he calls "extensive historical time," that is, history as the extensiveness of time in a linear and chronological fashion. This is time that is portioned out in units, time that lasts, and time that is organized and developed.[55] This is what Manuel Castells referred to as "Clock Time," which is characteristic of industrialism and capitalism, and is characterized by the "discipline of human behavior to a predetermined schedule creating scarcity of experience out of institutionalized measurement."[56] This extensive historical time, in which the linear time of minutes, hours, days, weeks, seasons, etc. was thought to generally exist outside of subjective experience, is being subsumed under what Virilio calls "intensive time" (and what Castells called "timeless time"). Basically, the "old-fashioned" understanding of historical time as duration is disappearing in favor of the *instant*. As Virilio puts it: "It will no longer be important to last, but to "get a thrill" – the quality of life will depend on the intensity of the instant, and not the stability of duration."[57] This is because with Real-Time internet technology people cannot be separated by physical obstacles or by temporal distances, thus durational distinctions of *here* and *there* and *near* and *far* lose much of their meaning when two people at other ends of the Earth can – in Real-Time – play each other or play together in an online game. This is because the World Wide Web, as its inventor Tim Berners-Lee pointed out, was designed as a tool in which to break away from the constraints of time and geographic space.[58] Significantly for Virilio, with the new instantaneous communications media, arrival now supplants departure; that is, without necessarily leaving, everything "arrives."

Thus unlike extensive historical time, this new a-historical technological intensive time has no relation to any calendar of events, rather it is pure computer time, and as such helps construct a permanent present, an unbounded, timeless intensity. [59] In short, this is the time, and by implication the existential experience, of the online gamer. And as everything is instantly – and intensively – arriving then to say that the gamer has been playing for six hours assumes that he/she experiences time as having a linear departure point (00:00) and an arrival point (06:00). But this is not how the online gamer experiences time, and so by overlaying an extensive historical conception of time onto the a-historical intensive time of internet use means that Tao Ran is, literally, out-of-synch or out-of-time with the activity he is trying to measure.

Anyone who has played online games knows how time appears to "fly" and so people are inevitably surprised to learn that what they thought was an hour of play has actually been three. But Tao Ran uses industrial Clock Time in which to analyze gaming time, which for him is both "normal time" and "productive time" simply because he privileges work over leisure. But when this is not the time of the online gamer then this calls into question both the reliability and validity of using a model based on extensive time to measure an immeasurable intensive time-based set of experiences. Because the actual temporal experience of gaming is one of intensity then it is perhaps more objective or valid to refer not to "addictive," "compulsive," or "excessive" internet use but rather to *intensive internet use*?

It is precisely this passion for living an intensive sedentary "unproductive" life that is so problematic for parents and the normal functioning of society. Authority figures see the only "real" life as a gradual historical life wherein school turns into work which turns into the creation of a nuclear family and the accumulation of wealth, and so on. Whereas the intensive gamers, if we can call them that, envision a new kind of life: a sedentary intensive life concentrated on the *now*. This we should understand as the central battle between them. This is also why this intensive life must be seen as abnormal, deviant, and polluting for it negates a historicistic view of life, and that is dangerous to Chinese modernity (i.e., social stability and historical economic development).

This historical time that is *not* the time of the gamer is also linked to Tao Ran's other main "symptom': harming social functioning.

Tao Ran's diagnostic standard for internet addiction disorder: harming social functioning

In the second part of his diagnostic standard Tao Ran focuses on a problem previously mentioned. In addition to time spent online (for non-work/study purposes), Tao Ran's second "large symptom" is the "social harm" that prolonged non-work-related internet use is said to cause. Generally speaking, if spending long periods of time on the internet harms the social functions relating to the ability to study, to work, and to socialize then this can be defined as internet addiction. In one context, Tao Ran has said that to "indulge" for a long time online can cause a person to experience the following set of manifest symptoms:

a)   Feel pessimistic towards one's schoolwork and one's work prospects.
b)   Have a low opinion of oneself.
c)   Feel down in spirits.
d)   Have no interest in doing things.
e)   Have reduced feelings of happiness.
f)   Reduce exchanges with other people, even to the extent that one becomes afraid of associating with people.[60]

And conversely, Tao Ran argues, if these "social functions" – which in reality are not actually social functions but rather overt symptoms whose origin cannot be fully determined – are not subsequently harmed from internet use then it cannot be regarded as internet addiction. If prolonged, daily, repetitive and monotonous activity on a computer that harms one's social functioning is defined as an addiction then why do we not apply this same model to the workers at Foxconn working in the computer assembly department? "We are extremely tired, with tremendous pressure," computer assembly workers told *China Labour Watch*. "We finish one step every seven seconds, which requires us to concentrate and keep working and working. We work faster even than the machines. Every 10 hour shift, we finish 4,000 computers, all the while standing up. We can accomplish these assignments through collective effort, but many of us feel worn out."[61] This exhaustion from monotonously and hurriedly assembling computers is accompanied by a sense of alienation and isolation because as they are working like machines they either have no time to, or are prevented by management from, communicating with each other, and so exchanges with others is reduced. As a result of this machinic environment many employees reported not even knowing the names of their fellow assembly line workers and even their roommates. Hence why worker Lin Fengxiang would make the following remark: "In here, nobody gives a damn about you."[62] The repetitive and generally uncontrollable nature of their work extends to their whole lifeworld within the confinement of the massive military-style factory in that every day they wake up, they eat breakfast, they go to work, they work a ten- or twelve-hour shift, they go back to their dormitories, and finally, they sleep. As Geoffrey Crothall of the *China Labor Bulletin* described the way the labor regime harms both their social functioning and their state of mind, "It's a very dehumanizing place, and the workers are little more than machines there."[63]

The fact that ten workers committed suicide in the first six months of 2010 indicates that Foxconn is harming the worker's "social functioning." Thus if employees were to answer Tao Ran's symptom list we could be fairly confident that many would report feeling pessimistic toward their work; have a low opinion of themselves; feel down in spirits; have little or no interest in doing things (other than sleeping or resting their worn out bodies); have experienced reduced feelings of happiness since arriving; and would have found communication with others reduced. However, Tao Ran is only interested in diagnosing those engaged in leisure activities and not work activities, for work, whether at the office or in the classroom, has a social value (i.e., exchange value) as it is seen as contributing to social functioning; in particular present and future economic development. While the leisurely use of the internet, and online gaming in particular, is perceived as having little or no social value and thus can only be conceptualized as harming, rather than in any way contributing to, social functioning. That's why Tao Ran has the following banner hanging up on the entrance of his clinic: "Concentrate on work, speak the truth, try real things ... and you'll achieve."[64] The implicit message being: "Work will set you free."[65]

Thus there is perhaps a simple reason why time is used to "diagnose" intensive internet use – which in reality is to control, discipline, and punish the bad "time waster." In a society where the latest Gross Domestic Product (GDP) figures are written in large bold characters on the front page of the newspapers, then "the people" must adhere to a new maxim: time is money and money is time. And so you can wreck your health either through over-work or over-study, for you are carrying out your "social function" by contributing to current and future GDP and generally maintaining "social stability." This is partly why "internet addiction" is said to inflict damage upon one's "social functioning," for to be seen to function in a social way is to be a productive worker in a factory or office and not an idle unruly youth on the streets.

The distinctions between the concepts of "work" and "leisure," as Elias and Dunning argued, are distorted by a heritage of value judgments. For instance, work ranks high as a moral duty and an end in itself, while leisure, by contrast, ranks low as a form of idleness and indulgence.[66] Or more specifically, that which has an *exchange value* is acceptable, while that which merely has a *use value* is unacceptable if done during "productive" time. And as Erich Fromm argued, the need for exchange is not an inherent part of human nature, but is rather a socio-historical outcome of the abstractification inherent in the social character of those living within capitalism. That is, the process of living is experienced, or ideally meant to be experienced, analogously to the profitable investment of capital, with one's life and one's character being the capital which is invested. In this way the felt need to measure acts of living in terms of something quantifiable appears in the tendency to question whether something is "worth the time."[67]

It is this inherent prejudice toward exchange value that Tao Ran rests his definition of internet addiction upon. It assumes time has an inherent (exchange) value, and that time spent playing games is not "worth the time" and thus a "waste of time;" while time spent in an alienated office environment online for 10 hours, for example, is "time well spent." He reduces the productive act of living to the profitable investment of capital by measuring living acts in terms of something *quantifiable*. So the real issue is not simply that internet gaming may lead to internet addiction, but more so that (amateur) internet gaming has no exchange value. The "internet addict" is not something that can be found in nature, not some naturally occurring poison, but is rather the product of the market-led reform period, both technologically and morally, and so expresses the inherent values that capitalism engenders.

The evidence for this lies in two related figures: the "gold farmer" and the professional gamer. Gold farmers are simply young people who make a living playing computer games, often working 10 hour shifts in labor conditions that are, as one gold famer put it, "just like working in a factory."[68] Gold farmers, who often earn similarly low wages to factory workers (e.g., 1200 yuan per month), are employed by internet-based companies to game so as to accumulate virtual weapons, tools, equipment, money, etc. The company then sells these in-game advantages to players in other countries for money. Thus like the factory, the company makes its profit from the surplus labor of the gold farmer. Despite the fact that the gold farmer is doing exactly what the internet addict is doing – daily online gaming in excess of six hours which could be said to harm their "social functions"[69] – the gold farmer is exempted from internet addiction because his/her online gaming has an exchange value: he/she accumulates virtual wealth in exchange for capital. Likewise, the professional gamer is often playing for more than six hours per day.[70] Even though objectively speaking the act is the same for both the professional and amateur gamer, subjectively speaking, however, the professional gamer is "competing" for prize money (and making money for technology companies) while the amateur gamer is "playing" for pleasure. As competing in a competition for prize money is a legitimized professional sport then playing for money, as opposed to playing for fun, pushes the gamer out of the (potential) category of addict and into the realm of a (potential) champion.

Alternatively, if the aim of the internet addiction disorder model is to be objective then if we apply the same model to work-related activities we understand how this so-called normal functioning of society is *itself* bringing suffering to young people and harming their social functioning, in particular, the impact upon interpersonal family relations. For example, many students who have to study monotonously and repetitiously for more than six hours per day are said to suffer from anxiety, insomnia, poor memory recall, vomiting, and even delusions resulting from the incredibly competitive and intense pressures of exams, in particular the crucially important national college entrance examination (the *gaokao*) – an exam that for many parents, as highlighted later, has become their "obsession" par excellence.[71] Even though many students may "pass" Tao Ran's symptom-based criteria if it was redesigned for "exam addicts," the suffering that excessive study negatively alters their state of mind and the harm it brings to their social functioning is dismissed as students *should* be studying excessively but *should not* be playing excessively.

Significantly, Tao Ran and his colleagues presented, in the February 2010 issue of the journal *Addiction*, an eight-point list of symptoms as criteria for assessing internet addiction. The clearly stated aim of this paper is to propose that the following diagnostic criteria are useful for the standardization of diagnostic criteria for "Internet Addiction Disorder". The reason why this statement is made overtly clear is that the findings from this paper can then hopefully be presented as "evidence" that there exists a *valid* and *reliable* diagnostic criterion for internet addiction and therefore this model can, or indeed should, be included in the fifth edition of the American Psychiatric Association's *Diagnostic and Statistical Manual*. The eight-point list used to diagnose internet addiction is as follows:

1) *Preoccupation*: a strong desire for the internet. Thinking about previous online activity or anticipation of the next online session. Internet use is the dominant activity in daily life.
2) *Withdrawal*: manifested by a dysphoric mood, anxiety, irritability, and boredom after several days without internet activity.
3) *Tolerance*: marked increase in internet use required to achieve satisfaction.
4) *Difficult to control*: persistent desire and/or unsuccessful attempts to control, cut back or discontinue internet use.
5) *Disregard harmful consequences*: continued excessive use of internet despite knowledge of having a persistent or recurrent physical or psychological problem likely to have been caused or exacerbated by internet use.
6) *Social communications and interests are lost*: loss of interests, previous hobbies, entertainment as a direct result of, and with the exception of, internet use.
7) *Alleviation of negative emotions*: uses the internet to escape or relieve a dysphoric mood. (e.g. feelings of helplessness, guilt, anxiety).
8) *Hiding from friends and relatives*: deception of actual costs/time of internet involvement to family members, therapist and others.[72]

In contrast to the first part of the criteria, wherein personal motivations are subsumed under the weight of a quantifiable amount of time spent online, Tao Ran and his colleagues now place full weight on the controllable-uncontrollable threshold said to underpin the internet user's relationship to the internet. In fact, in the first paragraph of this paper they lay out very clearly what, for them, underpins the behavioral mechanisms of the internet addict. They write:

> Behavioural addiction affects a vast number of individuals and occurs when people find themselves *unable to control the frequency or amount of a previously harmless behaviour* such as love, sex, gambling, work, internet and chatroom usage, shopping or exercise. Behavioural addictions are considered *impulse-control disorders* and share many underlying similarities to substance addictions, including aspects of tolerance, withdrawal, repeated unsuccessful attempts to cut back or quit and impairment in everyday life functioning.[73]

Not only do we see a claim that people can be "addicted" to love (and exercise), but Tao Ran is also now saying that people can in fact be addicted to work.

Thus should he not remove the work-related/non-work-related binary from his criteria? In this definition we also see Tao Ran now returning to the model that conceptualizes an equivalency between the internet addict and the so-called gambler, the drunk, and the druggie. It is not time spent online per see that is apparently central to defining internet addiction, but rather when internet users are unable to control the frequency of their use, and thus the amount of time spent online is auxiliary to, or a necessary by-product of, this uncontrollable behavior. So while on the one hand internet addiction is defined simply by time spent online that is for non-work-related purposes, irrespective of the user's personal and subjective motivations, at the same time we see that this is in fact not the case, and, instead, what defines internet addiction is precisely the subjective and *intra*personal "impulse-control" mechanisms which are said to drive the increased frequency of internet use and, more importantly, the assumed *inability* to reduce time spent online.

Simply put, the internet addict is a person who *thinks about* the internet too much; is *unsettled* in some psychological way when not online; feels a *need* to get online more and more; is *unable* to reduce this increased time spent online; *disregards* the harmful consequences presumably associated with getting online despite knowing them; *loses* interest in other activities; uses the internet as a *remedy* to negativity; and, finally, is in *denial* about their problematic internet use and so uses *deceit* to cover it up.

Put in this way, it is not at all clear whether the internet addict is psychologically *sick* or simply socially *bad*. That is, a naughty son who wants to do that which he is not meant to do, and so gets agitated when not allowed to do it, and so through rebelliousness not only continues doing it but actually increases his use, which *expectedly* impacts upon his other activities and on his social relationships, and so in order to continue defying societal norms and expectations acts socially in appropriately (i.e., "bad"). If we bring to the surface both the entire social context internet use takes place in and the lifeworld of the young internet user, which a symptom-based method tries to keep subsumed or compressed because it tends to negate the surface-level symptom list, then a very different picture emerges. The picture created by a sociological analysis of Tao Ran's mentally diseased internet addict is not of a psychologically sick individual, but rather of a socially deviant group of individuals we could call *rebels with a cause*.

It is no coincidence the criteria set out earlier seeks to conceive of the internet addict as equivalent to the gambling addict, the drug addict, and the alcoholic. This is because this set of criteria, which is in effect the search for the *signs* of internet addiction, was itself built upon the gambling addiction model by American psychologist Kimberly Young.

Kimberly Young and the birth of internet addiction

In 1998 Young published a book whose mere title, let alone its content, teaches us a great deal about both the birth of the internet addiction concept and the subsequent underlying frameworks and assumptions driving the biomedical-based internet addiction disorder. Not only did Young call her book *Caught in the Net: How to Recognize the Signs of Internet Addiction*, but in addition, the main question underpinning her search for the *signs* of people caught in the net, like small vulnerable ships caught in a turbulent undercurrent, was this moral-based judgment: "was there something *sinister* going on in cyberspace?"[74] From the outset of this psychological inquiry into problematic internet use, internet users are conceptualized as being caught or captured, and thus left "tingling," from the "cornucopia of electronic delights" of the internet. An experience she calls "mindthrill," as though their own will, volition, and motivation for getting online have been spirited away to the online world.[75] At the same time, the internet itself is assumed, from the very beginning, as some kind of sinister device with ulterior motives, for like Alice falling into the black hole of Wonderland, Young claims it allows users to "escape into a fantasyland."[76]

In short, if the unsuspecting internet user, in particular those with "weak self control," are not careful then they will quickly get "caught" by the inherently addictive qualities of the internet, and online games in particular.

For Young, people – as in anyone, but think of Xiao Wang – are susceptible to the "lure" and "addictive" pull of the internet's chatrooms and interactive games, and thus become both "hooked" and "psychologically dependent" upon the *feelings* and experiences they get while online. By becoming caught in this sinister black hole of the net, as it possesses "addictive potential with harmful consequences" (think of Xiao Wang's blurred vision) internet addicts are then said to "waste" away the hours in this "Terminal Time Warp."[77] In particular they are said to waste away precious work time and time spent socializing with "real" people in the "real" world, because the assumption is that (exchange value-based) productive time is good, and people offline are real.[78]

Conceptually, Young represents a particular social arrangement – conservative suburban heterosexual family life – as not only normative but also ideal. Not only does she subjectively privilege physical and geographically local relationships over digital communication, entertainment, and information-seeking, she also celebrates the suburban, conservative, and hetero-normative family as a social unit hermetically sealed off from alternative friendships, relationships, and communicative practices that occur through digital means and across distances. Rather than viewing digital media as something that emerges alongside and through social changes to the perception and functioning of family, friendship, communication, and ways in which leisure time is legitimated, digital media, on the contrary, is seen as facilitating the breakdown of "normal" social life per se. The solution Young offers to this breakdown of normal living that internet addiction is said to cause is grounded in a combination of extreme vigilance, alarmism, and a Foucaudian level of surveillance of both self and others.[79]

And so like the SARS virus, if "left undetected and unchecked," this inherently addictive internet will "silently run rampant in our schools, our universities, out offices, our libraries, and our homes."[80] And because of its power, stimulation, and excitement, the internet can seemingly strike "any internet user" at any time and in any place, and so Young, in what can only be described as a state of high paranoia, warns the reader to be extra vigilant because "an internet addict could be your best friend, your own child, your parent, your partner ... or you!" For Young, this existential threat to humanity is going to emerge as "the addiction of the millennium, surpassing even TV with its pervasive grip on our minds and souls."[81] This despite the fact watching TV has never been legitimately recognized as an addiction. Thus before the world spirals out of control by swallowing everyone up into the black hole of internet addiction, Young wants to help weak, dependent, captured, and susceptible internet addicts – whom she refers to as "information-hungry ... internet junkies" and "on-lineaholics"[82] – get out of the "black hole of cyberspace."[83] Presenting the internet as a kind of evil electronic opium is, for Young, a positive methodological step because "like Luke Skywalker in *Star Wars*, if you learn about the *dark side* right from the start of your internet training, you have a far better chance of not giving in to it later."[84] Therefore, drawing from the same criteria used to diagnose "compulsive" gambling and alcoholism, Young created the following questionnaire to pose to internet users:

1) Do you **feel preoccupied** with the internet (i.e., think about previous online activity or anticipate the next online session?
2) Do you **feel restless**, moody, depressed, or irritable when attempting to cut down or stop internet use?
3) Do you **feel the need to** use the internet with increasing amounts of time in order to achieve satisfaction?
4) Have you repeatedly made **unsuccessful efforts** to control, cutback, or stop internet use?
5) Have you jeopardized or risked the **loss of a significant relationship**, job, educational or career opportunity because of the internet?
6) Do you stay online longer than **originally intended**?
7) Do you use the internet as a way of **escaping from problems** or of relieving a distressed mood (feelings of helplessness, guilt, anxiety, depression)?
8) Have you **lied to** family members, a therapist, or others to conceal the extent of your involvement with the internet[85]

As is clear, while Young took from the gambling model, Tao has taken from Young's model, and thus we can now refer to this as the "Young-Tao model." After receiving the replies to these eight questions from 496 respondents, Young evaluated their answers and "discovered" that 396 (80 percent) of these respondents were indeed internet addicts. Thus speaking in the kind of language used to incite a moral panic, she rashly concluded: "I had tapped into a potential *epidemic*."[86] Or we could say, like Tao Ran and the hundreds of so-called treatment centers and military-style boot camps that use punishment-based practices international law would classify as torture and/or mistreatment, she saw a potential market of prospectus clients. Tao Ran's paper cited earlier also reports similarly high respondent rates for their eight-point symptom list.[87] The methodological purpose of the Young-Tao symptom list, which can only be said to capture the signs or overt symptoms of human behavior, are presumed by them to *reliably* illustrate or illuminate the "fact" that internet addicts, just like compulsive gamblers, alcoholics, and drug addicts, suffer major problems in the main categories of everyday life: work, school, family, and relationships.[88] Others, however, have called into question their gambling-based model and the assumption that assessing the overt signs of behavior around internet use actually offers us a reliable and valid concept called internet addiction disorder.

3   Critiques of the Internet Addiction Disorder model

The April 2008 issue of the *International Journal of Mental Health and Addiction* contained a series of articles by experts on problem gambling questioning whether such a concept as internet addiction or "videogame addiction" even exists. The center piece was an article by Richard T. A. Wood entitled *"Problems with the Concept of Video Game "Addiction": Some Case Study Examples."* Following Wood's article are commentaries by Alex Blaszczynski, Mark Griffiths, and Nigel Turner, respectively. These three commentaries are then followed by another article from Wood responding to some of the issues raised by the other commentaries. These exchanges, which are focused on online gaming more than simply internet use per se, make for an interesting discourse on a critique of the Young-Tao model, and so I use them later as a guiding principle in order to elaborate upon all the major conceptual problems stemming from the Young-Tao model. I begin by elaborating on more general problems associated with the Young-Tao model, and then I move to address each particular criterion in the Young-Tao model highlighted through these exchanges.

Misusing the World Health Organization for legitimacy

Richard T. A. Wood begins by pointing out an obvious but crucially important point touched upon earlier: there is currently no such clinical criteria called "internet addiction" that has been accepted by any reputable organization responsible for defining disorders of the mind or body (e.g., The World Health Organisation (WHO); The American Psychiatric Association; the Chinese Classification of Mental Disorders).[1] The fact that the internet addiction concept is not recognized has not prevented Young and Tao (and others) from using, and some would add misusing, this concept in order to "diagnose" and "treat" this mental disorder which does not, in effect, legitimately exist.

In order to justify his use of a clinical criteria that has yet to be accepted Tao Ran has continually claimed he is merely adhering to the guidelines set out by WHO defining what, in one context, he has called a "disease." For example, on the *Focus Point* TV program mentioned earlier, Tao Ran was asked to provide to his detractors justification for using a biomedical-based model for treating young people. "I would tell them the WHO has a regulation on what is a disease," answered Tao Ran. "Anything that gives oneself suffering or brings suffering to others, and wherein social functions are harmed, then this can be designated as a disease. This is not what I, Tao Ran, says, this is the WHO's disease concept." Elsewhere, he has simply substituted the term "disease" for the term "mental illness," as though they are equivalent and interchangeable, and argued that "internet addicts all possess these two conditions" (i.e., Their internet use a) brings suffering onto oneself and others, and b) harms social functioning).[2] But in explaining how to interpret the harming of social functions, Tao Ran neglects completely the theoretical underpinnings of the biomedical-based model and, using a subjective, moral-based judgment instead, argues that harming social functioning can be defined as someone who "*should* go to school but does not go to school, *should* work but does not work, and so normal social intercourse does not exist."[3] Someone not doing what they should, let alone the taken-for-granted assumption that someone should *naturally* want to go to work and school, does not indicate a person's impulse-control mechanism is dysfunctioning, but rather that the person is not adhering to societal norms and expectations (i.e., they are acting "badly'). In this way, Tao Ran has mistaken badness for sickness.

When we look at the WHO's conceptualization of the term "mental illness" (let alone disease) we observe that it is not simply premised upon bringing suffering onto oneself and others and harming social functioning. For example, under the heading "*Mental Health and Substance Abuse*" the WHO says mental disorders produce "disability" – and not principally suffering or harm – mainly in the following areas of a person's functioning:

1) Activities of daily living, including self-care – grooming, dressing, bathing, keeping one's body and the environment clean and looking after one's health. [Note the emphasis is on the *difficulties* of daily living, and not on bringing suffering onto oneself and others].
2) Social relationships, including communication skills, ability to form relationships and sustain them, social skills required for daily activities, and taking care of others. [Note the emphasis on problems relating to the *ability* at dealing with the normal functioning of society, and not on "harming" social functioning].[4]

Likewise, the WHO, in a section called "*The International Classification of Disease*," outlines "disorders of adult personality and behavior" (which both Young and Tao claim internet addicts possess). For the WHO, specific personality disorders:

1) [A]re deeply ingrained and enduring behaviour patterns, manifesting as inflexible responses to a broad range of personal and social situations. [Note the emphasis on inflexible responses and not on self-harm or social malfunctioning].

2) They represent extreme or significant deviations from the way in which the average individual in a given culture perceives, thinks, feels and, particularly, relates to others. Such behaviour patterns tend to be stable and to encompass multiple domains of behaviour and psychological functioning. [Note the emphasis on deviation from the average and their stress upon psychological, and not social, functioning].

3) They are frequently, but not always, associated with various degrees of subjective distress and problems of social performance." [Note the emphasis on "distress" and "performance" and not "harm"].[5]

Benefiting from a moral panic and parental concerns

After Wood makes this important point, which calls into serious question any treatment done in the name of "internet addiction," he makes another crucial observation. Wood points out that in this absence of any recognized criteria, professionals and clinicians often base their construction of internet addiction upon their observations of some individuals who have *concerns* about their internet use, or in response to *other people* (i.e., parents) who have concerns about another individual's behavior (i.e., children). The negative portrayals in the mass media around internet addiction highlighted earlier, which have greatly contributed to the internet addiction phenomenon in China being elevated to the status of a moral panic and which Tao Ran and many others have benefited greatly in terms of social and economic capital, has resulted in parents across China generally accepting the existence of the internet addiction disorder concept. These high-profile cases, which are the exception to the norm even before their content and context are distorted, have, on the one hand, increased parental fears and concerns around their child's internet use, while on the other hand, increased their willingness to send their child off to a clinic like Tao Ran's advertising to parents that it can successfully, and more importantly, *scientifically*, "cure" their child of this internet addiction.

At the same time, the Party-State's media apparatus and concerned parents have targeted internet bars as a space of deviance, vice, and violence spreading a kind of social disease that is supposedly infecting China's young population. We should note here that online games are equated with opium not only at the level of individual pathology, but also at the level of social pathology. A major concern with "internet addiction" is the way in which it will affect China's modern development, not only the moral and spiritual cultivation of the individual, but also the nationalistic rhetoric of breaking free of the shackles of foreign invasion. By evoking the internet bar as a kind of *opium den* moral entrepreneurs and medical crusaders draw a parallel between China's rapid modernization through the importation of foreign technology, and the foreign importation of opium that led to the spread of opium use and national humiliation during the Qing dynasty.[6] This is best encapsulated by a comment made by anti-internet crusader Zhang Chunliang. Very much like Young in the US, Zhang has said that if internet games are not properly controlled in China then they may become the twenty-first century's "electronic opium" and "spiritual opium."[7] To make his point that internet games threaten to effect the downfall of China, Zhang says that internet bars have spread with the speed of a "toxin" attaching itself to the "social body like poisonous tumours."[8]

But rather than conceiving of the internet bar as a dehumanizing electronic opium den, we could, on the contrary, take a more humanistic stance and think of it as a kind of Daoist monastery. The internet bar could be conceptualized as a kind of monastery for spiritually starved and ideologically deserted youth in that it provides, at a certain level of consciousness and sociality, a kind of sanctuary from the upheavals of China's modernization process. For example, Daoism is said to enable ecstatic spiritual journeys.[9] Like the monastery, it could be argued that the internet bar is a place that is a kind of safe haven from the dangers outside, which provides a cathartic experience and an arena in which to vent one's frustrations and worries. In this sense, a certain kind of gaming could be said to be driven by a desire to leave behind the (ugly) "human world." The central concept within Daoism is *wu wei*, which is often translated as meaning "action without action" or "effortless doing."[10] Are not "internet addicts" partly condemned because they are said to be doing "nothing" while obviously doing something?

In any case, Sun Hualin noted in her ethnography of internet bars in Wuhan that the popular daily newspaper the *Wuhan Evening News* ran a large number of negative portrayals of internet bars stating how the "poison of net bars" has caused harm to young people and simultaneously unnecessary worry to their parents.[11] On the front page of the January 3rd, 2003, edition they ran a story entitled "Net Bars Summoning the Soul of Our Next Generation," in which the article exposed a number of internet bars that allowed – illegally – middle and elementary school pupils to enter. These deviant, and not simply sick, young people reportedly played truant to go to internet bars where they "smoked, played games, and stayed overnight, forgetting about eating and sleeping."[12]

The following day the same newspaper published an article titled "Daughter, Where Are You?" The story was centered on a father who was looking for his 15-year-old daughter because she had not been home for ten days. Despite searching in internet bars all across the city the parents had still not found her. The story, which we will see is a common narrative presented by parents, claimed that their daughter used to be both a *good* child and *good* student, but that since she started going to internet bars she has been transformed into a different person. That is, her soul has been spirited away by the poisonous net bar to the online world. For example, she stopped calling home to let her parents know where she was, and she often skipped school and stayed in internet bars overnight.[13] In contrast to this letter, wherein we learn nothing of the parents' own role in their daughter's absence and involvement with the internet, the interpretation of the parents' letters I present in the following pages places full weight on the interpersonal relations within the family of this apparent internet addict. Unsurprisingly, then, Sun Hualin noted that the majority of the parents of those visiting internet bars also perceived the bars as unnecessary, harmful, and evil.

However, we must also ask if this negative perception, at the same time, does not serve a function for parents by attributing the blame of the breakdown of communication between parents and child to the pull of the internet and the internet bar and *not* to the actions of the parents themselves.[14] Later we will see that a child's increased time spent away from the family home, and subsequent increased time spent online, can only be understood if we bring the parents' own *intra*personal thoughts and *inter*personal actions into the picture.

While many parents may agree with the educational benefits computer technologies can bring to their child, using this same technology to play online video games is seen as detrimental to their schoolwork and thus diminishes their potential to enter university and may curtail a potentially successful career path. That is, internet use for leisure diminishes the child's exchange value. This parental fear is central in understanding the internet addiction phenomenon, for since it is almost always the parents, and not the child him/herself, that is forcing or deceiving the child to seek help, then we must analyze what is behind the very real parental fears, concerns, and worries that partly drives the internet addiction phenomenon.

Killing in the name of internet Addiction: the case of Deng Senshan

A counter discourse has emerged detailing a very different kind of horror story related to the internet addiction phenomenon. Instead of highlighting the way so-called violent video games turn young people mentally ill and violent, the media, and in particular China's burgeoning blogging community, have been writing about the way the methods used to "correct" the behavior of deviant youths are themselves violently harming the "social functioning" and state of mind of these youths through their disciplinary punishment-based methods.

The most obvious example of the harm done to youths in the name of the internet addiction disorder model is the case of Yang Yongxin mentioned at the beginning, who used illegal electric-shock treatment on 3,000 youths as a way to "cure" them of internet addiction. Likewise, we could mention the 13-year-old boy who jumped off the second floor of a boot camp after drinking four grams of a chemical used in disinfectants in order to escape the abuse he was receiving at the hands of the camp's "educators."[15] While the negative experiences from Yang Yongxin's victims (see Huang He at the beginning), which were made public through blog posts, investigative journalism, and TV exposés, eventually led to the Ministry of Health banning the use of physical punishment as a treatment method, this measure was still unable to prevent a number of deaths occurring at several military-style boot camps across China.

The tragic case of 15-year old Deng Senshan offers us an example of the way treatment centers and military-style boot camps feed into, and economically feed off of, the moral panic and parental fears they help to create in the first place.

In July of 2009, Deng Fei, Deng Senshan's father, saw a television advertisement one evening promoting the "Set Sail Rescue Training Camp" in Guangxi. The advertisement seemingly showed how successful the camp was in turning young people who had become "addicted" to playing online games, at the expense of their schoolwork, into *normal* children. Deng Fei, who had been desperately trying to get Deng Senshan away from the home computer he himself had bought him and back into the school books, was impressed with how the kids were seemingly transformed after being sent to the camp. Through the combination of the emotive power of advertising – in which the smiling family members in a fifteen-minute advertisement were actually paid actors – and the perceived scientific legitimacy of the internet addiction concept, parents like *Deng Fei* are able to project their concerns, fears, and desperation onto the commercial boot camp as being some kind of panacea for the child's and the family's problems. The boot camp, for its part, is fully aware that it is parental worry, more so than the child's mental and spiritual health, that is driving the industry, for the camp's own promotional pamphlet read:

"Let the parents worry less, let the children be happier!"[16]

However, one should question how a prison-like camp that was a three-story building with steel bars on the windows and verandas, attached to which was a small exercise area surrounded by a four-meter-tall iron fence, could in any way produce genuine happiness. In reality, treatment clinics and military-style boot camps are aimed not at the production of genuine happiness and self-realization, but rather obedience. But Deng Fei was seduced by the seemingly well-mannered students that greeted him upon arrival, which can be understood as a deceptive strategy the camp used on parents to convince them that their regime is effective and produces the disciplined subject parents so desperately desire. Believing that Deng Senshan had a minor problem with "internet addiction," Deng Fei therefore took his son – who was told he was going on a "vacation" – to the camp for private "re-education" at a cost of 7,000 yuan per month. His wish was that when he returned one month later Deng Senshan would be all brand new, just like the young people in the TV advertisement. That is, like the family car that is not running properly, many parents, who are living in an increasingly consumer-based *nowist* culture where interpersonal relations are partly patterned on the relations between consumers and the objects of their consumption,[17] believe that such boot camps offer a quick-fix disciplinary solution to a problem they have pre-emptively affixed upon the child as principally "the child's problem."

Fourteen hours after leaving his son in the assumed safe hands of the camp's "professional" staff, Deng Fei received news that his son was dead. The "educators" at the camp had beaten his son to death. But first they had tortured him so as to force him to obey the camp's regulations.

Like all the new recruits before him, Deng Senshan was immediately dragged off to a confinement cell upon arrival; or what the camp referred to as the "compulsory course for new students." According to ex-victims, this course of confinement generally meant being forced to stand two days and one night in the confinement cell with no food or sleep, while only being allowed several half-hours of rest coupled with a water-break. Refusal to obey this order resulted in being beaten by the instructor and having the period of confinement extended. Deng Senshan emerged all bloodied from the confinement cell that evening and was subsequently ordered to run hundred laps of the exercise field. At the thirtieth lap he apparently collapsed from exhaustion. The instructor hit him first with a stick stripped from a wooden chair, then he hit him with the chair. The instructor then kicked him down on the ground. Deng Senshan was subsequently sent to the local hospital, wherein he stopped breathing and was soon pronounced dead.

Reflecting on his deceased son's internet use, a grieving Deng Fei came to a new conclusion: His son was never addicted. "He didn't smoke, he didn't drink. The internet was probably his way to vent the pressure on him," he said echoing an argument I myself will make as constituting one of the main "pull" factors of online games. "We didn't know that then. But we know that now. It wasn't really an addiction. It was his way out of the pressure of being a student." Senshan's mother then added to her husband's revised interpretation by saying: "He didn't even play that much."[18] In many ways, Mr. and Mrs. Deng are emblematic of the countless parents across contemporary China who are driven partly by fear to seek help – any help – for a "bad" child they are unable to control and discipline. While more than a dozen people were jailed for Deng Senshan's death, the reality is that in the name of "curing internet addiction" boot camps such as these are often producing, rather than reducing or eliminating, what we could call *biopsychosocial distress* within youths labeled as internet addicts.[19]

Concept substitution: gambling becomes gaming

The next important observation Wood makes is the fact, as pointed out earlier, that the criteria used to label online gamers as "addicts" has been achieved by using either the *DSM-IV* substance abuse criteria, or, more frequently, pathological gambling screens, through substituting the word "gambling" for the world "gaming" (or "internet use").

Wood, pointing to other studies,[20] calls into question the validity of criteria such as the Young-Tao model because some of the criteria included may be only measuring *high levels of engagement* rather than addiction per se. Criteria in the Young-Tao model measuring high levels of engagement are: (criterion 1) being "preoccupied" with gaming; (criterion 3) increased time online related to seeking feelings of achievement/satisfaction; (criterion 5) staying online longer than originally intended; and, (criterion 8) using euphoric feelings from gaming to "escape" feelings of distress. Wood says that such criteria are "peripheral" to criteria for addiction and so cannot be considered as valid properties that identify addictive behavior patterns because they are also associated with aspects of "normal" play.[21] And because these aspects – i.e., thinking about gaming when not gaming; gaming more because it provides positive reinforcement; finding yourself spending longer than intended gaming; and liking the way negative feelings are replaced with feelings of happiness – are aspects of normal gaming, including these peripheral criteria to identify video game "addiction" results in a significant overestimation of its prevalence. Thus, the research Wood points to by Charlton found that using a similar check-list of criteria to the Young-Tao model resulted in a blurring between high levels of engagement and addiction.

And because Young and Tao load their symptom list with half of these periphery criteria it should not be too surprising that they report such high rates of prevalence, and thus around 80 percent of Young's respondents and those brought to Tao's clinic are "diagnosed" with internet addiction after answering the symptom list. To put it more simply, by using these criteria it cannot be made clear whether the gamer is engaging in gaming more than he/she *should* be, so that one's gaming is simply excessive relative to the normal gamer, or whether the gamer has in fact lost control over his/her gaming. In short, this points to gaming as principally being a habit and not an addiction.

Wood then points out perhaps the key aspect calling into question the validity of a model that attempts to substitute the concept gambling for gaming, and the fact that there are very distinct qualitative differences between gambling and online gaming. For example, gambling is premised upon the wagering of money in order to try and win back more. According to Wood, when a problem gambler loses money they will typically chase their losses as a way in which to try and win back their money. This often results in them invariably getting deeper into debt. Mounting debt usually leads to increased stress, and a need to gamble develops in order to alleviate that stress.[22] Or as Nigel Turner said concurring with Wood, gamblers often get trapped in a cycle that creates a downward spiral. They start out gambling because they *want* to win, but eventually they are gambling because they *have* to win.[23] This mechanism of debt, and the serious consequences resulting from it, does not generally occur in online gaming, and definitely not with internet use. Gamers start out wanting to win and have some fun, and this "want to" does not by necessity turn into "have to" even if they continually lose. While online gamers may spend money purchasing virtual goods so as to advance within the game, and as a result some get themselves into financial difficulties because they are often students with no income, such investments and the problems stemming from them are not comparable to gambling – where debt is absolutely central. In fact, gamers are not driven by increasing their economic capital or by trying to regain capital that has been lost, rather they are driven by the desire to gain social capital and more existential needs such as: the desire to avoid aloneness; the desire to be part of a world outside oneself; the desire to express one's individuality; the desire to be a *someone*; and the desire to feel like a winner by dominating others. As Griffiths significantly pointed out in co-authored research on the existential dimensions related to playing *EverQuest*, for some individuals the game fulfills particular existential needs. These include social contact with a virtual community that enables the individual to explore different ways of *being*.[24] In a similar fashion, central to the exploration by Chinese youth for different ways of being in the world is the search for freedom; and the internet is central to this exploration.

In responding to Wood, Blaszczynski adds that it is neither scientific nor logical to simply adapt and apply the set of diagnostic criteria used to define gambling to then define video game addiction.[25] Blaszczynski argues that it must be empirically demonstrated that similar and consistent etiological processes and principles apply across each related disorder, something which neither Young nor Tao has thus far achieved. As an example of the etiological non-complementarity, Blaszczynski points out that unlike either drug use or alcohol consumption, online gaming is a competitive skill-based activity designed to improve individual performance by competing against others in a multiplayer interactive game premised upon rules, objectives, and outcomes and is, therefore, driven by a different set of motivations, benefits, and costs. That is, structurally speaking, online gaming is complementary with sports such as tennis, golf, billiards, or basketball. In fact, it is this etiological complementarity to other sports which has allowed video gaming to have become accepted worldwide as a professional sport whose gamers are considered not mentally disordered but professional athletes and even *heroes*.

Moreover, Blaszczynski highlights the way gaming has personalized meanings for the gamer, in particular achieving intangible self-satisfying accomplishments through the goals set out in the game. I would argue that unlike psychotropic substances such as LSD, which are known to result in what is called ego-loss or ego-death, online gaming, on the contrary, is centrally related to the desire to inflate the ego or self.[26] As both the inventor and first user of LSD, Dr. Albert Hofmann, wrote of his experience: "Every exertion of my will, every attempt to put an end to the disintegration of the outer world and the dissolution of my ego, seemed to be a wasted effort."[27] The problem for gamers, according to the Young-Tao model, is that since this is taking place in an unreal fantasyland, and not in the real world, then the feelings of achievement and self-satisfaction are not considered legitimate. But as Griffiths highlighted in a co-authored paper with Chappell *et al.*, like taking up martial arts or learning to mountain climb, video games offer the gamer a challenging opportunity to grapple with and ultimately master what was previously difficult. Thus this experience not only appears to be one of a personalized liberation and freedom, but is also connected to expanding one's prior personal limits.[28] At this qualitative level we must disabuse ourselves of the notion that such activities are not real, even despite the fact that excessive gaming produces far reaching negative social effects upon the lives of the participants.

Next I deal with the criticisms relating to each individual criterion of the Young-Tao model.

Criterion 1: Young-Tao model – preoccupation

[A strong desire for the internet. Thinking about previous online activity or anticipation of the next online session. Internet use is the dominant activity in daily life.]

As noted before, Wood believes "preoccupation," or thinking about a pleasurable activity too much, is not a valid criterion for video game addiction as it is part of normal play and so tends to measure high levels of engagement rather than addiction per se.

Elsewhere, Rob Cover has uncovered an important hidden assumption underpinning a person's perceived "preoccupation" with digital media. Cover writes that in the moral panic over video gaming *passion* is re-written as *addiction*, which is supported by referring to the prolonged time spent both playing and thinking about playing. Cover argues that passion for and dedication toward one's career, sporting activities, and even politics is considered as "healthy," whereas passion for less physical, localized and normalized activities such as gaming online is represented as dangerous and addictive.[29] Unless such "preoccupations" are put into social context they remain, in effect, meaningless.

Criterion 2: Young-Tao model – withdrawal

[Manifested by a dysphoric mood, anxiety, irritability and boredom after several days without internet activity.]

Echoing Wood, Blaszczynski says that the "core" criteria underpinning the addiction concept are tolerance, withdrawal symptoms, and relapse. Echoing the Young-Tao model, he also believes that central to an addiction is the element of *impaired control*, in particular the recurrent difficulties in containing behaviors despite the genuine motivation to cease or cutback. But while there is enough empirical material to argue that the substance-based addictions produce serious physiological and psychological changes when use is withdrawn, Blaszczynski argues that much research remains to be done in showing that people experience genuine withdrawal symptoms when cutting-back or ceasing non-substance behavioral addictions such as video gaming. Elsewhere, Ng and Wiemer-Hastings found from their survey results that those playing the massively multiplayer online role-playing games (MMORPGs) for more than 25 hours per week would not feel irritated if they could not play for one day.[30] Thus Tao Ran's earlier claim that you may see a physical reaction in the person when gaming is stopped, "just like someone coming off drugs," is not substantiated by empirical research. It also fails to see the obvious differences between substance-based and non-substance-based forms of behavior.

Criterion 3: Young-Tao model – tolerance

[Marked increase in internet use required to achieve satisfaction.]

Wood questions the assumption that the internet addict is like the problem gambler in that "tolerance" to gaming results in a marked increase in internet use because the gamer feels an ever-decreasing sense of satisfaction the more he/she plays, and so needs to play more in order to "feel the same way." For Wood, tolerance in relation to problem gambling stems from the initial excitement and arousal gained by first placing successful bets, and then the felt need to place larger and larger bets in order to feel the same initial excitement, because small bets no longer produce excitement. He therefore finds it difficult to see how the excitement of playing video games can be increased in any comparable way. This is especially the case for the popular game *World of Warcraft*, for the initial feelings stemming from learning this difficult and complex game are more frustration and tension than satisfaction and happiness. In reality, gaming for longer periods or playing more frequently does not, in itself, increase the overall intensity of the gaming experience, let alone simply using the internet, and so comparing the action of problem gambling with excessive gaming is not comparing like with like.

This is even less of the case for using the internet to chat with friends, watch movies, read news, search information, buy/sell goods, and send emails. For example, how could someone chase the supposedly diminishing excitement of sending an email, searching information, or having a conversation? Tao Ran has argued that you can divide internet addiction into five separate categories: (1) online gaming addiction; (2) online pornography addiction; (3) cyber-relationship addiction; (4) internet information addiction; (5) internet trading addiction.[31] He claims that most of those "suffering" from cyber-relationship addiction are young females. Not only does such a claim problematically feed into the essentialist notion that females are "naturally" inclined to communicate, but it also assumes that females are only seeking cyber-relationships with other females, which obviously is not the case. Nevertheless, how can a female that is supposedly addicted to cyber-relationships experience *tolerance* to chatting and so needs to markedly increase her internet use so as to achieve (or exceed) the same level of satisfaction she experienced when she first started chatting?

We should also call into question the theoretical basis of the tolerance criterion. Griffiths, in a co-authored paper, referred to tolerance as a cognitive-based component that is premised upon the person having significantly stronger *positive outcome expectancies*.[32] This cognitive process is considered dysfunctional as it is said to maintain addictive behaviors. That is, the gamer is said to cognitively expect, the next time he/she games, to desire a more positive outcome than the previous gaming session. If video gaming, in and of itself, is not an inherently negative activity, then how can the desire for a more positive outcome be seen as dysfunctional? Ethically – and not simply cognitively – speaking, do not most people hope or desire for a positive outcome in almost everything they do? Thus, contradictorily, a positive seems to be a negative.

Criterion 4: Young-Tao model – difficult to control

[Persistent desire and/or unsuccessful attempts to control, cutback, or discontinue internet use.]

In relation to the question "Have you repeatedly made unsuccessful efforts to control, cutback, or stop internet use?" Wood argues that an answer in the affirmative does not necessarily indicate that the person is in fact "addicted" to gaming. Wood points out that there are many habitually formed behaviors that, while difficult to give up, do not constitute an addiction. For example, a young child may find it hard not to suck their thumb, many people find it difficult not to eat snacks between meals, limit the amount of Coca Cola that they drink, or the salt they put on meals, while some may drive the car to the shop when they *know* they really should walk. More importantly, this question contains a problematic assumption, and that is that repeatedly trying to alter one's behavior is premised on the assumption that the person, him/herself, wants to genuinely change. In reality, many young people do not want to limit or stop playing online games; instead they are forced to, often for good rational reason, by their concerned parents. And so being "unsuccessful" at doing so does not necessarily indicate they cannot control their "impulses" and so are "addicted" to online games, but rather that they refuse to obey their parent's expectations and societal norms. In short, the child may be "bad" (according to societal norms and expectations), but he/she is not sick. This component, wherein parents desire the child to change while the child does not, is important for learning why parents have to deceive their child into going to boot camps and clinics.

However, this situation negates the premise upon which the success or failure of treating problematic gaming, gambling, drug use, and alcohol consumption lies. It is generally agreed that accepting that there is a problem is the first step on a road to recovery, but the confinement cell that greeted Deng Senshan, for example, indicates that these young people first need to "learn" that they have a problem that needs changing. But as Senshan's father understood too late, sometimes concern over the child's gaming behavior is partly a consequence of parents misunderstanding the nature of their child's internet use because they have been bombarded by media hype, a moral panic, and marketing propaganda by boot camps masquerading as advertising and promotion.

While subjectively focusing only upon issues related to efforts of controlling the reduction of use, the Young-Tao model fails to see the other side of the coin. Feelings of (being in) control are a crucial "pull" factor of online interaction. But the desire to want to feel like one is in control of one's online world only makes sense vis-à-vis the feelings of not being in control in offline situations.[33]

Criterion 5: Young-Tao model – harmful consequences

[Continued excessive use of internet despite knowledge of having a persistent or recurrent physical or psychological problem likely to have been caused or exacerbated by internet use.]

Wood argues that the consequences of excessive gaming do not compare reliably to both problematic gambling and heavy drug or alcohol use. For example, excessive online gamers do not usually end up with huge debts, and it is highly unlikely that a 17-year-old in China will have his/her house repossessed because of any debts accrued while gaming. Likewise, contrary to Tao Ran's very serious claims of mental illness highlighted earlier, Wood says that excessive gamers do not typically suffer severe health consequences as would a heavy drug user, who unlike the gamer is ingesting directly into the body a psycho-active substance that is usually illegal and often mixed with toxic chemicals. While we could say that Xiao Wang's online gaming caused his eyesight to deteriorate, we could also enquire into the way excessive study prior to and concurrent with gaming deteriorates young people's eyesight, and their overall physical and mental health more generally. Thus any claims Tao Ran makes about internet addiction causing "network autonomic dysfunction, gastrointestinal disorders, eye fatigue and other somatic symptoms," let alone serious psychological problems, must be shown to *not* be related in some way to excessive schoolwork and other non-gaming-related activities.

Contrary to Wood, Griffiths claims that "very excessive" video gaming does in fact result in negative health consequences, principally around hearing, vision, and repetitive strain injury (wrist/elbow/neck pain).[34] This should not be particularly alarming as workers working in assembly plant factories such as Foxconn experience very similar harmful consequences from repetitive labor practices that effectively treat them as machines. Nevertheless, Griffiths also adds that after a review of relevant literature he concluded – in contrast to Tao Ran's claims – that the adverse effects of video gaming for all but a very small subgroup of players are generally temporary and relatively minor, resolving relatively spontaneously with decreased frequency of play (this also calls into question claims around withdrawal symptoms).[35]

Griffiths has also reported elsewhere in a co-authored paper that a consequence of excessive gaming is "neglect of self," in particular disregarding or ignoring personal hygiene and physical health.[36] But since many people do not adhere to standard norms of hygiene or physical fitness then how can such criteria be valid for a biomedical-based diagnosis of internet addiction?

While any repetitive action done with enough frequency will inevitably cause physical problems, as any professional athlete can attest to, it is also worth pointing out the reported positive effects stemming from internet use and online gaming.

The journal *Surgical Endoscopy* published research on how videogame experience affects the speed of surgical skill acquisition. Trainee medical students with gaming experience (more than three hours per week) were found to take significantly less time to reach proficiency than did non-gamers. This was attributed to gamers having acquired, prior to their formal medical training, the visuospatial and motor skills required to excel in performing surgery due to gaming relying heavily on hand-eye coordination.[37]

Likewise, researchers in California have found that internet use among middle-aged and elderly people helps to exercise and improve brain functioning, thereby partly counteracting the age-related physiological changes that cause the brain to slow down.[38]

Moreover, The Walter Reed Army Medical Center in Washington uses a virtual driving simulator, which is based on videogame technology, as a way to both help injured ex-soldiers learn to drive again and to give them a new lease on life?[39]

In contradistinction to Tao Ran's claim that excessive internet use causes depression, the National Health Service in England has offered an online computer program to internet users looking for ways in which to actually treat their depression.[40]

Finally, the European Parliament announced at the beginning of 2009 that computer games are "good" for children. Toine Manders, the Dutch parliamentarian who drafted the report, said: "Video games are in most cases not dangerous. We heard evidence from experts on computer games and psychologists from France, the US, Germany and the Netherlands and they told us that video games have a positive contribution to make to the education of minors."[41] In particular, the European Parliament recognized video games as stimulating the learning of facts and skills such as creativity, strategic thinking, cooperation, and innovative thinking, which it considered to be important skills for an individual to possess in an information society.

***Criterion 6: Young-Tao model – social communications
and interests are lost***

[Loss of interests in hobbies and entertainment as a direct result of internet use.]

For Wood, the primary consequence of excessive gaming is *time loss*, and so problems are created by spending too much time on one activity to the detriment of other activities. In China the central problem for parents, and by extension the central problem of the internet addiction phenomenon, is the way study time is lost through gaming, which then impacts negatively upon the users schoolwork, and school grades in particular (their "social functioning"). Wood, citing his own study of 280 videogame players, found that 82 percent experienced time loss frequently or all the time.[42] Significantly, more than half of the players thought this had some positive features. Contrary to the assumption that time loss or spending longer online than originally intended is inherently negative, some said they actually *liked* losing track of time because they found it a relaxing experience and a sign that the game was engaging and value for money. More importantly, it provided them temporary relief from the stress of everyday life. Experiencing time loss also showed to them that they were enjoying themselves so much that time passed quickly. Conversely, those who disliked time loss suggested that this was because it meant they missed appointments, which sometimes caused conflict with others.

Thus Wood asks an important question that points to the first part of Tao Ran's standard: "Does spending a lot of time doing something define an activity as addictive or problematic?"[43] In echoing earlier comments about Tao Ran's diagnostic standard making a subjective value-judgment around acceptable and unacceptable activities, Wood argues that on its own it does not. This is because there are many socially acceptable activities people undertake for long periods of time that are not regarded as inherently addictive; for example, study, work, reading, watching television, playing a musical instrument, or training for a sports competition. Somewhat similar in form to Tao Ran, however, Wood says there has to be some *negative consequences* before behavior can be considered a *problem*. And similar to Young, Wood says such a negative consequence might be that time spent playing leads to a conflict in the person's life through neglecting relationships, work, school, etc.

However, contrary to both Tao and Young, Wood argues that in reality it is difficult determining whether or not the time spent playing video games is having a negative effect, as it ultimately comes down to a question of value judgment rather than any objective scientific measurement. For example, due to subjective bias what is neglected is the positive relationships internet users obtain while online, thus helping us to see excessive internet use is not at all a zero-sum game. For example, Griffiths and Cole found that among the gamers they surveyed around 75 percent reported having made "good friends" within the game – two-thirds of which attributed this positive relationship to the game.[44] This shows they were socially active, thereby negating the criterion's assumption that social communications and interests are lost. This is because it fails to take into equal account the social communication and interests obtained while online. In reality, most parents see their child's internet friends not as good but rather as a *bad influence* on their child's schoolwork. While parents in China, and subsequently treatment centers, use a perceived negative effect – decreased study time, loss of interest, and even rejection of school – as the main reason for concern that the child has a problem with playing online games, Wood argues that this concern by others, in itself, does not constitute grounds for labeling the behavior an addiction. This is partly because this negates the social context in which their increased internet use and decreased interest in school take place, in particular the parent–child interpersonal relations and the highly competitive and often monotonous education system. By pulling the parents out of the equation and therefore downplaying their responsibility and the important part they play in their child's internet use, the parents (and school) are, so to speak, let off scot-free.

While the Young-Tao model suggests that internet addiction stems from prolonged repetitive behavior that results in negative consequences, in particular the way alternative activities and "normal" socialization suffer due to time loss, Blaszczynski argues that such a model creates confusion and overlap between the terms use, misuse, abuse, dependence, and addiction. For example, gamers may *misuse* their time gaming as determined by parental concerns and social norms, while parents may also express concern about excessive internet *use* negatively interfering with schoolwork. Likewise, parents may say their child has become *dependent* upon the internet for making friends, or say the child *abuses* the internet during the weekends when he should be doing his homework. But, Blaszczynski would argue, such judgments are not equivalent to an addiction because the distinctions between these terms have not been demonstrated.

Moreover, Mark Griffiths argues that excessive activity and addictive activity, while overlapping, are two very different things.[45] For Griffiths, the difference between healthy excessive enthusiasms and addictions are that healthy excessive enthusiasms *add to* life whereas addictions *take away from* life. But, again, we come back to value judgments, which never exist within a social vacuum, for who decides which activities are "adding to" and "taking away from" one's life? As I have argued, internet addiction disorder judges relations based upon exchange value as "adding to" life, while mere use value activities (i.e., playing for leisure) "takes away" from the child's "precious" study time.

To a certain degree the Young-Tao model is built upon the social (and not scientific) judgment that online gaming is so problematic precisely because it is seen to be taking away from important parts of people's "normal" lives. For Young it is principally in the realm of significant social relationships, in particular the breakdown of marriages – which internet use is said to *cause*. While for Tao it is taking away from youth's "precious" study time. But young people are attracted to the internet in China partly because *they* feel it adds to their life, in particular the social relationships they make and the feelings of enjoyment, achievement, and satisfaction they gain. But since cyberspace is seen as an unreal fantasyland then people like Tao Ran, and parents especially, conceptualize these relationships as also being of an unreal, and thus deviant and socially unacceptable, nature.

Criterion 7: Young-Tao model – alleviation of negative emotions (through escape)

[Uses the internet to escape or relieve a dysphoric mood (e.g. feelings of helplessness, guilt, anxiety).]

While recognizing that some people play online games too frequently and for periods of time that is unhealthy for them physically, psychologically, and/or socially, Wood, nevertheless, reminds us that it is common for people to become excessively involved in activities if the activity has the capability of offering them a distraction from other issues in their lives which they find stressful and difficult to deal with. Citing other research, Wood says the authors found that those adolescents labeled as "addicted" to online games gamed primarily as a means of coping with stress.[46] Likewise, Wood's own co-authored research found that those who gamed most frequently were far more likely than those who gamed less frequency to game in order to escape from other problems in their lives.[47] Conversely, other co-authored research by Wood found that half of the sample of non-problematic gamers reported that they often played games as a way of both relaxing and escaping from everyday stress.[48] The Young-Tao model assumes that escaping into the virtual world potentially indicates a sign of addiction and thus is an inherently problematic activity. Wood, however, says that the use of games for relaxation and escape is not necessarily a problem in and of itself, but rather is a central part of normal gaming.

In contrast to Tao – who by setting up a subjective binary between the good real world and the bad virtual world argues that Chinese youth use the internet as a way in which to *escape reality* – Wood argues that some gaming is used as a mechanism of escape *in order to* cope with a range of stressful issues affecting the individual and, I would add, in compensating for relationships and feelings unavailable to them in the real world. If young people in China are using the internet, and online games in particular, as a mechanism in which to deal with, and even avoid completely, problems arising from living in a world that is going through a huge disorderly social transformation yet often not providing them with their perceived existential needs, then how does it makes sense to blame either the internet or them for doing so? That is, if Chinese youth are having difficulties dealing with their personal and social problems, and so instead choose to immerse themselves in the internet, then surely their gaming behavior is first a *symptom* rather than the specific *cause* of their problems, and then secondly, once their intensive gaming produces interpersonal problems their gaming behavior constitutes *both* symptom and cause of their problems.

In response to Wood's argument that problematic videogame playing is symptomatic and a consequence of other underlying problems, and so cannot really be classed as an addiction, Griffiths counters this point by arguing that many "traditional" addicts such as alcoholics and heroin addicts participate in their behavior as a response to other underlying problems. Thus Griffiths says we can divide addiction into two types: (1) "primary addiction," where the person is addicted to the activity itself; and (2) "secondary addiction," where the person's addiction is symptomatic of other problems.[49] Put this way, addictions, for

Griffiths, should therefore be defined in terms of the resultant behavior of the individual and not the cause(s) of the behavior – as he said earlier, behavior that takes away from life. But, again, this would require us to make value – and not scientific – judgments upon what constitutes socially acceptable and socially unacceptable forms of behavior.

Nigel Turner also criticizes Wood on this point. Like Griffiths, Turner says that a large percentage of drug abusers and pathological gamblers also have pre-existing psychological problems, and so argues we cannot redefine addiction by dismissing all such cases where the behavior is a result of pre-existing problems. Referring to B.F. Skinner's cognitive-behavioral concept of addiction,[50] Turner says it could be argued that people develop an addiction because they experience either a positive reinforcement (e.g., the high, feeling great/excited, winning the game), a negative reinforcement (e.g., emotional escape from their problems), or both. Videogame game play is said to be both positively reinforcing (e.g., the thrill of winning, beating other players, and getting the highest score) and negatively reinforcing (e.g., fantasy, escape). As such it could be considered a candidate for a legitimate addiction. But if this was the case then we could include work and parenting as candidates for addiction. People feel "high" when they do well at work and/or may "bury" themselves in their work when they have personal problems, while parents feel great and excited about being with their child but may also use the child as an excuse (escape mechanism) in order to avoid social confrontations. The fact is, as Wood points out, claiming behavior that is rewarding is addictive fails to see that rewards are subjective – and I would add, contextual and historical.[51] For example, playing *World of Warcraft* throughout the night or running a marathon throughout the day can be, so to speak, one person's idea of heaven and another person's idea of hell.

Dismissing this cognitive-behavioral model, Turner says an addiction is not merely something a person has learnt, like Pavlov's dog, to do or not do. Differing from Griffiths who says an addiction is behavior that takes away from life, Turner conceptualizes an addiction as something that the person has come to *depend* on so strongly that he or she simply cannot stop doing it. The person is so strongly dependent that the addiction has become an additional problem on top of any pre-existing problems. But as Blaszczynski pointed out, this understanding creates confusion and overlap between the terms dependence and addiction. Later I present empirical data to demonstrate that those called an internet addict by their parents have not come to depend so strongly on online games that they simply cannot keep their hand off their joystick. This reduces the entire context their internet use takes place in to a one-to-one relation between internet user and internet premised on control-impulses and positive and/or negative feelings.

While Wood, Griffiths, and Turner bicker over the role excessive gaming *as a symptom rather than cause* plays in relation to the addiction concept, the main shortcoming of the Young-Tao model gets obscured. By generally focusing on the overt signs of problematic internet use the Young-Tao model tends to present symptoms as cause, and more problematically, fails to effectively address and change the actual underlying problems preceding or even causing increased and excessive internet use. Significantly, Tao Ran has said that two important "causes" of internet addiction are family and school, in particular, poor family educational methods, violent and critical parents, hostile and un-harmonious husband-wife relations, lack of fatherly love and authority, violent teachers with bad tempers, an unfair school evaluation system, and an excessive focus on individual grades.[52]

The Young-Tao model, with its focus on the overt signs resulting from a one-to-one relation between internet user and internet, necessarily ends up principally forcing the perceived *disordered* individual to correct or rectify their behavior rather than the disordered aspects of his/her life that underpins their internet use. Thus while the internet addict may have cleaned up his/her act, this method has in no way altered the disordered nature of family and school relations even Tao Ran has said lies at the bottom of the internet addiction phenomenon. In an off-hand remark, however, Tao Ran has expressed explicitly how his primary focus is on changing the overt symptoms of the perceived individual addict and not the root causes underlying problematic internet use, for he told a reporter that if his internet addiction disorder model is approved by the Ministry of Health then "it will be applied by hospitals, and all hospitals can then diagnose internet addiction and admit patients."[53] Yet how can hospital treatment of this kind, which would presumably consist of medicating the patient so as to alleviate symptoms, trans-form the root causes of the problems existing below these signs and symptoms that contribute to intensive internet use?

Criterion 8: Young-Tao model – deception

[Deception of actual costs/time of internet involvement to family members, therapist and others.]

While the Young-Tao model focuses on deception, dishonesty, and "hiding" from friends and relatives – which at best can only be said to capture levels of deviance rather than addiction per se – what gets lost or neglected is, conversely, the honesty expressed online and the new friends acquired. Not only have we seen earlier that many gamers make "good" friends while gaming, but Griffiths and Cole also observed a significant positive correlation between the number of hours played per week and the number of friends made within the game. In addition, some internet users reported being more "honest" while online. For example, Griffiths and Cole found that about 40 percent of respondents discussed sensitive issues with their online gaming friends that they would not discuss with their friends in the "real" world.[54] Thus, if dishonesty and hiding from offline relation-ships are assumed to capture internet addiction, then in what way does honesty and the flowering of online friendships cancel out these negative aspects? Relatively speaking, if negative relationships signal addiction then surely positive relationships signal non-addiction? Likewise, if Griffith and Cole report more than a third of gamers claiming they could be more "themselves" online than off, then this seriously calls into question the validity around deception, dishonesty, and hiding offline because this is not how they "really" feel. The problem is the inherent bias toward offline relationships and the undervaluing of online relationships.

An alternative line of questioning would be asking why people feel "more themselves" when online, because this phenomenon tends to signal there is not something principally wrong with the virtual world but more so the real world.

Summary of the Young-Tao model

The Young-Tao model is weighed down with hidden assumptions, subjective bias, and value judgments. Tao Ran misrepresents the WHO's definition of a mental disorder for legitimacy, discarding also his own biomedical interpretation by confusing badness for sickness. The Young-Tao model cannot make a clear distinction between high levels of engagement (a habit) and "addictive" behavior, because it overloads the criteria with "periphery" symptoms stemming from normal play and so produces a distorting and inaccurate overestimation of prevalence. Specifically, this cannot prove in any reliable way that their internet use is *not* a habit. The model is also unable to show consistent etiological processes apply across both gambling and gaming (let alone drinking and drug use), which is important because there are very distinct qualitative differences between the two activities (e.g., the mechanism of debt; gaming is comparable to sports). Moreover, unlike some drugs, gaming is not premised upon ego-loss but rather on ego-survival, maintenance, and inflation. The model also subjectively dismisses feelings of satisfaction and achievement gained online as "unreal." Likewise, thinking too much about gaming is negatively related to "addiction," while thinking too much about socially acceptable activities is positively tied to terms such as "passion" and "dedication." We also see that it is not at all clear that repetitive non-substance behaviors produce physical withdrawal symptoms that can in any way be compared to substance-based activities. Furthermore, the model misleadingly assumes tolerance to gaming, and much more problematically internet use in general, is equivalent to gambling, drinking, and drug taking. Quite simply, internet use is not premised upon the user chasing a supposedly diminishing sense of excitement. Moreover, unsuccessful attempts at controlling behavior does not necessarily measure addiction, but rather difficulties adhering to norms and expectations and/or refusal to do so.

Likewise, the harmful consequences of gaming do not compare to gambling, drinking, or drug use. The model does not succeed in validly demonstrating any perceived harmful consequences stem from internet use and *not* from other activities. In reality, the Young-Tao model, and Tao Ran specifically, seemingly distorts the physical and psychological consequences as other research has found they are generally minor and temporary, resolving spontaneously with discontinued play. Furthermore, time loss through gaming does not indicate addiction, because many users actually enjoy this normal aspect of play, as it is relaxing. Time loss is principally a value judgment and not an objective measure as it assumes time spent playing online games is time "wasted." By focusing only on what is "lost" while online the model does not take into equal account that which is "gained" while online (e.g., friendships, positive feelings). These criteria are driven by concern by others not doing what is expected of them, resulting not only in an ethical judgment upon behavior but also a confusion between terms such as use, misuse, abuse, dependence, and addiction. The model also assumes that using the internet to deal with personal issues is misdirected, and, by implication, using medication, psycho-therapy, and military discipline is correct. However, doing so tends to indicate their internet use is a symptom and not necessarily a cause of their problems. This obscures the real issues involved and generally forces the individual to change, thus failing to deal effectively with the root causes of one's problems. Finally, trying to measure "deception" merely captures levels of social deviance and not biomedical addiction. There is a bias toward only capturing perceived negative outcomes and not any positive outcomes, which could, if undertaken objectively, cancel out these negative aspects. But as we see, the Young-Tao model is designed to *highlight*, rather than downplay, any perceived negativity stemming from internet use, which ends up unreliably and invalidly misrepresenting the effects of internet use.

DSM-IV and the mental disorder concept

What is a symptom without context or background?

What is a complication separated from what it complicates?

Georges Canguilhem[55]

The criticisms offered point to the Young-Tao model lacking reliability and validity for diagnosing a certain kind of individualized relationship to the internet as constituting "internet addiction." But there is a larger, and perhaps more important, issue at work here. As mentioned, the ultimate goal of promoting the Young-Tao is its inclusion in the 2013 DSM-V. Being included in this diagnostic manual would legitimize the Young-Tao model and its current illegitimate use. The importance of this possibility cannot be downplayed for the *DSM-IV* is used by virtually every mental health professional in the United States (and commonly used throughout the world) to guide diagnosis and to justify third-party reimbursement for treatment (i.e., medical insurance).[56] But to be included in the DSM-V signals not only that gathering overt symptoms signals an "internet addiction" but that, more importantly, this internet addiction is, itself, a mental disorder. As Wakefield has noted, every specific condition listed in the *DSM* as a disorder must satisfy the logical requirements set out in the manual's own general definition of a mental disorder.[57] Thus, I propose to do to the Young-Tao model what proponents of the Young-Tao model must necessarily do themselves: *Does the internet addiction disorder satisfy the logical requirements set out in the* DSM-IV's *own general definition of a mental disorder*? If not, then internet addiction disorder is not a mental disorder, and should not therefore be included in the DSM-V.

Allan Horwitz, in his analysis of the *DSM*'s general definition of mental disorder, historicizes and contextualizes accurately the crucial problems relating directly to the Young-Tao model. Horwitz, a sociologist, notes that the publication in 1980 of the *DSM-III* marked a revolution in thinking about mental illness. The creators of the

DSM-III basically overthrew the broad, continuous, and vague concepts of Freudian psychoanalysis and reclaimed the categorical illnesses of pre-Freudian asylum psychiatry. This was achieved by importing a medicalized framework organized around specific disease entities to formulate the basic nature, causes, and treatment of disturbed behaviors. The fundamental premise of the *DSM-III*, and by extension the Young-Tao model, was that different clusters of symptoms indicated distinct underlying diseases such as schizophrenia, depression, panic disorder, substance abuse, and perhaps "internet addiction disorder."[58]

Horwitz notes that the growth in the number of diagnoses included in the *DSM* since the *DSM-III* was published in 1980 – which now numbers almost 400 apparently distinct mental disorders – was achieved through three different methods.

First, the *DSM-III* simply recategorized as discrete diagnostic entities the wide range of problems that Freudian psychoanalysis had already pathologized. Basically, the classifiers of the *DSM-III* took the problems Freudianism had defined as psychological disturbances and reformulated them in the language of categorical illnesses. This was undertaken not with the aim of using research and theory to advance the profession so as to better serve the interests of its suffering clients, but more so to maintain the existing clientele of mental health professionals, who requested a large categorical system that would include all behaviors clinicians encountered in their practice. Thus problems of ordinary life such as dealing with troublesome children (e.g., who only want to play online games and refuse to do schoolwork), poor marriages, frustrations in careers, personal identity crises, and general dissatisfaction were reconceptualized as discrete forms of individual pathology.[59]

Second, the *DSM-III* discarded etiology (the study of causation) by adapting an atheoretical method of focusing on observable symptoms only, *regardless* of the cause of such manifest symptoms. By disregarding causes or whether observable symptoms actually indicate a mental illness, the *DSM* could both encompass the conditions treated by all competing schools of psychopathology *and* expand the number of conditions that could enter the new diagnostic manual. Thus, acute dissatisfaction with life could be renamed "dysthymia"; distress arising from problems with significant others could be called "major depression"; and the disturbances of troublesome children could be renamed as "conduct personality" or "attention deficit disorders."[60]

The third method facilitating the growth in the number of supposedly distinct mental disorders in the *DSM* was through focusing on the issue of reliability while, at the same time, downplaying the issue of validity. Horwitz points out that an emphasis on reliability is a very useful method in which to expand a categorical system because, in the absence of a valid definition, there is basically no limit to the number of discrete criteria professionals can develop. Echoing the eight-point criteria of the Young-Tao model, Horwitz hypothesizes that if a person wants to create an entity called "compulsive television watching" (or "compulsive internet use") then one can easily come up with specific criteria, such as: "at least five hours per day, at least six days a week, limits outside activities, friends and family comment on the behaviour, etc."[61]

While such a criteria-list could train observers (e.g., doctors in hospitals throughout China) to "measure" the disorder in a consistent way, this high reliability, says Horwitz, would be meaningless without a demonstration that "compulsive television watching" is a *mental disorder*. That is, the high reliability of the Young-Tao model, wherein they can "diagnose" rates around 80 percent, is completely meaningless if the model has failed to establish validity in which to prove that "compulsive internet use" is actually a valid mental disorder. Thus what, according to the *DSM-IV*, constitutes a valid mental disorder?

Horwitz reminds us that the classifications of distinct disorders that underpin the *DSM*'s diagnostic psychiatry are useful when two broad criteria are met: "(1) that each constellation of symptoms is actually a valid mental disorder; and (2) that using manifest symptoms to distinguish diseases aids in establishing distinct causes, prognoses, and treatments for each condition."[62] Thus this text is designed to address this very problem: Does the so-called "internet addiction disorder" meet these two broad criteria; that is, is the constellation of symptoms identified to "diagnose" a certain form of internet use actually a *valid* mental disorder called "internet addiction," and is using these symptoms to distinguish "internet addiction" from "internet use" aiding us in establishing distinct causes, prognoses, and treatments for this condition?

In order for "internet addiction disorder" to be classified as a valid mental disorder in the *DSM-IV* it must meet three broad criteria. First, for a clinically significant behavioral or psychological syndrome, or pattern, that occurs in an individual, to be classified as a mental disorder in the *DSM-IV* the syndrome or pattern under consideration "must *not* be merely an expectable and culturally sanctioned response to a particular event, for example, the death of a loved one."[63] In addition to the behavior under consideration not simply being an *expectable response to a stress condition*, the *DSM-IV* adds that the following criterion must *also* be met in order for certain kinds of behavior to be classified as a mental disorder: "Whatever its original cause, it must currently be considered a manifestation of a behavioral, psychological, or biological dysfunction in the individual."[64] Thus according to the *DSM-IV* a mental disorder – that is not simply an expectable response to a stress condition – must also be shown to have originated from a dysfunction *in* the individual, and, therefore, it must be proven that there is something wrong with the *internal functioning* of a person. Finally, the *DSM-IV* is very clear on the third part of the definition: "Neither deviant behaviour (e.g. political, religious, or sexual) nor conflicts that are primarily between the individual and society are mental disorders unless the deviance or conflict is a symptom of a dysfunction in the individual."[65] That is, mental disorders, such as "internet addiction," must be distinguished from inappropriateness as defined by social norms (i.e., deviant behavior) as well as from expectable responses to stressful environments; while, at the same time, shown to be the result of an internal dysfunction. This is because the inappropriateness of behavior is not sufficient, in and of itself, to indicate the existence of a mental disorder. Rather, this merely indicates that the person is "*bad*" (i.e., a social deviant or rebel going against social norms) – and not *sick* (i.e., behavior that is an un-expectable response to a stress condition originating from a dysfunction *in* the individual).

We can observe the serious disconnect between Tao Ran's symptoms-based diagnostic methods and the social context of his "patients," and thus the failure to adhere to the requirements of the *DSM-IV*, by referring to how, in actual practice, he and his staff come to diagnose the person brought to his clinic. American writer McKenzie Funk faked "internet addiction" as a way to be admitted into Tao Ran's clinic, wherein he subsequently wrote about being force-fed unknown medication and subjected to pseudo-psychotherapy and military-style drills and exercises. Upon entering, Funk was first asked the eight-point criteria symptom list. He was then given a computer-based diagnostic test wherein he was required to answer ninety statements. He was to rate their "truth" on a scale from A (not true at all) to E (very true). The list included the following statements:

> You have headaches. You get agitated. You feel dizzy or faint. You have less desire for the opposite sex. You have no desire for food. You check things again and again. You hear things others cannot. You feel that others control your mind. You can't control your temper. You blame your troubles on others. You blame yourself. You are forgetful. You feel lonely. You feel scared. You feel bored. You feel sick. You feel irritable. You cry easily. You worry about your appearance. You worry too much. You can't fall asleep. You have a hard time breathing. You feel your brain is empty. Your heart beats too quickly. You have chest pain. You are afraid of open spaces. You want to smash things. You think about death. You want to end your life.[66]

Not one of the ninety questions mentioned the internet directly, let alone the actual social context and circumstances these symptoms stem from, therein sealing off these overt symptoms from reality and, validly speaking, making them all diagnostically meaningless. Despite failing to demonstrate that these overt symptoms are a) *not* an expectable response to a stress condition, b) *are* the result of an internal dysfunction, and c) are socially inappropriate actions, Funk was, nevertheless, told that his score of 1.50 indicated high marks for anxiety and depression. Likewise, his score of 2.00 indicated he possessed a worryingly high level of "paranoia," while his 2.20 rating for "obsessive-compulsive disorder" was said to be "bad." Funk noticed a score of 60.1 at the bottom of the computer read-out that looked out of place, and so asked what it signified. Without hesitating, the nurse answered, "that means you're an internet addict."[67] How can a set of statements such as these, that neither refer to the internet nor one's use of it, be said to measure internet addiction?

This is thus the task before us. The data that follow is designed to address this question of the internet addiction disorder being, or not being, a valid mental disorder according to the *DSM-IV*. Or to be exact, the narratives to be presented are designed to demonstrate that the person labeled an internet addict is, in reality, neither an internet addict nor an individual suffering from a mental disorder. Rather, the person conceptualized as an internet addict is, in fact, a rebel (social deviant) going against the normal functioning of society.

4 The humanistic intensive internet use model

Xiao Wang – life is violent

Let us return back to Xiao Wang's letter sent to Tao Hongkai, the first part of which was introduced at the beginning of Chapter Two. Doing so allows us to move beyond merely the overt symptoms he expressed in the first part, and which the Young-Tao model overly focuses upon, and toward both a more contextual understanding of Xiao Wang's social existence and the theory and method used in this book as a way to make sense of the offline *and* online lifeworld of these "cultural rebels" called internet addicts. Here is part two:

> I feel that the pressure in reality is getting more and more, I also cannot say specifically what this pressure is, I just always feel that this pressure is great! In summary, I am infatuated with "the internet" approximately because in the virtual world I can find a sense of satisfaction and freedom. Inside the internet I simply don't know what is pressure or worry. I am able to say and do whatever I like, and no one is going to discriminate against me as everyone online seems equal, and so in cyberspace you can feel like an emperor. I don't receive any restriction/obligation there. The friends in cyberspace really stick together through thick and thin, and so I feel that my friends online are the only ones I can consider to be real friends. But in reality? It is really difficult to accept! Like this I have broken away from reality.
>
> Oh, I forget to mention some things! This is my personal situation. My body is quite fat, my height is 180 cm, and my weight is 115 kgs, which is regarded as a "big fatty"! Fat people are a group where it is easy to be discriminated against by other people, so where can you go? You can feel people's abnormal looks towards fat people! But inside games this situation does not emerge. In the real world I absolutely don't love to show my face where there are lots of people, for fear that people will make fun of me. Even though there are people who speak nicely, people aren't perfect. Each has their own good points. I really don't know where my own good points are. Sometimes I quietly think about such things, and the more I think the more scared I get! I am about to be 20. I still have no special skill, later I will need to get married and start a career, and support a family to keep body

and soul together? But at the moment what skills do I have? What can I study now? I ask you to tell me, am I really a person that no medicine can save? Isn't it too late to study anything? Tell me!!! I am sorry, writing is making me agitated.

I feel that there is this nameless pressure that is too great, which also makes it hard to breathe, and sometimes I think that I am on the road to ruin! I really think it is worth dying! But I know that it cannot solve the problems. My mind is in a great contradiction!

Now I don't know what is good! Now I want to go to the internet bar.

Now we see Xiao Wang suffering not simply from "internet addiction" but from an ever increasing, yet mystifying, nameless pressure that appears to envelope him like smog. We also see that he is not using the internet simply to escape reality, but rather because he is seeking out feelings of satisfaction, freedom, peace, equality, and superiority there. Thus we see the interconnectedness of his "real" world and his "virtual" world, wherein the real world is full of discrimination – it is cold and dangerous – while cyberspace is perceived as a space of equality – warm and safe. This helps us learn why young people, who are relatively powerless in an authoritarian society, are so attracted to the internet, as it is a kind of safe monastery in a world out-of-balance. By feeling like an "emperor" the powerless Xiao Wang is also able to feel in control of his actions and the center of the universe. That is, he is able to express his individuality and to feel like an authoritative figure himself (as opposed to constantly feeling the pressure from authority figures such as his parents and teachers). We also see Xiao Wang attracted to the freedom and non-restrictions the internet offers. This is why it is so dangerous and revolutionary to parents, the school, and the Party-State, as it is a massively popular tool that allows individuals to do as they please. It is unstructured and there is no centralized power structure, rather power is disseminated among every user. Its power structure is not vertical but horizontal, as it was invented as a technology to eliminate the possibility of a central and hierarchical control mechanism.[1] This is why it is so attractive, as they are free to do as they please and there are no parents or teachers imposing obligations, tasks, and restrictions upon them within cyberspace.

In contrast to many parents of "internet addicts" who see their child's online friends as "unreal" and "bad," we see Xiao Wang referring to online friends as even more real than any friends in the so-called real world. Significantly, we also learn that a discriminatory society "pushed" him away while the facelessness of the internet "pulled" him in by allowing him not simply to escape reality but to partly overcome it. Nevertheless, his sense of failure at not having "made it" at school has seemingly left him facing a serious existential crisis, wherein he feels deep regret at not having adhered to social norms and expectations. Unsurprising that he desires to go online as it is here, and nowhere else, where he is able to experience a sense of happiness and freedom from the knots that bind him so tightly he feels unable to breathe and is thinking of death. Whether it is the correct method or not is another issue, but what seems obvious is the internet – as his only hobby – has become his weapon in fighting this "nameless pressure that is too great."

Retreat from reality or advance in a different direction?

Video games ruined my life. Good thing I have two extra lives.

(Read on a t-shirt)

Tao Ran has said that "under heavy pressure in life or work, some internet users hope to escape reality or release their emotions in cyberspace."[2] This is because they are said to "lack self-confidence and often don't have the courage to continue their lives." And so in the real world, according to him, "they become depressed, upset and restless," while at the same time, "believe the virtual world is beautiful and fair."[3] Griffiths has described this escape from reality as an in adequate stress-coping strategy, which is premised upon the gamer "playing the hurt away."[4] Xiao Wang, and more importantly the narratives that follow, offers us an alternative understanding of the aims and motivations underpinning excessive internet use. Through the theory of Norbert Elias we can see that far from the real and virtual world being part of a binary opposition, they are, on the contrary, intimately interconnected and thus we cannot understand the one without the other.

The notion of "compulsivity" that underpins all the behavioral addiction concepts, wherein addicts "cannot help" but act compulsively because their use is caused by forces largely beyond their control, removes from the outset the motivation and will of the user and, instead, locates it in their body or mind.[5] This particular conception of human behavior overlooks the fact that Xiao Wang was so attracted to the internet not simply because it allowed him to escape or retreat from reality, but more so because it allowed him to *advance* toward a new and different social reality. It was not simply that Xiao Wang had failed at life and so he drowned himself in games as a way to escape his difficulties and avoid his problems, but partly that *life had failed him* and so, like a migrant seeking new lands, he migrated to cyberspace in search of biopsychosocial solutions as a way to prevent him from drowning existentially. This *intra*personal (psychological) and *inter*personal (sociological) process that gives back personal motivation and will to the young person can best be understood with reference to the words of Major General Oliver Prince Smith at the infamous battle of Chosin Reservoir during the Korean War: *"We're not retreating,"* declared Smith, *"we're just advancing in different direction."*[6]

But this view – wherein internet use is a socially active process – is only possible if we move away from the value-laden real/virtual and work/leisure binaries currently underpinning the internet addiction disorder, wherein Young considers the online world to be "make believe."[7] For example, criterion-6 of the Young-Tao model assumes that the real is equivalent to the social and the virtual to the non-social, and so the internet addict's life is said to become both less real and less social the more time spent online. But since the internet is premised upon the meaning-making interplay between subjects and texts/images then internet use must be understood as a communicative (and thus social) practice.[8] As Ng and Wiemer-Hastings pointed out for example, social interaction in MMORPG games such as *EverQuest* is essential as you must collaborate with other players in the game in order to succeed in more complex goals. Actually, to advance further in the game the player must join a "guild" or "clan."[9] Proponents of internet addiction overly focus upon how the gamer has become a "failure" within so-called "real" society as they make a sharp distinction between the real and the virtual world, thus overlooking how the gamer is obtaining success, or at least personal feelings-of-success, through internet use. According to the Young-Tao model such achievements are not considered successes as they possess no social value. Likewise, we must ask why the gamer desires to join a clan or guild, for like almost everyone, the gamer also wants to be part of a collective affiliation and if "real" Chinese society is not providing such affiliations then it is rational, logical, and normal (i.e., expectable) for a young person to seek solutions to such an existential need online – and so does not indicate some kind of internal dysfunction.

Ng and Wiemer-Hastings also point out that such games provide internet users such as Xiao Wang anonymity, or what we could call "facelessness," allowing them to both create new social identities and the possibility of raising their self-esteem. Nevertheless, this is said by them to be a "substitute for real-life social interaction" that offers them an "escape from reality."[10] But as we see with Xiao Wang, the friends he made online were not considered by him as "substitutes" for "real" friends, rather these friends were more real than any friendships he had in the real world. That is, it is on the internet and *not* in the real world where Xiao Wang and others like him are able to make "real" friends. As we will see, many claim it is in fact the real world itself that is harming their social functioning because, for example, it is difficult to make real trust-based friendships centered around equality. Thus it is online, through applications such as QQ, where they are able to communicate their true feelings, for in this "faceless" space of sociality a "big fatty" like Xiao Wang is not discriminated against by feeling the "abnormal looks" he encounters in the real world. His attraction to this space of perceived equality only makes sense if we understand the authoritarian space of inequality that is his "normal" world. How can we say he has some mental illness for rationally choosing to evade an environment that is hostile to him and instead seeks out a safe space free from hostility? How is that harming his "social functioning" as it relates to freedom from discrimination? On the contrary, he is actively attempting to reduce the harm done to him by societal discrimination by *choosing* to advance in a different direction – an option that has been offered to him by the Party-State and the marketplace.

Norbert Elias and the quest for excitement

In order to move away from the binaries the Young-Tao model sets up between both the real/virtual and work/leisure we can refer to the work of sociologist Norbert Elias. For Elias, the world of work and the world of leisure are intimately interconnected because leisure activities partly serve an important function for the "serious" business of complex modern life, or what is called the normal functioning of a society. While the daily routines of life – going to work or school – demand that people keep a check on their moods and emotions, leisure activities (basketball, online gaming, karaoke, etc.) allow such feelings to flow more freely in a setting specially created by these activities – and which are also partly reminiscent of, or mimic, non-leisure reality. Basically for Elias, leisure pursuits can provide sufficient *complementary correctives* for the unexciting and suppressed tensions produced by the recurrent rational routines of non-leisure life. Thus while excitement is often severely confined and restricted during the serious business of life, as many over-worked-and-under-relaxed students in China will tell you, leisure activities are specifically designed to appeal to and arouse people's feelings directly. Eliciting excitement and creating tension through leisure pursuits is achieved by imitating that produced by non-leisure life situations, yet most importantly, without its more serious dangers, risks, and consequences. In this way, imaginary danger, mimetic pleasure, fear, sadness, and joy are all produced and potentially even resolved by the setting of the leisure activity. This is why Elias refers to the feelings aroused during leisure activities as the "siblings" of those aroused during the serious business of life.[11]

This can be understood by referring to the words of "Kim" (the son of a policeman and ex-colleague of Renfei). While enjoying karaoke with his work colleagues in Dalian I asked Kim what his favorite online game was, at which he replied *"Counter Strike"* (*CS*). I therefore asked him what it was he liked about this "violent" game. He said he enjoys playing *CS* because he can *"fa xie"* (give vent to; let off) feelings of anxiety stemming from his work and feelings of loneliness stemming from him being a migrant worker in an unfamiliar city. Quite simply, through being able to *fa xie* their feelings online gaming allows Chinese youth like Kim to *blow off steam*. However, their desire to blow off steam only makes sense if we understand the pressure cooker that is their so-called normal life. "Sometimes I feel like a prisoner," bemoaned 13-year-old Karmapa Lama, the No. 3 Lama in Tibetan Buddhism. In order to deal with his frustrations this young man likes to play so-called violent video games, despite the fact he abhors violence. He reportedly likes to play these games as they help him to get rid of "bad energy."[12] Likewise, while observing research subject *Renfei* study for an important university exam in Dalian, I saw him constantly watching a movie online or playing online snooker as these online leisure pursuits, according to him, made him feel "new" and "fresh" about preparing for an exam he said was "like my imprisonment." Far from being a kind of *poison* that was polluting his mind the internet functioned, conversely, as a *remedy* to his existential imprisonment. Renfei's critique of an education system that he said fails to understand the mood or feelings of students because it turns them into a kind of memorizing machine, and, conversely, the student's own desire to introduce both cathartic affect and self control into this process, indicates that there is an important humanistic *spiritual* dimension to online games vis-à-vis the sometimes dehumanizing "real world.'

In this sense the pleasurable play-excitement which young people seek in online games thus represents, at the same time, the complement and the antithesis to the recurrent emotional restraint and monotony, routinization, orderliness, and staleness of their purposeful rational routines encompassing their school/work life. As a complement to the world of purposeful, task-directed, and often impersonal activities, leisure activities, according to Elias and Dunning, are anything but representatives of an "unreal" fantasy world. On the contrary, the mimetic sphere of the world of leisure forms a distinct and integral part of social reality, and therefore it is necessary to move beyond a strict binary division between the "real" world of work and the "fantasy" world of play.[13] Such a conceptualization points in the direction of socially problematic internet use being premised not upon *category* (addict/not addict) but rather upon *dimension* (levels of intensity/ degrees of effect upon entire lifeworld).[14]

The division bell

In order to best visualize the way non-leisure life and leisure life form not a distinct binary opposition but rather are two sides of the same coin, we can refer to the famous cover diagram on Pink Floyd's album "The Division Bell."[15]

The picture on the cover seemingly of two metal heads facing each other is an optical illusion. This is because the two metal heads in profile facing each other also form, at the same time, the image of a larger third face looking directly at the viewer. We can simply say that the face on the left is non-leisure life (work/school), the face on the right is leisure life (internet/karaoke), while the third face looking directly at the viewer is the incorporation of work and leisure that constitutes "social reality" or the lifeworld of the intensive gamer. Thus while work and leisure appear distinct, they are actually integral to each other and thus form a larger whole. Subsequently, non-work-related internet use can only be understood in its relation to work-related activities. In this sense the internet connects the real and the virtual, for it is an apparatus that links processes of the real to those of the virtual, and thus inserts itself into everyday life, culture, and community in a seductive way.[16]

Gaming and scientific habits of the mind

We can observe the way games mimic the normal functioning of society by referring to the operations and functions of many of the video games themselves. For example, the structure of many MMORPG games, like the structure of the education system, the workplace, and the military, is partly premised upon the player being given a set of objectives for which he/she then has to individually, or in a group setting, engage in a large number of rational and logic-based tasks – sometimes simultaneously – in order to successfully obtain both the goals set and rewards offered within the activity.

Elias' basic premise is the quest for excitement in our leisure activities is in some sense complementary to the discipline, control, and restraint of overt emotionality in our non-leisure life, and thus we cannot understand the one without the other.[17]

Such a perspective helps us understand why one of the most popular video games in China (and throughout the world) is *World of Warcraft*. Quite simply, *World of Warcraft* is the mimetic electronic form of "socialism with Chinese characteristics" (i.e., authoritarian State capitalism). What is fascinating about *World of Warcraft* is not the way it is opposed to real life but rather how it mimics it. Within *World of Warcraft*, when you move your character and "his" troops, the character always says "with honor." And when asked to carry out a task, one of the characters will say "Certainly. I will go straight away." This obedience to given orders is just what school is asking of the student; however, the crucial distinction within the game is that the order-receiving student has become the order-giving teacher or master. In the game the player is asked to build up the population so that these "peasant workers" can build a town. The peasant workers, under orders from the master, obediently say when they appear, "Ready for work," and when ordered to chop down trees they answer "More wood." The operation here mimics the construction industry wherein migrant peasants are ordered to always be "ready to work" and ready to get more of whatever is asked of them. In this sense, the player, through the main character, is carrying out the operations of a Chinese entrepreneur – using a disposable workforce to build an object, and at the same time, his/her wealth.

Thus the premise or ethic of the game, like the global economic system in which we live, is based upon speed and efficiency, but perhaps most importantly of all it is centered upon excess and expansion. The player must extract the maximum amount of resources (gold and wood) in order to build up an army/work-force, that then goes out into "the world" in order to expand their empire, killing whatever comes in one's way (specifically one's competition) so that the player can continue the cycle of extraction, consolidation, and expansion. In a way the game is designed to teach the user about the fundamentals of imperialist-style global capitalism, especially the ethic of competition, and the operations involved in being "successful." It is a kind of learners' manual for how "socialism with Chinese characteristics" works, as the underlying message is "to get rich is glorious."[18] The capitalist-ethic is a highly valued ethic in China today, as it is throughout our globalized world, which is expressed through the desirable figure of the entrepreneur. We have seen how the Communist Party, beginning with Former President Jiang Zemin, now appropriates successful entrepreneurs into their ranks, while simultaneously the Party-State has been rapidly expanding its military apparatus. At the same time the Party-State has been expanding into Africa and other places in order to conduct trade (say with Burma for wood) so as to fuel its economic and social expansion. Thus by playing *World of Warcraft* the gamer is not simply getting further away from reality but, on the contrary, touches against the ethical heart of China's market-driven economic system.

Because video games are simulated or mimetic worlds that the gamer is continually trying to master by using techniques to uncover the hidden rules that govern such worlds, researchers are now beginning to realize that gamers, without them often even realizing it, are involved in scientific thinking while playing. After all, is not the basis of the scientific method a technique used to uncover the hidden rules that govern the world?[19]

The way gamers of MMORPG games are, literally, doing science while playing has been uncovered by research carried out by American scholars Constance Steinkuehler and Sean Duncan. Through both playing MMORPG games for 12 hours per day and through textual analysis of the forums gamers use to communicate with each other while gaming, Steinkuehler and Duncan discovered that such video games were fostering what they called "scientific habits of the mind."[20] For example, their research found that 86 percent of the *World of Warcraft* discussion forums (that were not simply social banter) consisted of talk described as "social knowledge construction" – i.e., the collective development of understanding through argumentation and joint problem solving. Moreover, 86 percent of these forum posts built on ideas that previous posters had raised, while roughly another third used counterarguments against previous posters' ideas. As another illustration of scientific argumentation, Steinkuehler and Duncan found that in 28 percent of the posts individuals used data or evidence of some form in order to warrant their claims. Gamers are undertaking what they call *systems-based reasoning* because in such games individuals collaborate to solve complex problems within the virtual world, such as figuring out what combination of individual skills, proficiencies, and equipment are required to, for example, conquer an in-game boss dragon.[21]

Most important off all, however, is that the students engaging in these science-based conversations and operations are precisely the same ones who are tuning out of science in the "real" classroom. Steinkuehler and Duncan think video games are the way to reverse this trend because students get bored by science as it is too often presented as a stale collection of facts for memorization. They therefore argue that schools ought to be embracing games as places to show kids the value of scientific scrutiny and the *quest* for knowledge. Former President Jiang Zemin, however, referred to such online games as being part of the "flood of trash" on the internet which he defined as being "anti-science, false science ... and downright harmful."[22] But this research is important because it shows that gaming is complementary to formal education and not simply opposed to it, and that the gamer – far from escaping reality and becoming poisoned by information pollution – may enhance the cognitive skills that are deemed the most important to the normal functioning of society. However, they are getting their science in a fun way and not in a creativity-sapping rote-learning fashion (as Renfei bemoaned). This, therefore, shows just how close MMORPG gamers in China are to the CCP's guiding ideology of "the scientific outlook on development." Thus far from taking them further away from reality such games, on the contrary, touch against the beating heart of the Party-State's political machinery. Quite simply, playing *World of Warcraft* not only allows youth to *fa xie* their suppressed tensions and to feel like the center of the universe, it also, without them being fully aware of it, forces them to cultivate a (fun) scientific outlook on development. From this perspective The Ministry of Culture's regulation issued on June 22, 2010, stating that online games must be free of content that can lead to the imitation of behavior that violates social morals, must be much more specific about the morals these gamers are supposedly violating.[23] In actual practice many gamers are engaged in activities which are pro-entrepreneurial and pro-science and thus it is difficult to argue that online games stripped them of morality.

As mentioned earlier, Griffiths described excessive gaming as an inadequate stress-coping strategy premised upon the gamer "playing the hurt away." Such a perspective assumes that, like drowning oneself in drink or drugs, gaming simply alleviates tension by "numbing" them to their hurt or pain. Not only does this overlook the fact that gaming partly functions for the survival, maintenance, and inflation of the ego or self, but Elias also demonstrates that leisure pursuits such as video gaming function by actually *creating* tension. Elias argues that sports are designed to stir the emotions and to evoke tensions so as to produce what he calls an "enjoyable and controlled de-controlling of the emotions."[24] Elias has described the process of sport as a controlled and generally non-violent mimetic battle which begins with a phase of struggle centered around battle-tension and excitement. Such tension and excitement is often demanding in terms of physical exertion and/or skill, but is also often exhilarating in its own right as a kind of liberation from the recurrent routines and stress-tensions of non-leisure life. This is usually followed by a phase of decision and release from battle-tension either in triumph and victory or in disappointment and defeat.[25] This central function of online gaming was clearly expressed by Xiao Kang (see later), who wrote: *"infinite pleasure comes from the battle with others."*

And so it is the creation of these tensions and the battle with others, and not simply in the drowning of them, that have a liberating, even cathartic effect for the player, because such activities can loosen and even free stress-tensions. The mimetic tensions of leisure pursuits and the related excitement which are generally free of the danger, risk, or guilt one experiences in the serious business of life can therefore serve as an antidote or remedy to the stress-tensions being produced within the person by a society like China going through profound social transformations and often disorienting upheavals.

In fact, Elias's insight into the cathartic quality of leisure activities comes from the ancient theory of Aristotle. Aristotle's theory of the cathartic effects of drama and music derived from observations of physicians cleansing the body through purgative. Aristotle suggested, figuratively, that drama and music could have a similar curative effect upon the body – not through the movement of the bowels but, so to speak, through a *movement of the soul*. Thus Aristotle surmised that if a person was tense or overexcited then exciting music could help them to calm down. Or if a person is feeling numb with despondency and despair they could seek relief in the stirring-up of their emotions through mournful tunes. In this sense the essence of the curative effect of these leisure pursuits is that the excitement which they produce within the person, in contrast to the excitement in seriously critical situations, is *actually pleasurable.*[26]

Turning such a theory toward the young online gamer we can think of it in this way: if an adolescent in China is frustrated by the competitive and repetitive nature of his school life then he can play a competitive and repetitive online game in which to calm him; or if he is sick of the serious task-oriented nature of the education system then he can play a task-oriented online game in order to relax.

This is because, unlike many school-based activities, his online activities, which mimic his non-leisure life, give him pleasure and excitement. For example, one afternoon I chatted on QQ to a student at Jiaotong University in Xi'an who likes playing basketball and computer games with friends. I therefore asked him why he thinks many young people like to play computer games. He replied, "Maybe only in computer games can they relax themselves and get what they want." So I asked him what is it that they wanted. He said they want "crazy," "excitement" – meaning intense feelings of fun. Thus through the infinite pleasure that comes from the exciting battle with others, the stressed person is able to deal with these stress-tensions through a cathartic experience such as playing *World of Warcraft*.

China's *pharmakon*: poison or remedy?

Aristotle used the concept *pharmakon* as a way to understand how something can be said to act as both a poison and a remedy. Thus while we have seen how video games are said to *pollute* the mind of young people, and so they are said to require medication, psychotherapy, and military-style discipline in order to cleanse or purify them, through the idea of the pharmakon we can see the opposite: gaming, figuratively speaking, is itself a kind of bodily cleansing that attempts to purge or rid the body of the socially produced "impurities" or "bad energy" young people encounter during the serious business of life – in particular, the pressures stemming from school and family life.

In understanding that online gaming is sometimes an inside remedy to outside "poisons," and that, in addition, such gaming is not necessarily the root cause of a person's problems, we can refer to a conversation I had one day with "Fan." While chatting on QQ to "yuan" (Fan) about his leisure activities in Zhengzhou he said he likes to play the online game "Red Alarm."[27] He likes playing this game partly because it can "make your thinking more meticulous." In addition, he also likes to listen to music and take photos while living in a city he described as "not good" (read: chaotic) because according to him there are "so many people coming and going." Fan particularly likes Korean and classical music because "when I am listening to it I can feel cozy and so your troubles can float away." When he is upset he also chooses to play Red Alarm as it can help him deal with his troubles, even though he knows his troubles will not disappear. I therefore asked him where his troubles come from. He replied: "From money." He added that we worry about "how to spend it, preserve it, invest it, and shopping." "Trouble," he surmised, "is like a cloud which comes without notice, anytime, anywhere, and so then the game goes on and the music plays." What he is saying is that playing games and listening to music can be a kind of cathartic experience that functions to make the "clouds" go away, and that gaming, rather than simply being the problem, is, for him at least, part of the solution (or a strategy) to resolving his non-leisure life problems.

In this way, online gaming can be understood as a way of dealing with, rather than simply escaping from, China's fraught modernization process. It is only in this way that we could approach gaming as a kind of "drug" in a metaphorical sense, but it is a drug as a remedy or antidote and not – as is commonly understood when the term "electronic opium" is used – as a poison. As Derrida noted in his famous essay "Plato's Pharmacy," the pharmakon is ambivalent because both "remedy" and "poison" already bear its own opposite within the term itself, and therefore the term constitutes the *medium* in which these opposites are opposed.[28] It is this medium operating between remedy and poison that is one of the keys for uncovering the secrets of the internet addiction phenomenon.

We can observe the pharmakon of internet addiction in operation by referring back to the TV program *Focus Point* both Tao Ran and Tao Hongkai appeared on. Also appearing on the program was a person who works within the gaming industry for *Sina.com*. Speaking as an industry insider defending the gaming industry against Tao Ran's claim that such games are a kind of poison polluting the mind of youth, "*Bai Ma*" said that "within the industry there is a point of view that sees online games as "chicken soup for the soul," and therefore they can be a remedy."[29] Fellow panelist and well-known sports program host, Liang Hongda, interrupted him by asking rhetorically: "You mean "poison chicken soup'?"[30] In this short dialogue we see through the medium of online games how the pharmakon operates with games being seen, at the same time, as both cathartic chicken soup for the soul and as a chicken soup containing poison.

Interestingly, pharmakon in ancient Greek religion was a kind of human scapegoat, in which a deviant or "outsider" was first chosen and then expelled from the community during times of disaster and/or crisis as a way to purify the city. The pharmakos – the scapegoat, the deviant, the outsider, the rebel – was sacrificed by being led outside the city walls and killed in order to purify the "evil" that had infected the city from the outside.[31]

In a way the "internet addict" is the pharmakos of contemporary China. The internet addict – the deviant, the rebel – is a kind of scapegoat for the "poison" that China's modernization process has produced during a time of moral crisis. This deviant must be led away to a treatment center so that they can be purified of this poison contained within this electronic opium said to be imported through video games from the West. But the so-called internet addict is being sacrificed, by being forced to turn his/her problems into an "individual pathology," so that the more significant creator of these problems, China's modernization process itself, can be absolved of blame through what amounts to a societal catharsis. The question then arises: Should deviant and rebellious Chinese youth be treated as scapegoats for socially and structurally produced problems? Instead of seeing how online games poison both the mind and social functioning of the gamer, we should, instead, see in which ways the gamers' whole social existence – or lifeworld – is itself being "poisoned.'

Tao Ran claims a prolonged and "preoccupied" usage of the internet poisons young people like Xiao Wang by causing them to "have a low opinion of oneself," "feel down in spirits," "have no interest in doing things," "have reduced feelings of happiness," and "have reduced exchanges with other people." First, how can it be proven that these possible outcomes are symptoms directly caused by internet use? In any case, Xiao Wang's feelings of satisfaction and freedom he had online are not simply "substitutions" for "real" feelings of satisfaction and freedom, but should instead be seen as real feelings in and of themselves – *as experienced by him*. As I will highlight, many pessimistic feelings toward schoolwork precede internet use, and so rather than internet use simply causing a pessimism toward schoolwork it is also the case that, on the contrary, pessimism toward school-work, and life more generally, is contributing to internet use.

Moreover, "internet addicts" such Xiao Wang show us that rather than internet use resulting in one undervaluing oneself and causing one to be down in spirits, that on the contrary, internet use and gaming may actually increase their self-worth and make them feel happier. Later we will see how Xiao Kang said with pride how his gaming made him popular, and how Huang He said that the thing he liked the most was the self-respect he gained from the 40–50 fellow gamers calling him a "big brother" (*laoda*). Earlier we also saw how Xiao Wang felt like an "emperor" in cyberspace. This experience is a central pull factor of online games as they are able to feel in control of their *own* actions and the center of their *own* universe. That is, powerless individuals living in an authoritarian society who are constantly under attack by authority figures such as parents and teachers are able to express their individuality and experience feelings of power and authority. This is because games provide an opportunity to demonstrate one's mastery over oneself and others and to potentially obtain (relative) fame and acceptance within the gaming subculture.[32]

Videogame play is personally meaningful precisely because playing such games means making choices and taking actions, while the game assigns outcomes to those choices and actions. For youth whom feel they have little choice over their actions, then engaging in an activity that is designed to support meaningful kinds of choice making is a highly desirable object indeed.[33] Tao Ran narrowly focuses on the possible negative or poisonous outcomes relative to the "real world" and does not take seriously into account the positive that internet use engenders relative to their entire existence. This is partly because he assumes that the cause of excessive internet use is to "escape reality" and so once mired in this virtual reality the internet addict will "lose touch" with reality and so will somehow forget how to associate with "real" people, thereby becoming afraid of socializing. But for many their "fear" of the real world preceded their internet use, and so their internet use is partly a remedy to this dangerous and mistrustful real world where strangers are sometimes seen as potential thieves, parents as enemies, and classmates as rivals; therefore they seek out more positive social relations on the internet. The question is not that the internet has made the individual fearful of the real world by poisoning him/her, but that the threatening real world has caused the individual to reject this "sick" society, or society out-of-balance, and instead attempt to remedy this negative situation by migrating online where they can encounter relations based not on mistrust and suspicion but rather mutual respect and equality.

Pathology of normalcy and culture of excess

Tao Ran refuses to entertain the idea that contemporary Chinese society *as a whole* may be lacking in "sanity." He, like psychiatrists the world over, holds that the problem of mental health in a society is only that of the number of "maladjusted" individuals – paradoxically millions of "internet addicts" in particular – and not that of a possible maladjustment of the whole social system itself. Following German social psychologist Erich Fromm in understanding the crucial social conditions underlying the young "internet addict" in China, we should perhaps focus on the latter problem. Not the problem of individual pathology, but rather the *pathology of normalcy*, particularly the pathology of so-called "normal" contemporary Chinese society.[34] Fromm forces us to think about what is the more important generator of mental distress: the individual organism or the socio-economic organism? For example, Tsinghua University and *Xiao Kang* magazine (*"Well-off"* magazine) conducted a survey among a segment of China's middle class. 88.9 percent of those surveyed said they were over-fatigued, while 53.3 percent said they were not satisfied with their physical and mental condition. In addition, more than 60 percent of the respondents said they were sacrificing their health for money.[35]

But authority figures like Tao Ran, and the Party-State itself, have difficulty confronting the possibility that its capitalist reforms and political system may be making people "sick," for this would call into question the very legitimacy of their authority, power, and right to govern (let alone the "right" of boot camps to create wealth and power off "sick" individuals). And so the strategy is a simple but incredibly effective one: *"individuals are forced to seek biographical solutions to socially produced problems."*[36] The effect of this socio-political strategy can be simply understood by reference to the QQ name of a young man I chatted to online one day about his life and internet use. He went by the name of "one person's battle."[37] Quite simply, their battle with the *World of Warcraft* is, simultaneously, also their battle with their own *lifeworld of warcraft*.

Fromm argues that a "sane" – or perhaps more specifically a healthy – society would promote individual development and (democratic) self-expression within the context of a vibrant communal life. To do this, however, individual communities, cities, and society as a whole, must find ways to address certain universal human needs, including needs for: 1) Relatedness; 2) Transcendence; 3) Rootedness; 4) A sense of identity; and 5) A framework of orientation and devotion.[38] In trying to unravel the underlying mechanisms driving the internet addiction phenomenon we should therefore keep this question close at hand: Has the Party-State created a society to address these needs? Only by understanding the "sick" aspects of the so-called normal functioning of contemporary society does the mass migration to the internet in general, and online games in particular, become fully comprehensible. For example, through the letters we can observe there is a certain kind of pathology of normalcy, and not simply individual pathology, which is leaving some young people feeling separate, rootless, fragmented, frustrated, confused, and uncomfortable. Therefore a (cyber) space which seemingly offers relatedness to others, the transcendence of aloneness and separateness, a sense of rootedness, orientation, comfort, and even spiritual nourishment is going to become highly sought after and desired. Only then does their "devotion" to the internet really make empirical sense.

In order to gauge the underlying "sickness" of a society, Fromm argues that a high suicide rate in a given population is expressive of a lack of societal mental stability and health.[39] According to the Beijing Municipal Bureau of Health, suicide in China has become the top "killer" of young people aged 15–34 (significantly, the same age cohort of the "internet addicts'); and also the fifth largest cause of death among the entire Chinese population.[40] Citing United Nations' statistics, journalist Ding Gang says that 250,000 people commit suicide in China per year, which is a rate of 22.23 per 100,000. This rate is said to be 2.3 times higher than the global suicide rate. According to the WHO, a country is a "high suicide rate country" if it is above 20 per 100,000.[41]

In interpreting these figures, Chinese journalists point to the rapid social transition brought about by the opening-up reforms, which while creating economic growth has also created a "tremendous pressure and *disorientation* that Chinese have never experienced before."[42] Significantly, of the top ten countries in the world for high suicide rates, nine are (like China) ex-communist states going through rapid market reforms and social and structural transformation. The WHO's own interpretation of the high suicide rate in China is attributed to three leading factors: social, economic, and cultural changes. Cannot the same be said for "internet addiction," in that the cause of excessive internet use does not lie with the maladjusted and pathological individual but rather a maladjusted social system?[43]

We should ask why the very small number of deaths that are (misleadingly) attributed to internet addiction – which are themselves being quickly surpassed by the deaths relating to the "cure" of internet addiction – has received more public and media attention than this extremely serious and problematic issue affecting Chinese youth? Part of the answer lies with the fact moral entrepreneurs and medical crusaders such as Tao Ran and Yang Yongxin can create wealth directly from "internet addiction," yet cannot from suicide. Likewise, is it a coincidence that the increase in suicide among the young and the rapid increase in socially problematic internet usage – along with the rapid increase in religious and spiritual seekers and followers – is occurring simultaneously; for are not these threads all intimately related? While the number of online gamers now exceeds that of the 70–80 million Communist Party members, the same exponential growth has simultaneously been occurring within Chinese citizens seeking out Christianity, which according to some estimates already exceeds 70 million followers. Echoing Fromm, Pastor Jin from the Protestant Zion Church in Beijing reportedly said "Our church offers people a feeling of *belonging* to a family. There are more and more contradictions in our society as different interest groups emerge and gaps open up between regions and between social groups. Christianity can help by providing comfort and spiritual strength."[44] For Jin's followers, as for followers of online games, many of them have family problems and so find warmth in belonging to a religious affiliation. The thirst for video games, spiritual anchorage, and even suicide, it could be argued, are all related to the outcome of the *dangers of modernity* and are, in effect, kinds of weapons used during the individual's confrontation with an often *excessive* and *dehumanizing* modernization process that is attempting, for example, to turn Chinese youth into *grade-making machines*. Gaming, religion, and suicide are, in a way, particular remedies employed by young people living within a *culture of excess*.

Fromm argues that another gauge of pathology of normalcy, and I would add a culture of excess, is excessive alcohol consumption. During China's opening up and reform transformation there has been a striking increase in alcohol consumption and related problems associated with excessive alcohol use. While alcohol has traditionally been part of social life in China, commercial production has increased 50-fold since the mid-1950s. According to Cochrane *et al.* there has been over the past 20 years a marked increase in the prevalence of what they call "alcohol dependence."[45] Leaving aside the issues associated with such a term, the point is that as we have seen a rapid increase in internet use, we have also seen a simultaneous rapid increase in alcohol (and legal and illegal drug) consumption.

Moreover, China, like many of the post-industrial economies, has seen an accompanying increase in hypertension. One study looking at the relationship between hypertension and premature death attributed a marked increase in hypertension, or high blood pressure, to excessive alcohol consumption, excessive smoking, excessive salt intake, excessive body-weight (obesity), and lack of exercise.[46]

Alongside hypertension brought about by burgeoning excessive living, or living out of balance for those with the economic capacity to do so, there has also reportedly been a rapid rise in diabetes in China with 10 percent of adults apparently having it and another 16 percent said to be on the verge of developing it. A rate that has surpassed many so-called developed economies. Increases in wealth and greater choice has led to sweeping changes in diet, with urban residents in particular eating heavily salted foods, fatty meats, and sugary snacks, which while boosting obesity rates has also boosted rates of type 2 diabetes.[47]

Another indicator of the "pathology" of contemporary China is the rising rate of infertility. For example, The 2009 Investigative Report on the Current State of Infertility in China found a significant decline in the average sperm count of men on the mainland, from about 100 million sperms per milliliter of semen 40 years ago to about 20 to 40 million in recent years. While for women there has been a rapid rise in rates of infertility brought about through abortion-related complications. As with computer technologies and alcohol, abortion in China is heavily marketed, with ubiquitous advertisements featuring stylish and beautiful young women plastered on billboards, TV, and computer screens. Couple this with the "sexual revolution" in contemporary China where premarital sex has become common as sexual mores have loosened – yet where a general lack of sex education around contraceptive methods still prevails – then many young females resort to abortions following accidental pregnancies.[48]

Accompanying this sexual revolution (and new found emphasis on individual desire[49]) has been a reported 10-fold increase in syphilis cases over the past 10 years, with cases now apparently growing by 30 percent a year. This rapid increase in syphilis is generally attributed to the boom in prostitution, wherein migrant workers in cities along with businessmen and government officials all seek their services.[50]

There is likewise the rapid rise of cancer rates in China since the 1990s, which was said to be responsible for one in five deaths in 2007, up 80 percent since the start of the opening and reform 30 years ago and now China's biggest "killer."

The explosion of cancer rates has been particularly acute in areas close to chemical factories as they release carcinogens into water supplies and the food chain. Thus while there are hundreds of military-style boot camps operating to bring an unruly population under control through medical and military purification, there are now hundreds of infamous "cancer villages" dotted across the country that are, literally, killing people.[51]

Thus excessive use of the internet, like all the other excesses selected earlier for comparison, is a *product* of China's modernization process, or culture of excess. And so making sense of this phenomenon requires us to contextualize excessive internet use within a much broader culture of excess and excessive-living that permeates, following the rise in consumerism, many aspects of contemporary Chinese life (and life in post-industrial consumer-driven societies). When we examine excessive internet use within the context of the consumer revolution taking place in contemporary China, wherein Chinese consumers want it *here and now*, then this deviant behavior turns out to be paradoxically consistent with one of the important aims driving Chinese society that could be conceptualized thus: *to get as much as you can as fast as you can.* The so-called internet addict is living for now or today, much to his/her parent's concern as they plan for the child's tomorrow, not simply because they are rejecting their society's values, but, on the contrary, precisely because they are responding more automatically and more hurriedly to its subliminal call: *consume baby, consume.*[52] While America's rapid economic and modern industrialization process is referred to as "The Gilded Age," perhaps we can refer to China's rapid economic and modern industrialization process as "The Age of Excess?"

Existential needs, social functioning, and individual happiness

A large part of the political legitimacy of the CCP is premised upon providing what Deng Xiaoping called a "well-off society" (*xiaokang shehui*) to its citizens through economic development. But the data offered here raise the question as to whether there is something fundamentally problematic with the economically dominated "normal" way of life and with the aims toward which "normal" people are striving. The narratives offered later of seemingly normal Chinese families is principally designed to demonstrate that there is something rather abnormal with their "normal" way of life, and with particular reference to the parents of so-called internet addicts, something fundamentally misguided with the aims – and the means to reach these aims – toward which they are striving. Could it be that excessive internet use, excessive drinking, excessive eating, excessive strivings for sex, love, and spiritual connection tell us that people cannot, so to speak, "live on economic reforms alone?" And that, most crucially, the Party-State is falling short of producing a social system that can satisfy profound needs in its citizens because it has been "addicted" to fast economic development at any cost.

In short, when trying to understand the psychology around internet usage I propose that, following Fromm, we base our analysis upon Chinese youth's material, mental, and spiritual needs stemming from the actual social conditions of their existence (and not just from the overt symptoms stemming from their existence).[53] When we do so we learn that it is actually the specific conditions of China's modernity that compels citizen's to find ever-new consumer-based biographical and individual solutions to the social and structural contradictions in their existence. In this way I follow Fromm in arguing that the necessity to find ever-new solutions for the contradictions in one's existence, and to find ever-higher forms of unity with nature, with one's fellows, and with oneself, is the source of all psychic forces such as passion, affect, and anxiety which motivates people.[54]

Thus we must ask: what function does the internet play in the life of China's (urban) youth in helping them find these ever-higher forms of unity? Conversely we must also ask: are the particular conditions of young people's real-world existence providing for their material, mental, and spiritual needs? This text, again following Fromm, therefore works from the premise that while many of today's youth have their basic physiological needs satisfied (food, clothing, shelter) such satisfactions do not, in any way, solve their *human problems*, for their needs are not simply those rooted in their body, but are also rooted in the very peculiarity of their incredibly complex social existence.[55] We must therefore locate Chinese youth's passion for and devotion toward the internet within this search for answer to their existential needs.

The question we should therefore be asking is: has contemporary Chinese society provided spiritual solutions to the existential and emotional problems faced by young people who have grown up in a period of excessive capitalism and materialism?

Fromm argues that normal or healthy can be defined in two main ways. First, from the standpoint of a functioning society, a person is called normal or healthy if they are able to fulfill the social role they are *expected* to take in that given society. More specifically, fulfilling one's social functioning requires a person to study and/or work in the fashion which is expected of them.[56] The Young-Tao model, with its focus on internet use harming social functioning, is partly a disciplinary sanction against the person *not* fulfilling their social role; in particular those whom refuse to devote their existence to a *life-of-study* and, instead, devote themselves to a *life-of-leisure*. On the other hand, Fromm argues, normal or healthy can be approached from the perspective of the individual, and so we can look upon normalcy or health as the optimum of growth, happiness, and satisfaction of the individual. If the structure of the society was built in such a way as to offer the optimum possibility for individual happiness *and* satisfaction then both perspectives would coincide.

However, this is arguably not the case in contemporary Chinese society due to factors such as living out of balance and the larger culture of excess that passes for normalcy. As a result there is often a disjunction between the aims of the "normal" functioning of society and of the full development of the individual. This excessive fast growth and "development" of the economy coupled with the consumer-led culture of excess may arrest the young person from being able to reach positive growth and happiness because they are required (by their parents, their school, and the market) to study-to-excess if they hope to become a saleable commodity in the marketplace after graduation.

These two different concepts of health, wherein the former is governed by social necessity and the latter by the values concerning the aims of individual existence, are central to understanding the internet addiction phenomenon. According to Tao Ran's and the parent's perspective of "health," the child should submit to the normal functioning of society, and so their existential needs and their (consumer-society produced) desires and wants should be subsumed under this priority. In particular, pressurized and fearful parents living in a social system lacking in comprehensive social safety nets such as public healthcare and old-age pensions, problematically neglect the mechanisms that could lead to the optimum health and happiness of their child by focusing "compulsively" upon the child's schoolwork so that the child will obtain the relevant qualifications needed to "get ahead" in a hyper-competitive system. The Young-Tao model, the treatment centers, and the military-style boot camps take the structure of their society for granted, and as a result the young person who is not well "adapted" to it assumes the stigma of being in need of "rectification" and "correction." The treatment centers and boot camps are, therefore, generally working in the service of this normalcy, and so are tasked with trying to force the deviant child to adapt to the normal functioning of society. But as Fromm emphasizes, often such people are adapted only at the expense of having given up existential needs in order to become more or less the person he/she is expected to be. For Fromm, this deviant person can be understood as someone who was not ready or willing to surrender completely in the battle for their individual autonomous self. It is at this point, in the "internet addict"'s' battle for his/her individual self, that the rebel (with a cause) appears.

In being willing to fight the pathology of normalcy the intensive internet user, from the standpoint of human values, can be considered less "disordered" than the ideal normal person who has handed over completely his/her individuality to this pathology of normalcy. It is precisely at the level of human values that Fromm says we could call a society pathological, as its members are partly crippled in the growth of their whole personality. But since the term pathological is used to indicate a lack of social functioning then pathology of normalcy can be understood to mean a social structure that is generally adverse to genuine human happiness and self-realization.[57] And because some youth feel that normalcy is adverse to producing genuine happiness and self-realization, and is thus harming their *individual functioning*, millions of them are deciding, for better or worse, to seek it out in cyberspace.

Applying the theory of Erich Fromm and R.D. Laing

In order to fully contextualize this striving for individual freedom from the pathology of normalcy, then I frame it within Fromm's main theoretical threads. The first is to locate internet use within what Fromm calls the individuation process, whereby the adolescent begins to break away from the primary ties of parents and, at the same time, begins to orient and root oneself to a world outside of these primary ties. For example, they begin to spend time within a peer group after school socializing at the local internet bar where they come into contact with the aptly named *World Wide Web*. The main reason for taking the analysis to this processual level is because, as Tao Ran has pointed out (yet then denied), and as my own data confirm, "internet addiction" is primarily happening to adolescents aged around 17 years (i.e., the period leading up to the college entrance exam). Therefore, we must understand the *intra*personal and *inter*personal changes taking place during these crucial years.

Stitched to the individuation process is what Fromm refers to as a *search for freedom*. In particular the search for freedom *from* preindividualistic ties and disciplinary mechanisms (i.e., parents and school) and the search for *freedom* to control one's own life, especially the desire to devote less time to school and more time to play. However, the normal functioning of society, as experienced through the parents' violent disciplinary response toward the child's rebelliousness, functions to thwart the individuation process from taking place until the child has (hopefully) graduated from university. It is in the thwarting of this expansiveness, which is experienced by the child as the suppression of freedom, where so many hostilities arise, such as the breakdown of communication between child and parents and, more importantly, where we see time away from home and internet use increase.

But this interpersonal individuation process is comprehensible only by seeing how it is connected to the structural process of *individualization* taking place in China during the market reforms. On the one hand, the generation born after the coming of the opening up and reform period has been *freed from* the bondage of the repressive big brother-like economic and political mechanisms that exemplified the Maoist era (e.g., the *danwei* system[58]). And thus the subsequent retreat of the Party-State from the private lives of normal and obedient citizens, alongside the reintroduction of capitalist ethics, has engendered a *freedom to* become more independent, more self-reliant, and more critical. However, at the same time, Chinese citizens were also "freed" from those ties which used to give them security (e.g., the iron rice bowl[59]) and the sense of belonging (e.g., as a "comrade" living in a *danwei*); and as I highlight later this "freedom" makes many feel alone, anxious, and powerless.[60]

In this sense, the "freedom" that Chinese citizens have gained from the collapse of the welfare aspects of Maoism is not necessarily a positive freedom because the subsequent process of individualization – what one does, how one does it, and whether one succeeds or fails is entirely one's *own* affair[61] – has enforced a sense of separation between one individual and the other; and thereby isolated and separated many individuals from his/her fellow citizens. While, at the same time, it has left some, especially those born after the opening up and reforms, "at sea" without sufficient institutional, social, and/or intrapersonal coping and relief mechanisms.[62] And so internet use is a mechanism taken up in order to deal with issues such as aloneness, separateness, rootlessness, disorientation, and anxiety while living within a period of excessive authoritarian and state-managed capitalism. Individuation is, we could say, a necessary process during modernity, but individualization has been a structurally-produced process brought about by the privatization and deregulation of social institutions during reform and opening up – i.e., handing over the individual to state-managed market forces. In this sense citizens are partly condemned to individualization and so must constantly adapt to changing social conditions, and are forced to find ever-new biographical and individual solutions to the social and structural contradictions in their existence. And so individualization is, as Bauman put it, like a "fate," in which individuals are patted on the back when they succeed yet labeled as "mentally disordered" when they rebel or fail.[63]

In addition to the very serious hostilities that arise within the family over an increasingly resistant and rebellious (i.e., individualizing) child are the actions of the parents toward the child – often beginning long before the child ever picks up a computer mouse. In order to understand one of the root causes of socially problematic internet use we can refer to the actions of the China Youth University for Political Sciences in Beijing. At the beginning of the 2009–2010 academic year the university offered a material reward, in the form of 100 yuan, for each freshman who registered alone on campus administration day. The university apparently presented this "bonus" as a positive means in which to cultivate "independence" within the post-1980s/90s only-child who are often criticized for being both "spoilt" and "selfish." However, in reality the university was offering this material reward not to encourage independence but rather because, as the head of the student department put it, "thousands of freshman and several times their number in parents cause disorderly traffic on campus every admission day."[64] The key here is not the thousands of freshman but rather the "several times their number in parents" who descend upon university campuses across China every year. As one student said, she would have actually liked to have registered alone but her parents were *more excited than her* about going to Peking University and so they had planned the details of the trip one month beforehand.[65]

That is, many parents, but usually the mother, invest more emotion in the child's education than the child themself. Or as Yang Xiong from the Shanghai Academy of Social Sciences said of today's parents living within the confines of the one-child policy: "Parents have to put all their dreams onto one child – they can't say if this one doesn't do well I'll put my hopes on another."[66] And like the university mentioned earlier, they offer material rewards to the child as a means in which to get the child to comply with their wishes and fears – wishes and fears which stem partly from the market reforms. But this inadvertently teaches them that "good behavior" will be rewarded with a monetary and/or material rewards and that money and consumption can solve all problems. It also teaches them that money is the commodity of the highest value, thereby fostering money-mindedness, materialism, and consumption. In responding to this university's new policy sociologist Li Dun said that the one-child policy has drastically changed the basic family structure, with the child, instead of the parents, now becoming the center of attention.[67]

This very shift in power relations and control mechanisms within the contemporary Chinese family is central for unpacking the mechanisms driving the internet addiction phenomenon. This drastic change in the basic family structure can be understood with reference to Fromm's concept of *filiarchy*. Quite simply, we can define filiarchy as children making family choices and decisions, as opposed to matriarchal-centered or patriarchal-centered decision-making processes.[68] Filiarchy, as I explain later, is the traditional patriarchal family structure flipped on its head, as parents hand over part of the power, authority, and decision-making process to the child by giving them what they want from an early age as a material reward for getting them to devote their whole existence to schoolwork. Dictating consumption from such an early age instills into the child – but the son especially – a sense of empowerment over their leisure world and the family environment. The slogan or mantra we can highlight for understanding filiarchy comes from the words of one child's mother: *No sacrifice is too great to give my child all the things I didn't have in order to insure her happiness.*[69]

But what is regarded as a sacrifice on the part of parents may be experienced in less benevolent ways by the child. "Giving my child all the things I didn't have" is partly the result of parents having come of age during the Cultural Revolution where their youth was materially, culturally, and educationally deprived. These "children of Mao," as Anita Chan called the generation of Red Guards,[70] but which I specifically mean those who came-of-age during Maoism, are now tasked with socializing and educating the current generation of youth whom we can call "the children of the market." The post-1980s/90s generation are not only being "paid off" by their parents with material rewards for adhering to the normal functioning of society (study, study/achieve, achieve), but they are also being bombarded – through advertising, the media, and the culture industries – by the full machinery of the consumer society in which they are coming of age within. It is this consumer society, in particular online games, that is enticing Chinese youth away from the normal functioning of society, especially "boring old" home and school. As one of the "internet addicts" mentioned later so poignantly put this battle for the hearts and minds of the consumer-driven individualizing child: *I was reluctant to return home, instead I wanted to play outside where I have lots more freedom.*

Two main factors why rebellious youth are reluctant to return home can be understood with reference to the work of psychiatrist R.D. Laing. The post-1980s/90s generation in China is considered to be spoilt. This is seemingly backed up by parents expressing their "love" for the child by showering them with gifts as a way to give the child everything they didn't have and by making them the center of the family nexus. However, when the seemingly loving mother says that no sacrifice is too great to give her child everything, what this actually means in practice is the following: no sacrifice is too great to give my child everything *so that* the child, in turn, will sacrifice their own autonomy and individuality for school and school grades. R.D. Laing, in his extensive investigations into the problematic interpersonal relations between parents and child(ren), helps us to learn that by smothering or *engulfing* the child in this way the parents are not simply spoiling the child materially but, more dangerously from an existential and emotional perspective, *loving the child to death*.

In relation to the parents of the so-called internet addict, the parents' *deathly love*, or *chained love*, stems from their "addiction," so to speak, to the child's schoolwork in general and school grades in particular. As I will demonstrate with reference to the parent's own narratives, rejection of school and the attraction to online games partly stems from the child's *reaction* to their parent's engulfment (as Laing calls it), who partly chain their love to academic performance. Feeling suffocated and blocked off from acting autonomously, we see the child rebel by retreating from the family thereby detaching themselves from the pathology of normalcy.

The central component here is the way the parent's engulfment produces within the child *fan gan* (a rebellious psychology).

This retreat from normalcy and advance toward the freedom of the internet, the internet bar, and one's peers, is partly done in order to *preserve* one's autonomy. As we saw with Xiao Wang, contact with "reality" is avoided not because one desires to simply escape it but rather because this reality is itself threatening, and so this social "implosion" is itself related to reality feeling implosive and a threat to one's autonomous self.

In addition to *fan gan* being produced by the parent's chained love, we also see how the parents' over-investment in the child's school grades is producing *fan gan* of a depersonalized nature. When we looked at the interpersonal relations within the family of the so-called internet addict we observe a process Laing called depersonalization. Quite simply, by focusing almost obsessively on the child's school grades the parent's actions, in the eyes of the child, reduce him/her to a kind of *grade-making machine*. As one young "internet addict" said to his mother: *All you – and my teachers – care about is school grades, school grades, and school grades. I hate you and I hate school.* By turning the son into a grade-making machine, by depleting him of his personal aliveness, the son, in turn, experiences the parents as treating him like a piece of machinery because they want to reduce the child – impoverish him – to a kind of individualized factory that spits out school grades. The child's "health" is often not based upon his happiness and satisfaction with *the quality of his life*, but rather on whether he is studying hard or not. Or as one parent so significantly put it: *I always hope that my son, when he changes his mind and corrects his conduct, is able to study well.*[71]

But to return back to my argument that the Young-Tao model is underpinned by a bias toward exchange value-based relations, we see a similar operation being carried out by the parents toward the child. The parent's engulfment and depersonalization toward their child – which later I frame as constituting the "push" factors of intensive gaming – are partly an outcome of the market reforms that are increasingly turning Chinese society into a consumer-focused society. The opening-up and reform policies have not only altered the Chinese citizens' relation to the economy but, much more significantly, their relation to themselves. Fromm argued that with the emergence of a market economy comes the emergence of a new social character he called "market orientation." Fromm invented the marketing orientation character structure to indicate that people living within a consumer-based society experience themselves as a thing to be employed successfully on the market.[72] More recently Bauman has added that people living in a consumer-based society must first *recast themselves as commodities*. That is, the children of the market must market themselves as *products* capable of catching attention and attracting *demand* and *customers*.[73] Because one's sense of value greatly depends on one's success vis-à-vis the market, his or her sense of self may not principally stem from one's activity as a loving and thinking individual, from one's *human qualities*, but rather from one's socio-economic role.[74]

Quite simply, the child becoming an un-saleable commodity on China's hyper-competitive marketplace is the great fear of parents whose child loses interest in school, while, simultaneously, gaining interest in the internet and its multiple applications and pleasures. Parents are afraid, in the very deepest sense of the term, that their child will be unable to be sold profitably on the market. Through the narratives offered later we can observe how the parents valuate the "quality" of the child (*goodness* vs. *badness*) against the "quantity" of the school grading system, therein showing us that what effectively amounts to a *war-machine* within the family is partly one between quality (use value) and quantity (exchange value). In this way the parents should never be simply blamed for some perceived parenting "failures," because they have not been provided with the necessary tools in which to effectively socialize and educate a child who is, existentially at least, living in another world.

I conceptualize the family of the "internet addict" as a "war-machine" because if there is something clear about this family it is that it has descended into a kind of war zone with two fiercely opposed sides violently fighting and striving to defend their position and advance their own interests. The family has become a war-machine because it is driven by a hostile conflict stemming from differing aims, wishes, and fears.

All in all, excessive online gaming is not principally about the correlation between individual and technology, but stems more from the individual's *inter-*personal relations to significant others and the structural conditions of his/her existence, in particular the conflict over autonomy and social order.[75] Moreover, Fromm tells us the challenging problem for investigations into the individual and group is finding out what the specific interaction is between a given character structure and a given social structure. This is, in a nutshell, the overriding concern: how, and in what ways, is this "internet addict" a product of the reform and opening up?

Turn on, boot up, and log in: the consumer revolution

Xiao Wang's experience helps us understand not simply the virtual world but, more importantly, the real world, or more correctly the relativity or "push" and "pull" factors operating between the two. Like a coin the internet – or its attraction – could be said to have two sides. Similar to migration, one side contains push factors while the other contains pull factors. For example, we should ask why Xiao Wang could not get this satisfaction and sense of freedom from his real-world life. Instead of focusing upon the presumed failures of the individual gamer we should focus upon the failures of Chinese society in not being able to satisfy the young, for we are not dealing with isolated cases here, but rather a group of young singular individuals who collectively, simultaneously, and in huge numbers, keep dropping out of the central, normal social structure. Tao Ran and others mask this *search for freedom* by claiming these young people migrate to the internet in order to simply "escape reality." But this washes over the political nature of their actions and the fact that intensive gaming is, itself, a critique of the status quo. Likewise, this also washes over the important fact that we cannot simply drop out of society or escape reality, rather, we can only drop out of social roles – i.e., one's role as a filial child or as an obedient student; that is, a *good* boy/girl.[76]

Like youth in America in the 1960s, who through drugs such as LSD choose to "turn on, tune in, and drop out," many young people in China today are deciding to *turn on, boot up, and log in*. While American youth were resisting and rejecting conventional society in favor of a youth-created counter culture, authority figures were bombarding them with shouts of "drugs are bad, drugs are escape, drugs are dangerous."[77] Today we are hearing the authoritative voices in China cry out "gaming is bad, gaming is escape, gaming is dangerous." But is it not strange that an experience which is regarded with such distrust, fear and loathing by those who have not experienced it is regarded so highly by those who have? The internet addiction phenomenon in China and the psychedelic movement in the US are connected not because video games are a kind of drug like LSD – despite the fact gaming is like the LSD of the internet age as it allows the participant to go on a spiritual "trip" or existential migration – but rather because of the contentious relationship between the users and the authorities. American youth in the 1960s, like Chinese youth today, experienced a sense of alienation from conventional "straight" society and so young people rebelled against the Protestant work ethic and traditional patterns of deference to authority.[78] In short, the internet addiction phenomenon is about the moral panic relating to youth seeking freedom – through resistance and rebellion – from authoritarian control mechanisms as they feel disconnected from straight society, and not simply about the object they have chosen to use for their rebellious journey.

They are also rebelling against a capitalist work ethic (even while partly adhering to it through gaming) and deference to authority figures such as parents and teachers. So the question is: why is gaming seen as bad, as escape, as dangerous? Bad and dangerous to whom? And escape from what? Since one group thinks it is bad and another thinks it is good, then we know that this is much more than simply a biomedical issue, rather it is a moral battle over the disciplinary boundaries demarcating the normal functioning of Chinese society. For if it was simply a demonic poison then video games would not be so highly regarded by gamers, the majority of whom suffer little or no harmful physiological consequences. Likewise, the games themselves would not be licensed to operate legally and there would be no large world-wide professional gaming industry. While China hosted the World Cyber Games in 2009, has anyone ever heard of "The World Opium Smoking Games?"

In this collective sense, Chinese youth today, like their parents before them, are also going through a kind of "Cultural Revolution" – or rather we should call it a *Consumption Revolution*. Both cohorts – the children of Mao and the children of the market – had and have rejected school over "revolution." The major difference being that during the Cultural Revolution rejecting school was endorsed by the Party-State, who closed them down, and therefore rejecting school was normalized and sanctioned. However, now 40 odd years later a group of young consumer revolutionaries are also rejecting formal education for excessive pop-cultural activities. The difference now is that the Party-State has not sanctioned this activity and so it is seen as deviant to do so, with the revolutionary activity undertaken to replace school becoming medicalized as a mental disorder. But the premise of their actions is the same: the rejection of formal education and the acceptance of excessive activities. However, no one was calling the Red Guards "revolution addicts," rather those who the Red Guards were labeling "counter-revolutionaries" and "capitalist-roaders" were seen as mentally ill, for they (like Tao Ran today) had the power and authority to do so.[79] But today's young revolutionaries lack this power and authority to define and to name. However, it is the same relation – Self-Other – yet it has turned on its head, for the powerful and violent Red Guards have become the relatively powerless and non-violent internet addicts.

At the same time, however, today's youth have recaptured this power within the home, over their parents, and so the rejection of school is occurring on an individualized and private basis, which is only possible in an individualized and segmented society. In this way, the revolution has retreated into the family and become personalized, with dropping out of school becoming the ultimate form of rebellion. While the Red Guards were involved in "the production of Maoism," the internet addicts coagulate around "the consumption of objects," for both cohort members are products of their time. Thus, the generational divide, and by implication the family war-machine, is related to the parents having grown up in an era of *producing society* while the post-1980s/90s generation are growing up in an era of *consuming society*. But when parents are criticizing their children for rejecting school they wash over the fact that their generation had rejected the formal education system, and instead played political games to violently excessive degrees. Both the Cultural Revolution and the Consumption Revolution are based on excess and the rejection of school, but only the Cultural Revolution was based on actual physical violence.

By presenting the second part of Xiao Wang's letter at the beginning of this chapter I have sought to highlight the motivation and will of the intensive gamer by showing how the presence of the internet and internet games allowed him to not simply drown himself or play the hurt away by escaping reality, but rather to advance in a new direction. By introducing the work of Elias we are able to conceptualize the lifeworld of people like Xiao Wang as a "Division Bell," wherein there is an intimate interconnection between their non-leisure and leisure lives. Or more specifically, the pleasurable play-excitement which young people seek in online games represents, at the same time, the complement and the antithesis to the recurrent emotional restraint, repetitiveness, orderliness, and staleness of their purposeful rational routines encompassing their school/work life. In this sense we can see how online gaming provides a cathartic or even spiritual experience vis-à-vis the sometimes dehumanizing real world. With reference to the pharmakon we can understand how internet gaming does not poison the gamer but, on the contrary, can serve as an remedy to stress-tensions being produced within the (individualizing) person living in a transforming society. By turning the pharmakon on its head we also turn Chinese society on its head and see that what is "poisonous" is not the internet or the pathological individual but rather the normal functioning of society, or what we can call the pathology of normalcy. And so the mass migration to cyberspace is partly premised upon seeking out more positive and healthy social relations as a way in which to counter a world out-of-balance that is largely driven by a culture of excess and contains engulfing and depersonalizing relations. Because they are coming of age not in a "harmonious society" but more so in a "harming-me society," the particular structure of their society is forcing them to seek individual and biographical solutions to their social problems. Since this social structure is generally adverse to producing genuine human happiness and self-realization, then in being willing to fight for autonomy and self-realization the intensive gamer comes crashing against this pathology of normalcy. This collusion centers around authority figures trying to get the child to submit to the normal functioning of society and the child, partly through *fan gan* (rebelliousness), deciding instead to turn on, boot up, and log in to a life online. By deciding to drop out of the normal social structure we see, in this collective sense, a segment of the children of the market seeking freedom – through resistance and rebellion – from authoritarian mechanisms of control and discipline. And because this consumer revolution is generally taking place within the walls of the family unit, then we need to take the analysis to the interpersonal relations within the home. This is our next task.

5   The family war-machine and the search for freedom

Intensive gaming and the family

The following discussion of the parent's letters functions to demonstrate the disordered nature of the family nexus, thus calling into question the assumption that "internet addiction" is an individual pathology. We need to contextualize norm-violating behavior such as increased internet use after one or more of the following situations occurs: a) the death of a father; b) the divorce of parents; c) a child subjected to acts of violence, absence, and neglect by one or both parents; d) feelings of intense pressure due to examinations and schoolwork; and e) feelings of depersonalization and engulfment due to parental pressure and over-investment functioning under the pretext of "love." This is because these factors are the common characteristics of the letters that, when taken together, constitute the parent's narrative. This contextualizes the lifeworld of the person labeled an internet addict, and when we filter this discussion through *DSM-IV*'s definition of a mental disorder we ask if it is more appropriate to conceptualize their reactions as being closer to a normal – rather than abnormal – response to their stress environments?

The following narrative is a letter (known as Letter-1) sent to Tao Hongkai from a person who had developed computer software that was designed to a) restrict access to games, b) to enforce rest, c) to manage time, and d) to filter sites. The objective of the software was to "put parents at ease by gradually guiding youth to cure internet addiction and get them far away from online violence and pornography." Once this was achieved then the software would hopefully allow them to "absorb beneficial internet resources, let youth continuously increase their knowledge and widen their horizon, and allow computers to become a good teacher and a helpful friend." This outcome can be understood as the parent's ultimate aspiration vis-à-vis their child's internet use. The following narrative basically contains a summary of the main points of the parent's perspective toward internet use. We begin here as this outlines the main problems we need to address in relation to "intensive gaming and the family."

I am manager Chen from the Jingxi computer science and technology company in Nanning, Guangxi. Young people's excessive enthrallment in internet games is leading them to idle away their youth and to lie to waste their school work, and so examples of harming their health can be found everywhere. Internet addiction has made lots of families lose their gentle and fragrant harmony, and makes it difficult for many anxiety ridden parents to sleep at night! My neighbour has a young child in the fifth grade. Before he became infatuated with internet games he was intelligent and showed filial piety and respect to his parents, and his school grades were in the top-five in his class. All the neighbours were full of praise for him. Since he has come down with internet addiction, he is simply no longer one's old self: he is always absentminded, and his grades have declined greatly. The parents have advised him in earnest, yet he just curses them loudly and his language is intolerable to the ear. He is already deeply immersed in this mud! To force him to change was unavoidable, and so the family tied up his hands and feet and locked him in a room. But he did all that he could to break loose, and then jumped from the second floor of the building, which led to him severely damaging his skull. This "internet addiction's" poison is too deep, and so it is devouring young people's frail mind and body. We have a responsibility to get them away from this abhorrent "internet addiction" so that they can find salvation![1]

Contained within the parent's "internet addiction narrative" we have the following rationalizations: first, the "child" becomes excessively "enthralled in" internet games, or like a child catching pneumonia "comes down" with internet addiction. This most often occurs during junior middle school at around 15–17 years of age. However, due to the parent's own attempts of trying to make sense of their child's internet use, we can find in their letters a whole range of vastly differing interpretations being employed to signify the child's relation to what they disparately refer to as "the computer," "the internet," "online games," "games", or even just simply "play." And so a parent speaks of the child being "infatuated with," "immersed in," or "addicted to" the computer. Or the child is thought to be "indulged in," "becomes a fan of," or "plunges into" the internet. Or the child "comes into close contact with," "has fallen in love with," or is "obsessed with" online games. Or the child is seen as being "poisoned by," "intoxicated with," or "a fan of" games. Or, finally, the child may simply possess an "insatiable desire for" play. While we can clearly see that many parents do not apply a one-dimensional biomedical-based model of mental illness upon the child called "addiction" while searching in the linguistic dark for terms that best explain their observations, we do see, nevertheless, that this particular configuration – child and technology – has "caused" the child to idle away their youth and lie to waste their schoolwork. For as Wu and Zhang so dramatically framed it: Having weak self control this abundant online information causes youth to suffer from *information pollution*, and therefore they waste their golden time and precious youth.[2] In short, child encounters internet = internet takes over child's life.

The apparent result, as the parents highlight, again and again, is a sharp decline in both the child's interest toward school and, most important of all, his/her school grades. For parents the alarm bells ring not when they observe unhappiness, stress, anxiety, or loneliness within the child but rather when their school grades begin to plummet. These declining school grades, in turn, are said to cause a harmonious family to morph into a kind of war-zone. The antagonistic relations that follow then results in the parents, but especially the mother, becoming riddled with feelings such as anxiety, desperation, powerlessness, exhaustion, and helplessness. The parents try to advise the child "in earnest," but almost always to no avail. What then follows is the breakdown in communication between child and parents, which is made more difficult because the apparently "weak" and "vulnerable" child used to be "intelligent," "good," "kind-hearted" and "lively" before coming down with "internet addiction." No matter what the parents try to do – scoldings, beatings, locking the child inside the house, asking family and friends to "reason" with him, sending him to a boarding school, sending him to a boot camp, or sending him to a psychiatrist – nothing seems to be able to pull the child out of the virtual mud. On the contrary, the more they try the worse the problem becomes. With nowhere in sight, except in some cases thoughts of death, the parents often turn to a military-style boot camp. When this fails some turn to the one person they believe can bring salvation to the family and transform a child who is simply no longer one's old self: Mr. Tao Hongkai.

Letter-6 – an ideal type

The following letter, Letter-6, is an exemplary example of the parent's narrative. Or rather we should say that Letter-6 offers us what Max Weber called an "ideal type."[3] Ideal types are useful cognitive tools for analyzing social reality, and so help us put the chaos of social reality in order.[4] The ideal type does not refer to some perfect idealized phenomenon, but rather is employed to stress certain elements common to most cases of the given phenomenon; in this case the common elements within the letters. Here the ideal type is used, vis-à-vis the parent's narrative, to highlight a certain common pattern of conduct and to order several phenomena so as to paint a collective picture of the family war-machine. And so to Letter-6:

> Please can you save my son and also save me.
>
> Since the first year of junior middle school my son started playing the game "*Legend*" on the internet. At the very beginning he would come home late after class was over and say the teacher had held them back. I did not think that in the second year I would discover that he was addicted to playing. His school grades subsequently declined. Later on I would go and collect him everyday from school, however, he was still able to go behind my back, as at three in the morning he would climb out of bed and sneak off to the internet bar. I then locked all the doors and hid the key. However, at midnight he got up and broke the screws on the lock and ran off to the internet bar. Since the son has become a fan of playing *Legend* his school grades have declined, he tells lies, he steals money, he fights, and he curses people. I have found lots of people to help persuade him and educate him but this has had no effect. I think that if it continues like this we can't

control it. I had to find a good school that I could shut him away in where he could lodge at. According to his test scores I chose a school with quite good control and management.

During vacation I said that he could relax by playing on the computer, but he again became addicted, which was even worse than before. He also learnt how to smoke and fight. Likewise, he was impious towards parental authority, and was able to not eat, not drink, not sleep, and instead spent from morning-till-night in front of the computer playing games. When you tell him to have dinner he will argue with you, curse you, be annoyed with you, and he will suspect you are trying to influence him.

According to everyone's methods and suggestions I went to talk with my son properly and to reason with him, but he paid no attention and just carried on playing. If you do not let him play computer games then it is like you are wanting to take away his life, and he exerts all his strength to resist, becoming irritated, and rambles on saying such things as I hate you. He completely does not listen, and if you speak lightly then he does not listen at all. If you speak forcibly he will argue with me, and even hit me. He will say you are a fake and a cheat. At the moment we are arguing over money, in order to buy weapons in the game *Legend*. He only finds me when he wants money.

I am a single-parent family, and it is very difficult taking care of him on my own, but because I am really capable therefore he doesn't feel it. How is it possible to tell him that he doesn't understand it at all? *His father passed away the year before last*. I am really tired, my body and mind are exhausted, and my brain is about to explode, I really want to die. I am a useless person, I cannot even educate my own son properly. At the moment I am afraid of him.

I have absolutely no choice but with a thick skin beg you to help me. Professor Tao please say you will definitely save my son, you are my only hope, this family has arrived at the moment when one's fate hangs in the balance, help me to walk out of this mess.[5]

Addicted to play

The first comment we can make about Letter-6 is the mother's initial comment that the child is "addicted to play."[6] "Play," as Johan Huizinga argued, is far from some kind of drug that the individual can easily become addicted to, rather play is deeply imbedded into culture – and is thus socially-constituted history. Specifically, Huizinga argues that not only does culture arise in the form of play – i.e., all society is a game, or a range of different games with different rules – but that to a certain degree the core elements of play (contest, performance, exhibition, challenges, showing-off, etc.) may actually precede culture. Huizinga directs us to think of the way woodcocks perform dances, bower-birds decorate their nests, crows hold flying matches, and song-birds chant melodies.[7] His point being that there is something *inherent* in humanity in regards to play, and so contests – whether the Olympic Mathematics Competition or the World Cyber Games – means a form of play. Actually, Tao Ran partly bases his treatment method upon the notion that life is a kind of game. Presumably in addition to the "confession" letters already discussed, Tao Ran has written that before discharging his patients from his hospital he gets them to sign an agreement stating that they understand the "games" in life are also the same as online games, in that there are rules. Following these rules – that is, being good – will result in being rewarded, while violating these rules – that is, being deviant by going against the normal functioning of society – should result in them accepting punishment for doing so.[8] Thus if life is a game then we cannot say they can be addicted to "play" for this would mean one could also be "addicted" to life.

Huizinga also notes the primary importance competition plays within the play-element. Instead of claiming competitive attitudes spring from a desire simply for power and domination *per se*, he rather argues that what is central to play is the desire to excel others, to be first in whatever game is being played and finally to be honored for this excellence. In short, the main thing is to have won, and so play is driven by a desire for victory and the subsequent spoils that emanate from such a victory.[9]

Thus it is no surprise that the mother in Letter-21 praised the son's pre-internet addiction spirit of "loving to excel others." That is, when the child is competing in the game of school examinations then "play" has the highest social value, and parents revel in the child being in the "top-five in the class"[10] or in "top of his class"[11] or "feel very happy" when the child is deemed one of Beijing's "three good students."[12] Little surprise also that the mother in Letter-29 said the son had "ideals" and "ambition" when he got three prizes in the province's Olympic Mathematic Competition, yet after he said he was unwilling to go to school, and instead just wanted to *play* online games, the mother became suspicious that he must have a "psychological impediment." Then to the child's disagreement, and the parent's dismay, a doctor at the local psychiatric hospital diagnosed him with "schizophrenia," making them admit him for (expensive) treatment. Likewise, the first feature the mother in Letter-27 mentions is the son obtaining a gold medal in the All China Cup Mathematics Competition, yet when he planned some years later to abandon study in order to become a professional gamer this was attributed to some negative "reasons relating to schoolwork and his body."

The point being that to excel in the competitive play of schoolwork is victorious – valued – and so one will be rewarded for complying. While desiring to excel in the competitive play of online gaming is disastrous – devalued – and so one will be punished for non-compliance. Thus mothers feel anxious, worried, and despondent when the child's grades have declined to "20th in the class,"[13] or have become "average."[14] Or worse yet, ranks more than 60th in the class,[15] or most disastrously of all, has slipped down to the bottom of the class.[16] But as Tao Hongkai told a group of about thirty parents at the "Shandong Healthy Internet Training Base," many parents put immense pressure on their child to be the first in class and to have the best grades, but in every class there can only be *one* "winner." His argument being that the parents' expectations and "love" toward their children are too excessive. And this excess, itself part of a much larger *culture of excess* that underpins contemporary Chinese society, has led to the children undertaking excessive activities like gaming.[17] The logic being that "like creates like" or "excess begets excess," which then makes "excessive gaming" not a so much a value judgment but rather the logical outcome of a child being brought up in a culture of excess.

This apparent "enthrallment" in school grades by parents, teachers, and the education system can have disastrous results for those students caught on the wrong side of the grade fence. For example, the mother in Letter-24, who claims the cause of her son's deviance and epilepsy resulted from him watching a horror film on TV when he was eight, attached a short paragraph her son wrote explaining how he himself understood his problems with school. He writes:

> Because I have never received the teachers and parents approval and my classmates help then I have been randomly labelled. Because my school grades were no good then this met with corporal punishment from my parents and cursing abuse from my teachers. Likewise, my brain reaction is a bit slow and so I was humiliated and insulted by classmates and teachers. Because of this I suffer from spiritual torture. Therefore, I really feel myself to be inferior and also my self-confidence cannot rise up, and so my character has become introverted. I hope you are able to communicate your thoughts with me, and communicate with me what you have learned, and make my spirit obtain purification and education.[18]

This demonstrates the negative consequences of both the parents and the school through *depersonalizing* the child/student by turning him into a *grade-making machine*. While it may be shown, with reference to the *DSM-IV*, that he has a physiological "internal dysfunction" (slow neurological response rate and epilepsy) his psychological and social behavior cannot necessarily be considered *socially inappropriate* for such thoughts and actions – i.e., distrust of others/non-communicative/desocialized – could arguably be understood as generally *expectable responses* to the stressful conditions he has to constantly face and endure. The central problem may not necessarily lie with him, but with others and his inter-personal relations with them, so that it is not him that is "mentally disordered" but rather the symbolically-and-physically-violent social environment in which he finds himself being spiritually tortured by. This demonstrates how his perceived psychological problems result not primarily from some internal psychological dysfunction but rather from the negative and violent social relations he is caught up in, which when he connects them all together has resulted in a retreat into himself, for that is the only perceived safe haven. Others, in a similar position, find this safety in the internet. It is also a good example of the negative results of the excessive attention paid to schoolwork and school grades, for instead of focusing on his extra-schoolwork issues, he is being judged, criticized, insulted, and tortured because he cannot *compete* with the other students; who in turn mock and tease him for being "slow."

Likewise, the son in Letter-33 bemoaned that fact that he is always failing in the real world, and so told his father, "*only through playing on the computer am I able to find a sense of achievement. I want to dominate the world, and I want to let people in the world listen to me/obey me.*"[19] This statement is perhaps exemplary for understanding the mechanisms and the character structure of some labeled as internet addicts. On the one hand we have what Laing calls the *ontologically insecure* person feeling isolated,[20] alone, and powerless because they are blocked from realizing their emotional and intellectual potentialities. That is, they are having difficulty adhering to social norms and highly prized social values. There is a feeling of being threatened by an outside world, and they feel their life is being thwarted, curtailed, and suppressed. On the other hand, there is a strong desire for a sense of power, domination and even a kind of destruction over others, the underlying mechanism being the struggle for freedom and independence. These two energies – the withdrawal from the "normal" world and the desire for domination and even destruction over others – are part of the same process. That is, the inflation of oneself through a desire for domination, expressed in intense and competitive online gaming, may itself be rooted in feelings of individual failure and powerlessness – within a system that over-values individualized success and power. And so the ontologically insecure person can *escape* these feelings of failure, isolation, and powerlessness by attempting to dominate others or even oneself, which can be understood as an attempt not simply to escape reality but rather to save oneself from being crushed by it. In short, says Fromm, "*domination and destruction is the outcome of a thwarted life.*"[21]

Or for our purposes: *excessive online gaming is often the outcome of a thwarted life* (and not a disordered mind).

As Fromm explains what he calls a *mechanism of escape*: "Those individual and social conditions that make for suppression of life produce the passion for destruction that forms, so to speak, the reservoir from which the particular hostile tendencies – either against others or against oneself – are nourished."[22]

Tao Hongkai understands this thwarted life, and the domination and destruction stemming from it, as principally the result of parents "spoiling" their often only-child (loving him/her to death), and so these ontologically insecure children become a *tiger* while at home in private, but a *mouse* when they are out in public.[23] We must understand this tiger-and-mouse distinction as being an important component of the production of intensive gaming and the production of ontological insecurity. Understanding this important aspect of the war-machine in the family contextualizes their intensive gaming, for it is understandable that they would retreat into the "hole" of the dark internet bar, as the internet bar is the safe hiding place of the "mice" where they are safe from "predators." This safety, in which the internet bar is like a kind of secular monastery, allows them to also continue to be the tiger they are at home, for they can become the master of their universe through gaming by dominating either other players or the computer game itself. That is, they can become a *laoda*.[24] Thus, intensive internet use makes sense if we grasp

Erich Fromm's and Tao Hongkai's main point: social conditions that make for the suppression of the young and dynamic life produce the passion for domination and destruction. Or to put it another way, intensive internet use cannot simply be reduced to the perceived failings of the individual because this negates the particular social and structural conditions from which such use stems.

Yet instead of understanding how the son's computer play is connected to his self-perceived failures at playing the school-game and the life-game, the father in Letter-33 simply took such words as signifying the son as having "delusions," "bizarre opinions," and possessing "weak self control." If the son had said something like "only through winning mathematics competitions am I able to find a sense of achievement. I want to dominate the World Mathematics Olympics, and I want the whole world to see my mathematical formulas," then we can be confident that the father would have said something like the successful son possesses ideals, ambition, and love at excelling others. Quite simply, there may be only a *social value* – and not a mental illness nor an "addiction to play" – that separates the "math champion" from the "internet addict." That is, if the child plays the piano or violin for three hours per day (on top of their "normal" schoolwork) he or she may be described by parents and teachers as a "dedicated" musician. Or if the child knows the statistics, trivia, and history of Olympic athletes such as Liu Xiang or Guo Jingjing, and has collected memorabilia from the Beijing Olympics then this child may be considered a "true fan" and a "good young patriot," for these are *socially acceptable* hobbies. But if the child takes the same approach to playing online games, spending hours each day online and reveling in the strategies, skills, details, and knowledge of the game then parents worry about the child being "addicted" to the internet.[25]

The exemplary example for understanding the way social value functions is the 9-year-old boy in Wuhan who could apparently recite 100 bus routes. Zhan Xingrui became a minor celebrity as a "walking bus information desk."[26] The parents allowed Xingrui to continue dedicating his time to reciting Wuhan's bus routes only after they saw that it *did not impact* upon his formal studies. It is significant that these parents would endorse their son's recitation of bus routes but would almost certainly be unwilling to endorse him if he decided to memorize all the characters in the online game *Legend*. Reciting bus routes, whose use value his parents measure in relation to them believing it to be an aid, and not a hindrance, to his studies, is considered a "hobby." But if he had devoted the same time and energy to gaming, then the parents, who see it as a hindrance and not a help to his schoolwork, would label him as being "addicted to" or "enthralled in" the internet. But Xingrui would arguably learn more important cognitive and spatial skills playing online games than he would by simply reciting bus routes, for he is already learning how to recite information at school, but he is not generally being taught the strategy, multi-tasking, and problem-solving skills one learns through gaming. For example, one study found that after only 10 hours of training with an action video game subjects realized substantial gains in both spatial attention and mental rotation, with females benefiting more than males.[27]

Just as significantly, on the same page as this article was a photo of about twenty-five kindergarten students, at Liu Yuan Kindergarten in Suzhou, dressed up in mock university graduation robes while holding a "diploma" and flinging black caps into the air mimicking a real graduation ceremony. This mimetic activity reflects the excessive nature of the education system and parental norms, because these 4- and 5-year-olds do not merely mimic adult tertiary education, but more importantly we see how competition is forced upon them and how Pavlov-based discipline-control-and-reward mechanisms are socialized into them even before they reach primary school. Quite simply, the beginnings of "internet addiction" can be located at this early stage of socialization in which *hurried* children are being forced to play miniature adults before they are physically, psychologically, and/or socially prepared to do so. While being trained in the academic regimen hopefully results, for the parents at least, in a child who can "hit the ground running" when it comes to important examinations later on, the question that arises is the following: is forcing young people to run this fast in the best interests of the child's all-round development? Or, conversely, does being put on this kind of treadmill lead to nowhere except to hurried, yet spiritually and psychologically undernourished, lives?[28] Under this pathology of normalcy it is little wonder that many young people are deciding to *turn on, boot up, and log in* to a life lived electronically.

To sum up this section we can say that *attributing* their son's deviant behavior to "internet addiction" implies that the son uses the internet because some mechanism over which he has little control forces him to do so, and his subsequent behavioral change is a function of the internet and not that of the user. The parents tend to not take seriously the fact that the son may have his own reasons that are worth mentioning – e.g., that he feels like a lonely failure and so seeks feelings of success and achievement through online games; feelings he was taught from 4 years old to over-value. For excessive internet use is seen as a function of outside forces (i.e., he *comes down with* internet addiction), and not of the person concerned. The son is, instead, conceived of as "unripe fruit" with weak self control who simply does not know what is best for him. This reveals that the term "internet addiction" is a good illustration of how attribution works. The explanations given are sometimes functional, even if unconsciously so, in that they are not designed to explain behavior in any scientific or objective sense, hence the large number of disparate terms ascribed to internet use by parents. Quite simply, the explanations function to a) justify their problematic actions (e.g., locking him up; beating him), b) reduce culpability (thus deflecting responsibility away from the parents), and c) to simply try and make sense of a seemingly un-sensible situation.[29] With respect to using "internet addiction," the parents must then demonstrate that the "addict" operates according to a set of principles or attributes that do not apply to the normal person – e.g., that he possesses delusions, bizarre opinions, and weak self control.[30]

Being locked up and being lonely

Rewards and punishment are the lowest form of education.

Philosopher, *Zhuang Zi*[31]

The second comment to be made about Letter-6 is the mother's two-pronged education-based strategy of locking up the son. First she locked all the doors and hid the key to prevent him from escaping. Then, because she had lost control over the son's behavior, she, like a quarter of the other parents, decided to find a school with strict management that she could "lock him away in." However, like manager Chen's young neighbor in Letter-1 whose family thought it "unavoidable" to tie up his hands and feet and lock him in his room, the son escaped quite easily. Similarly, the mother in Letter-32 had also lost control over her youngest son after his father died when he was 10 years old. In an effort to cleanse him of his gaming and deviant friends the mother lied to him by claiming that the family's small company had encountered difficulties and so they had to sell the house and move to the coastal city of Xiamen; where besides the family members he did not want to be with he would be completely friendless and alone. To prevent him from running back to their hometown to hang out with his friends, the mother locked him inside the apartment for the first ten days. He subsequently, and rather expectantly, "randomly smashed things."

Likewise, the son in Letter-26, who had been strictly controlled by both his father and teachers, slowly rejected both school and communication with his parents, to the point where the father – out of frustration and loss of control over the situation – allowed him to suspend his schooling. While his parents were both busy working, he consequently spent his days at home eating, sleeping, and watching TV as they did not permit him to go out. One evening he secretly went out to surf online, and when his father discovered this he told him to come home. However, like almost all the other sons in the letters, when the parents spoke he did not listen, and so his father locked the door when he went to work. Initially threatening to jump out the second floor window, the son, instead, waited until the mother came home and then walked out the front door, not returning until ten days later. Meanwhile, the mother spent her evenings after work searching internet bars, main streets and back alleys, stopping occasionally to cry angrily. At the same time she also admitted that the atmosphere at home had been oppressive, and this had influenced the son's mood. After returning home the son said something significant: "*I was reluctant to return home, instead I wanted to play outside where I have lots more freedom.*"[32]

What we observe when a parent employs the strategy of imprisoning or confining the child inside the apartment and/or sending him off to boarding school – as a last resort to prevent them from rebelling – is the opposite result from that intended. Instead of "softening up" the son, confinement, on the contrary, makes him harder by producing *fan gan* (resistance and rebelliousness). He is further hardened or made more resistant by the "pride" and "stubbornness" many parents say their children possess, but which may be more accurately understood as part of their socially produced "tigerness." The confinement is just a defensive and mitigating strategy – in the art-of-war between parents and child. It is just a suppression-based method used to control and not to fix the problem, which just leads to more resistance from the child thereby effectively creating even more problems within the household. In practice, using a kind of privatized imprisonment and physical force signals to the child that violence is an adequate method of conflict resolution. Thomas Mathiesen's work on the prison system and prisoners is revealing here. Mathiesen points out that the functioning of the prison system implies, for the prisoners, that they are being *rejected* by mainstream society. Their reaction to this rejection may be to *reject their rejectors*, which expresses itself in the commonly observed effect of punishment producing resistance.[33] In a similar way, punishing the son by locking him up – either at home, at a private school, or at a boot camp – may be experienced as being rejected by the parents, and so their reaction may be to reject their rejecters: to *fan gan*.

At the level of existential and emotional needs, Fromm would argue that the son does not want to be locked alone in a room because this act goes against the two needs rooted, not in instinctual physiological drives, but in the very essence of the human mode and practice of life: *the need to avoid aloneness, and the need to avoid isolation by being related to the world outside oneself*.[34] Fromm indirectly warns parents by saying "the possibility of being left alone is necessarily the most serious threat to the child's whole existence."[35] This is because aloneness and isolation prevent the person from being able to relate themselves to any system which would give meaning and direction to their life, and therefore feeling insignificant, or like a particle of dust in a dusty city, subsequently produces doubt, insecurity and an inability to act – that is, to live a meaningful and enriched life.[36] As Griffiths and his fellow researchers crucially pointed out, part of the appeal of multiplayer online games such as *EverQuest* is that they are based around cooperation and provide opportunities for new meaningful and emotionally resonant relationships and friendships to develop both within and outside the game, which they attribute to the human need for affiliation.[37] We must therefore not downplay the important role loneliness plays as an important "push" factor attracting young people in China, especially only-children, to the internet.[38] In fact, Guo Tiejun, a school headmaster-turned-psychologist who runs an internet-addiction research center in Shanghai, has based his treatment method upon loneliness being the root of intensive internet use and so believes the most effective method is to treat teens like "friends." Significantly, part of his "soft approach" to the problem was itself driven by encountering youths whose parents brought them to him after they had "suffered" under Tao Ran's "hard" regime without any positive outcome.[39]

Likewise, educator Mrs Fu Xueyu who works with families dealing with children labeled "internet addicts," told a group of parents that many of the adolescents she has seen share a common characteristic. Teacher Fu, who herself locates the source of deviant internet use primarily inside the disordered nature of contemporary family relations, says that these young people's "*inner being is like a deserted island*."[40] Some of the social conditions that she says engender such isolation and alienation are: family relations that are cold; the child having no friends; or, the child being unable to make friends. This is a remarkable analysis as these young people live in the most populated nation on Earth and in large cities surrounded by a sea of people, including usually having around sixty fellow classmates. Yet they feel as though they are alone on a deserted island (see Xiao Kang's narrative later). Therefore we must ask a very basic question: what is wrong with social relations in urban China? In highlighting the important role productive family relations play in warding off their inner being becoming like a deserted island, Fu Xueyu tells the parents that "communication is like a dose of good medicine, while the family is the child's safe harbor."[41] However, the young people I spoke to at the Shandong Healthy Internet Training Base, wherein they used the computer for communication as their family relations were as cold as an uninviting harbor, indicated that it was the internet, and not home, that was both a good dose of medicine, a cathartic experience, and a safe harbor (in an unsafe world).

While the letters point to an obvious crisis in young people obtaining direction and meaning in their life – and so use gaming as a means to try and obtain security, happiness, satisfaction, and excitement – this condition is not simply confined to a few "bad apples." In a kind of mirror image of the content of the letters, the China Population Communication Center carried out a survey by conducting face-to-face interviews with 133 "normal" students throughout schools in Beijing. The findings are worrying:

> 60 percent said they felt isolated.
> 60 percent said they felt lonely.
> 50 percent said they lack a sense of security in social interactions.
> 50 percent of respondents claimed they were not content with their lives.
> 20 percent felt like they were trapped in a state of emptiness.
> 80 percent experienced feelings of social injustice.
> 30 percent said they "never" communicated with their parents, while
> 25 percent did so only if they experienced a conflict.

And finally, yet not surprisingly if we apply Fromm's theory that "individual and social conditions that make for suppression of life produce the passion for destruction," a number of students surveyed said they developed an "intense anger."[42]

In interpreting the findings, the Center claims that these feelings find expression through "irregular behavior" such as skipping class and rebelliousness, which then leads to "psychological problems" like "internet addiction." This, however, tells us nothing of the cause and origin – that is, the producer – of these feelings. Instead, young people who are experiencing socially-produced *life* problems are chastised for having *psychological* problems. It is, I would argue, a way in which individuals are forced to seek biographical solutions to socially produced problems. Hu Deng, a member of the Chinese Psychological Society and a professor at Renmin University, argues, however, that the solution to these problems resides in "instilling the students with an ability to resist frustration."[43] Or as Renfei used to say: "Just suck it up." In fact, such students already have a tool they use to help them resist the frustration being produced by the so-called "normal" functioning of society: this *self-medication* that helps them *fa xie* (give vent to) such feelings is called online gaming. This is partly why the internet must be thought of as a remedy and not simply as a poison. The real issue is not having the ability to resist frustration, for this is more than likely to simply lead to repressing hostility and anger, thereby producing more emotional problems, but rather uncovering the source of this frustration. To do this we need to return back to what the son in Letter-26 said. "I was reluctant to return home," he confessed to his mother, "instead I wanted to play outside where I have lots more freedom." In this way an important component of the war-machine in the family is a two-pronged approach to freedom: 1) freedom *from*, and 2) freedom *to*.

It is no coincidence that the survey noted that "problems seem to increase as children get older," nor is it a coincidence that the child's internet usage, that is, their problems with school and home, often begins around the age of fifteen or sixteen (second or third year of junior high school). In order to answer why "internet addiction" is most often taking place around sixteen, or in the case of Tao Ran's "patients" around seventeen, we can refer to Fromm's "individuation process."

The individuation process

Society, crazy indeed...

I hope you're not lonely, without me

Society, have mercy on me.

I hope you're not angry, if I disagree.

"Society" by Eddie Vedder[44]

Fromm's individuation process pivots around an axis of differing forms of freedom, and a general summary of the *ideal* model of this process can be the following. During the early stage of individuation the child is still not yet completely severed from what Fromm calls the "primary ties," which are basically one's parents and other important family figures. Submission to parental authority during this early stage has a different quality from the kind of submission that exists once the child has become really separate from these primary ties. Nevertheless, because of his or her submission to and *dependence* upon guardians the child lacks freedom. But while the child may lack freedom, this is not generally experienced as negative freedom because these primary ties usually give the child a feeling of belonging, rootedness, and security. But the more the child slowly grows and changes, to the extent to which these primary ties become slowly severed, the more the child tends to develop a quest for freedom and independence.[45] The individualizing child is then confronted with a new, and potentially daunting, task: "to orient and root himself in the world and to find security in other ways than those which were characteristic of his preindividualistic existence."[46] Consequently freedom then has a different meaning from the one it had previously. One may have gained freedom *from* primary ties but this has been accompanied by a loss of security and *growing aloneness*. This is because as the child emerges from that world of primary ties it becomes aware of being alone, of being an entity separate from all others.[47]

During this process of individuation the child begins to increasingly experience a world both outside of oneself and outside of the primary ties. Therefore, as the letters highlight, the son begins to spend time within a peer group after school socializing at the local internet bar where he comes into contact with the World Wide Web. Expectedly this process entails a number of frustrations and contradictions concerning the interpersonal relations between parents and child. For example, the child wants to *play* online while the parents want the child to *work* at home. Consequently, we see the internet and the internet bar not being in conflation with school aims, but, on the contrary, in competition with the school over who can more "successfully" capture the attention, enthusiasm, time, energy, and passion of young people. In this sense the school is in competition with the market, for the parents and school want the child to be a *student* while the internet bar and its owner want the child to be a *customer*. But how can China's formal education system compete with the bright lights of the internet for the student's energy, passion, and time? Through the letters we see that this reorientation of the child's priorities, in turn, changes the role of the parents into that of a person with different aims which conflict with the child's wishes, and can result in the authority figure being seen in the child's eyes as a hostile and dangerous person. Basically the child interprets the parent's "love" as emanating from the thwarting of expansiveness, and of breaking the son's attempt to assert himself. This hostile environment, which the child interprets as the suppression of freedom, creates in the child the feeling of powerlessness. And so the child wants to spend decreasing amounts of time inside the home, which is like an uninviting harbor, less time at school, which is like a pressure cooker, and more time at the internet bar *where I have lots more freedom.*

Through the individuation process clearer breaks appear within the family as the child tries to "break out on his own." That is, he begins to seriously *think for himself and question authority.* The breakdown of communication, a common and central feature to all the letters, is emblematic of this rupture within family relations. What we see is the son decides to stop studying and instead decides to seek "freedom" in a new activity that he, himself, can have control and domination over and gain feelings of achievement and satisfaction from. The way in which online games provide them with this sense of freedom was nicely captured by a respondent in research looking into the phenomenological "pull" factors drawing people into the game *EverQuest.* "I felt free," said "Martin," "free of constraints and guidelines, free to create my character's own path instead of following in the footsteps of some strategy guide...every accomplishment was my accomplishment, and every accomplishment brought true satisfaction."[48]

In this sense, the family war-machine over internet use is a battle over the child wanting freedom from primary ties and his subsequent desire to accommodate issues of aloneness, and the parents desire to prevent this individuation from taking place before the child has passed the *gaokao* (college entrance examination), and ideally made it to university.

In fact, even Tao Ran acknowledges this vitally important element relating to the thwarting-of-individuation within the family nexus during what he refers to as their critical period in life. Tao Ran says that during the growth of the child the parents submerge the self-interests of the child under excessive academic requirements, which results in children often learning in a fatigued state in a one-dimensional world. He argues that with increasing age and self-conscious development – i.e., individuation – this suppression of the child's original self-interest (for play), which has not been raised to the level of consciousness, becomes activated.[49] This desire to do what one wants, as opposed to doing what he/she has been told to do (study, study, study), finds expression or release through internet use. Because the child has been effectively funneled through an education-only tunnel, the remedy Tao Ran, in theory, puts forth as a mechanism for them to achieve a "good mental state" is to train and mine children's interest so as to give them full opportunity to display and play to their own singular diversified development, in which entertainment is part of their "daily work activities."[50] Therefore in his hospital he has, inside room no. 8, toys and other figurines that the "patients" can play with while psychologists watch on. Likewise, room no. 10 contains rows of fake machine guns that the patients use for role-play scenarios that are supposed to bridge the virtual world with the real one. For Tao Ran youth running around a hospital courtyard in which there are metal grates and padlocks on every door and bars on every window shooting plastic guns at other "patients" is *real*, while playing with their friends in an internet bar is *fake*. These patients are well aware, however, that such "entertainment within daily work activities" function like the ten locked "treatment rooms" (i.e., solitary confinement cells) on the floor below that are geared toward *correcting* their assumed disturbed sleep, lack of motivation, aggression and depression.[51] That is, a "good mental state" is one where they are willing, through soft and hard coercive and disciplinary measures, to return back to the normal functioning of society.

The search for freedom within a hyperculture

In this sense "internet addiction" is centered around the coupling of freedom *from* parental and school disciplinary control and freedom *to* do as one pleases, which in this particular historical junction coagulates around internet use and online gaming while living within what later I call a *hyperculture*. Professor Yang Xiong has historicized the differing relation freedom has to the socio-political climate of the reform period, by arguing that freedom in the 1980s through rock 'n' roll music was about political demands stemming from social or moral repression, whereas today he says "it's totally individualistic – the kids want freedom, but the freedom to express themselves, to perform, because that makes them happy."[52] This changing relation to freedom, to society, to each other and to themselves can be understood as the historical change from the "we" generation of the 1980s to the "me" generation of today.[53] As it was for American youth in the 1960s, the issue for Chinese youth today is personal power, expression, and freedom.[54]

The parents, however, are so alarmed of this desire for personal power because they think this is happening to "a child," but today's youth are "growing up" more quickly (and in other important ways more slowly) than their generation, basically because the society in which they are embedded into is individualizing too. Or more specifically, the history of reform China is the history of growing individualization, but it is also, in a relative sense, the history of growing freedom.[55] In order to understand these intertwined twin processes we can refer to a survey conducted on one of China's biggest internet portals, *Sina.com*. Of the 54,000 (presumably mainly young) people who responded to the online poll 59 percent said "citizens have the right to do whatever they want to themselves."[56] The "character structure" of youth, if we can be so bold, is an outcome or outgrowth of this historical process from the we-to-the-me generation. It is a character structure that is increasingly being shaped by the internet, for through it young people are being empowered to seek freedom and independence. "China may not have free speech," imminent economist Huang Yasheng noted, "but it has *freer* speech, because the internet has provided a platform for Chinese citizens to communicate with each other."[57]

Without doubt youth today in China are more personally "free" than their parents and grandparents, and so are attempting to construct new social forms, and are having new experiences and exploring new social frontiers, with online gaming being the exemplary example. At the same time, the internet addiction label signals the boundaries of this new found freedom, for the concept acts like a kind of moral judge indicating when the "freedom fighter" has over-stepped the threshold of social acceptability. In this sense the "internet addict" must be thought of as a *rebel* and not as mentally disordered.

This process is made all the more confusing for the parents because no matter how many relatives and friends attempt to "persuade," "reason with" and "educate" the child no one is able to "get through to him." That so many people are unable to help comes as a shock to the parents, which both elevates the problem and tends to be interpreted by them as a sign that the son must really be *unable* to control his internet use. But attributing his aversion to school to an "excessive infatuation" with online games and *not* the opposite, in that his intense relationship to playing online games is itself partly "caused" by a distaste for school, blocks off an important avenue for comprehending why no one can get through to him. While there is an internal logic in arguing that only an abnormal activity like intense internet use – and not an apparently normal activity like school – could possibly be a causal factor in the son's problems, nevertheless, this view will fail to adequately deal with the son's very real detestation for school. And so for the transforming son, who genuinely detests school, all these people are an extension of his parents – fellow thwarters of freedom – and considering the entire context it is not that shocking such talks would have little or no effect.

When the son is sitting in front of an uncle, a teacher, or a psychiatrist we could ask the following: is he being urged to explore, experience, take risks, gamble, *open up* to a voyage of discovery? Or is he being told to *close off*, play it safe, protect his gains, and accept the authoritative voices of those who "know best?"[58] The "internet addict" is constantly under intense pressure to accept the authoritative voice of someone who seemingly know best, even though they themselves have never been through an experience quite like the one today's young are going through. Chinese society is going through such rapid, even hyper, change that those only a few years older, let alone a whole generation, may be unable to comprehend the "inner feelings" of today's intensive gamers. For example, a university student wrote to Tao Hongkai expressing his sympathy for those with an "insatiable desire" for gaming, but when it came to understanding them he came unstuck. "I once attempted to communicate with some high school students who have an insatiable desire for playing games," he wrote, "but I can only understand their inner feelings just a little bit."[59]

Nevertheless, this individuation process is not in reality the beginning of the family war-machine, rather the makings of the war-machine, as Tao Hongkai tells parents, was put into gear when the child was born. For according to his observation, the parents have spoilt the child by making the child the center of the family nexus, which in turn has "failed" to produce independence and self control within the child. And so when the child demands expansiveness and the escape from suppression then the fall into cyberspace is that much deeper because the child, in the eyes of Tao Hongkai and others, has not been provided with the appropriate tools and resources to engage with these new found freedoms in a "rational" or sober way. Yet laying the causation at the feet of the parent's supposedly poor educational and socialization methods misses another important element.

In another sense the character structure of the "internet addict" discloses the full contours of the shattering impact of modernity upon the Chinese population. In Europe, as Žižek pointed out, modernization took place over several centuries, and so there was time to adjust to this break and soften its shattering impact through the work of culture. China, however, has been exposed to this impact directly, so their symbolic universe has been perturbed much more brutally. Arguably, China lost socio-cultural ground during the destructive Maoist period and no time was given to establish a new socio-cultural balance.[60] In this way, the mass migration to the internet by Chinese youth can only be clearly grasped if we understand the way the post-1980s/90s generation and their parents have had capitalism thrown at them almost instantly, and so were not provided with adequate symbolic cushions to help them soften the blow and give them time to adjust to this "hyperculture."

By hyperculture we can refer to the impact of the rapid leap-frog economic model of the reform period where the political economy of wealth exists side-by-side with a political economy of speed[61] – not only the speed of delivery through 8 percent-plus GDP growth rates the Party-State has implicitly promised in exchange for political legitimacy and power, but also the speeding up or intensification of lives being lived *in-the-now*, and of which the culture of excess is partly a logical outcome. Because of the Great-Leap-Forward-like hyperactivity around China's hurried desire to play "catch-up" with the developmental model of the post-industrial economies, we are seeing a "pathological" socio-cultural state induced by high speed. Bertman has defined a hyperculture as "a society of "busy bodies," frenetically striving to keep up, not simply out of economic necessity but out of psychological preference. Time – unstructured, unused – hangs heavily on its head."[62]

The ideal character qualities engendered under Maoism – the compulsion to work, the readiness to make one's life a tool for the purposes of an extrapersonal power, a compulsive sense of duty – are actually also character qualities valued by a capitalist system and without which China's hyper-economic development is unthinkable. However, it is the perceived absence of these qualities that is partly driving the moral panic over excessive internet use by the post-1980s/90s generation, for without these qualities – strong work ethic, giving one's life to the market or the State – China's rapid 8 percent-plus per annum economic growth will not continue. "Internet addiction," which is said to be antithetical to these ethics because it is based on time-wasting selfish pleasure and consumption, and not selfless work and production (and then consumption), drives at the heart of China's growth model. Or more specifically the potential arresting of this growth, which is un acceptable for the Party-State because their legitimacy largely depends on them being able to continue delivering *fast* and *high* economic growth. This is why internet use for "non-work-related purposes" is seen as "useless" and as a "waste of time" (this even despite the fact that the gaming industry reportedly had sales revenue of 27.5 billion yuan in 2009[63]). But the fact is that ethics such as ambition, competition, aggressiveness, self-assertiveness, problem-solving, etc, are also central to gaming. That is partly why video gaming so easily became a global sport and its gamers' legitimate competitors, because its values are in line with the values of the market. The problem for the "internet addict" is that he is playing the wrong game: the game of use value and not exchange value.

Under this hyperculture-of-excess the internet is a protective screen and a tool in which they can establish new symbolic balance into a life out-of-balance.[64] The CCP, after failing with "socialism," imposed, seemingly overnight, the market upon the Chinese population and then expected them to simply "adjust." This can be thought of in the way that a person drains a swimming pool of its water – for during the Cultural Revolution the CCP tried to drain China of its culture – and then tells the swimmer to jump into the pool. In this sense, today's youth have been forced to try and swim without water. Little wonder that many of them are "drowning', or trying to maintain "air" by migrating into cyberspace – a space in which they can find a sense of security in an unsecure world.

Mao Zedong may have famously said power comes from the barrel of a gun,[65] but the current dilemma authority figures in China face (parents; teachers; government) is with the millions of young netizens who are showing that a virtual gun is also effective in bringing about the questioning of authority and the "normal" functioning of society. Through the letters we can gain an important insight into the particular social conditions that exist within certain families and is producing a large group of young people who are dropping out of the central and so-called "normal" social structure. In this sense, the "internet addict" offers us an example from contemporary Chinese society of the "canary in the coal mine" metaphor. Just as the death of the canary served as a warning to miners of poisonous gases by functioning as a biological indicator, the lifeworld of the person labeled an internet addict functions not to teach us of individual pathology but rather functions as a *sociological indicator* highlighting more general and more extensive social problems brought about by the opening up and reforms. The canary in the coal mine metaphor symbolizes sensitivity to a more general "pollutant," and so by studying the extremes or the margins (the deviant) we are, in fact, creating a picture of the center (the normal). Thus the internet addict is, in reality, a harbinger of both the present and the future.

Filiarchy

As already mentioned, one of the important social conditions existing within the family that underpins excessive internet use is the emergence of filiarchy. Professor of marketing, James McNeal, has used Fromm's term filiarchy to describe advertising in China increasingly *targeting* children as highly sought after and valued consumers, in particular the way parents, under intense pressure to conform, are catering to their child's newfound desire for this market-produced material consumption.[66] McNeal and Chan argue that children have become exceptionally valuable customers for the market in contemporary China, and thus possess much *market potential*, specifically because they wield a considerable influence on their parents' decision-making with regard to family expenses and the ways families spend leisure time.[67] They basically define filiarchy as children making family choices and decisions, as opposed to matriarchal-centered or patriarchal-centered decision-making. In relation to leisure pursuits they present the following data:[68]

Item	Age								
	4	5	6	7	8	9	10	11	12
Videogames	73	98	94	92	90	95	93	93	94
Movies	74	98	94	92	90	95	93	93	90
Toys	93	93	92	92	90	91	90	86	86

What this chart demonstrates is that beginning around age five the child is influencing the purchasing of video games, movies, and toys more than 90 percent of the time. And dictating play from such an early age instills into the child a sense of empowerment over his leisure world and the family environment, which is generally a controllable situation for the parents while the child is still attached to the primary ties, but comes back to haunt them in very serious ways when the child is going through both individuation – becoming a tiger – and the search for freedom from those mechanisms blocking him from realizing his life of consumer leisure. The parent's decision-making capacity is complicated not only by their social need to make sure the child is competing within a hyper-competitive education system, and so is not drowning academically, but they are also constrained by their general mystification with technology. Parents, who as the *psychic agency of society* are tasked with transmitting the requirements of society to the growing child,[69] recognize that their children have a knowledge and understanding of technology and computer-based goods that they themselves usually do not. Therefore the child's requests for such items, which many parents feel are essential in contributing to the child's academic development and success, are likely to get more serious consideration from parents. As highlighted earlier, this is also driven by the following parental desire: *"No sacrifice is too great to give my child all the things I didn't have in order to insure her happiness."*[70]

Yet as the letters so painfully describe, this is a sacrifice or Faustian pact that some wish they had never made, for the making of the "internet addict" is often conceived at that moment when the mother wants to give the child everything she didn't have. And when the child becomes accustomed to receiving "everything she wants" then in what sense is it irrational for the child to want to stop going to school and instead live a life of play and consumption; for this is what the child now believes is the pursuit that will bring her "happiness." The problem is that one child's perceived happiness may be one parent's nightmare – and vice versa. And so we read of 11-year-old Mengmeng who had "persuaded" her mother to allow her to purchase lipstick, nail polish, and wedge heels by using classic *fan gan* strategies such as going on "hunger strike" and locking herself in her room. When her mother protested that a famous labeled strapped dress Mengmeng desired was both too expensive and too revealing, Mengmeng reportedly retorted: "Mum, you have no right to interfere with *my* choice."[71]

The current family war-machine over internet use that began to appear around 2003 was somewhat predicted by Shao and Herbig around the mid-1990s in a paper on the "marketing implications" of what they, like many others, called China's "little emperors."[72] Shao and Herbig inadvertently warn – because they are actually celebrating the great market potential of the middle-class only-child – that a "generation of spoilt only-children" is in the making, because their parents are showering them with toys, clothing, and "anything they want." A major reason they give for this mass parental showering of luxurious consumer goods upon their only-children is the upbringing of these parents during the chaotic and materially-scarce Cultural Revolution as *children of Mao*. They therefore argue that the children of Mao "lost their childhood during the Cultural Revolution and are, to a considerable degree, living vicariously – that is, living their dreams through their children. The child's tyrannical rule over the household provides a hint of things to come."[73]

Since 2003 this market potential has transformed into market reality in China's first tier megacities. While per capita disposable income for China's urban residents in 2008 was reportedly 15,781 yuan, surveys have shown that the average annual spending by children in Beijing, Shanghai, Guangzhou and other major cities had exceeded 10,000 yuan.[74] Thus, Letter-6 provides us with more than a hint of what results when the family comes under the apparent tyrannical rule of the child, for as the desperate and despondent mother wrote: "My body and mind are exhausted, and my brain is about to explode, I really want to die. I am a useless person, I cannot even educate my own son properly, and so what other use can I have?" And so the term filiarchy is useful in rethinking the power relations between parents and only-child, or more specifically the consumer society-based condition that has emerged when the parents have either partly lost control over the child, and/or have handed over a certain kind of decision-making power and authority to the child, thereby turning him into a tiger at home and, potentially, a mouse outside. The internet addiction phenomenon can only be fully grasped through the filiarchal nature of parent–child relations and the parent's subsequent desperation and despondency stemming from the intensification of this relation.

From a historical perspective this is the Chinese family nexus flipped on its head, in that the child, who traditionally was "guided" by the strict rules relating to filial piety, has become part of the negotiating process over their education, sometimes to the point where unless their demands are met they will not go to school. In part, they are holding their parents to ransom by exploiting their "weakness" – i.e., the mother's over-investment of emotion in the child's educa-tion and the father's sometimes under-investment in the child's life. In part, however, the parents are simply trying to adhere to social norms, so that the mother's over-investment stems from trying to make sure the child can obtain the exam grades required to "get ahead," while the father's under-investment often stems from him having to work excessively so as to provide for the family. However, parents who hand over part of the power, authority, and decision-making process to the son by giving him what he wants from an early age as a material "reward" for getting him to devote his whole existence to schoolwork – a Faustian pact – may confront a tiger-like child saying "if you don't let me get online at home then I will not go to school."[75] The result is the son getting what he wants: freedom *from* authority and control. That is, he is not retreating (from reality), but simply advancing in a new direction toward an electronic-life of freedom *to* do as he pleases. While there is obviously a class dimension to this condition, as there are many parents who cannot afford to provide material rewards to their child, what is noticeable about the families seeking help at boot camps and clinics is that many of them are prepared, despite the fact they are from upper working-class or lower middle-class backgrounds, to do "whatever it takes," as one mother told me, to turn their child's life around.

Mothers often put these demands down to his "stubborn personality" and/or "pride," and so the mother in Letter-16, for example, said she could not even mention study matters with the son at all, for doing so would be like "lighting a barrel of gunpowder." Or like the family attending Tao Hongkai's four-day course wherein the mother told me over breakfast that the son had not been going to school for three months, and instead had been playing online games throughout the night and sleeping during the day. I therefore asked her where he was getting online. At home she replied. I asked her why she and her husband – who suffered from a physical ailment – allowed him to play online games at home throughout the night. She replied if they did not let him play then he would curse them and throw things around. The son, who just sat there nonchalantly like a mouse mum-bling to his parents and joking with a another mother's son, got up out of his seat, walked outside to the small store, brought a bottle of Coca Cola, and trotted off down the street drinking contentedly. It was 7:50 am. The parents had seemingly lost control over the son's actions. Likewise, the mother in Letter-6 bemoaned:

"If you don't let him play computer games then it is like you are wanting to take away his life, and so he will exert all his strength to resist." We should understand his resistance and rebelliousness as the lynchpins coupling freedom *from* school and freedom *to* play online.

I surmise that attributing this behavior to a "stubborn personality" partly functions to deflect attention away from the role their own actions and decisions play in helping to produce the family war-machine. That is, they choose, perhaps unconsciously, to believe in such personality "traits" because they want to believe in them, and because such beliefs serve functions for them.[76] In a more general sense, the same can be said of attributing their child's internet use to "internet addiction," for arguing that evil internet bar owners entice their kids into gaming, who, in turn, become enslaved to the games, deflects attention away from the role their own behavior – in particular the violent over-invested mother and the absent, neglectful, and violent father – plays in pushing the child into wanting (and not simply needing) to play games with friends away from home and school. But these factors do not seem to be addressed, and only a few parents in the letters were willing to admit their own "defects."

Likewise for the son, he has his own motives and intentions for being partly willing to be framed by his parents (but not others) as being enslaved by forces beyond his capacity to control, whether his personality "defects" or his "internet addiction." In practice, there is partly a strategic quality to these ways of acting, which has the underlying goal of being able to get out of having to go to "boring" school – a school regime whose boringness and dislike is made all the more clearer when compared to the exciting bright lights of online gaming. In almost all the letters the parents write of a son who "promises" to stop playing and start studying, but who never follows through with these promises and, instead, continues to go against the wishes of his parents; thus signaling to the parents that he must not be able to control his behavior. These are part of the strategies he employs in his search for freedom from school, and so exploding like a barrel of gunpowder is his way of building a "great wall" or shield between him and his parents. In this sense, the son is willing up to a point – i.e., the gate of any camp or facility wanting to "treat" him using discipline and punishment – to attribute his problems with school to "internet addiction" for this implies that he is *sick* and so should not be going to school. Instead, he should be "resting" at home, which means playing online, preferably at the internet bar with friends. And so through the prism of the family war-machine over schoolwork and leisure we can learn how much the traditional virtue of filial piety has been transformed during China's modernization, and now within some families we find an almost opposite situation being played out that we can describe as filiarchy.

Significantly, research by the Medical Faculty at Tongji University claimed that 90 percent of "internet addicts" have encountered problems in family education (i.e., that the parent–child relation is of a disordered nature).[77] This particular research divides disordered parent–child relations into four main categories. These following categories constitute "the family reasons for youngsters' internet addiction":

1) Laissez-faire style parenting

Busy parents who ignore providing family education for their children. If parents "let it be," or do not interfere, children with weak self control might easily become addicted to internet.

2) Naive style parenting

Some parents do not learn knowledge related to computer technology and so do not provide strict supervision to children's use of the internet.

3) Improper style parenting

Most of the youngsters are only-children. They are being spoilt at home by their parents.

These children become stubborn, unruly, and selfish. Subsequently, the educational measures and remonstration from parents do not work on these children.

4) Strict style parenting

Parents who are too strict on their children, and so may forbid their children to use the internet. When these children go through rebellious adolescence, they might resist their parents through prolonged use of internet.[78]

What this research argues is that "internet addiction" is the outcome of a dis-ordered family dynamic – in particular, as we see through the letters, because of parents who are absent, neglectful, unengaged, violent, over-indulgent (engulf-ing), and excessively strict. Likewise, Tao Hongkai's assistant, Cai Peng, said that he has noticed, after observing thousands of parents, a common pattern in relation to parental education and the occupation of the parents. He has observed three occupations that appear more dominant than others among the parents seeking help for their child's "internet addiction." Interestingly, these parents resemble somewhat the kind of parenting style highlighted in the research earlier. They are, in order of frequency:

1) *Business person*: Cai Peng's interpretation on why many "internet addicts" have a businessman/woman for a parent (or both parents) is that such parents are always away from their child on business trips. Due to them working long hours then they spend little time with their child. That is, the kids are neglected by one or both parents. However, this is usually the father. Moreover, when this (under-invested) parent discovers a problem with the child then they are more likely to use symbolic (scoldings) and physical violence as a tool in which to attempt to solve perceived problems. This method, in turn, produces resistance and rebelliousness (*fan gan*) within the child; or what Tao Ran conceptualizes as "oppositional defiant disorder."[79] These laissez-faire and strict parents are also inclined to blame the child for causing the problems within the family.

2) *Teacher*: This is especially so if both parents are primary or middle school teachers. These parents can be placed into two sub-groups that exhibit different characteristics:

    (a) These teacher-parents are usually very strict and are always forcing their kids to study excessively (i.e., engulfment and depersonalization). This parent basically desires to turn the child into a grade-making machine.

    (b) The teacher who can see other kids'/students' problems clearly, but cannot see their own child's problems. They are, according to Cai Peng, too emotionally caught up. They are rational and strict to their students while at work but do not use these professional methods on their own kids at home, which Cai Peng says is irrational. That is, they have trouble bringing work home with them, despite their best intentions. So the child is like the half-finished project – they want to produce that "dream child" but also want to keep their work at work and not have to bring it home with them.

3) *Doctor*: This parent, which can extend to nurses, creates a large number of excessive restrictions and rules upon the child around what they should and should not do – i.e., what is healthy and not-healthy, what is right and wrong, what is good and bad. For example, Cai Peng recounted the story of the son of a doctor at a camp who refused to eat anything that had pepper in it as pepper, according to his father, is bad for your stomach. He also refused to eat peanuts as peanuts, according to his father, are bad for your teeth. The result, according to Cai Peng, is that such kids are often overly anxious and cautious about everything they come into contact with. Consequently, these kids are seen as strange by their classmates so that it is difficult for them to make friends. Therefore they go online to make friends and to release this built up anxiety and tension over all the excessive rules and regulations put on them by their parents.

And so when Tao Ran claims that "about half" of the "internet addicts" need medical treatment because in addition to their internet addiction they also supposedly suffer from mental disorders such as attention deficit hyperactivity disorder, oppositional defiant disorder, affective disorder, personality disorders, and conduct disorders, then we should be suspicious of attributing these perceived problems to the bio-medical model, for this negates the whole family dynamic that contributes to the child's behavior and internet use.[80] Tao Ran claims that drugs can effectively control the assumed withdrawal symptoms, emotional disturbances, anxiety, depression, and other neuro-endocrine irregularities supposedly stemming from these apparent disorders, but what both Tongji's research and Cai Peng's participant observation are saying is that the child's problems principally stem not from a break down within their mind but rather from a break down within the family; in particular, the disordered nature of the parent's educational methods. Thus attacking the child's psychology with tricyclic antidepressants, selective 5-HT reuptake inhibitors, anti-anxiety drugs, and mood stabilizers in no way attacks or transforms the

disordered nature of the child's parental education that played an important contributing role in relation to the child's internet use. Nevertheless, if we read Tao Ran's
co-authored book we learn the real functional role of using medicines such as
amitriptyline, fluoxetine, diazepam, and sodium valproate. Tao Ran claims that
these drugs can gradually make their mood become more balanced, and therefore
this "balance" (read: docility) will hopefully increase their *compliance* to his medical,
psychological, or behavioral interventions.[81] Quite simply, he aims not to cure sickness but to control behavior.

Death and punishment

While filiarchy plays an important contributing factor underpinning socially
problematic internet use, this is not the whole story for explaining the perceived
tyrannical child. The mother in Letter-6 may have had thoughts of death, but just
before saying this she mentions, in an offhand way as though it is not all that
significant, that the son's father had passed away a few years ago. Should we find
it at all coincidental that the son's gaming, declining school grades, lying, stealing,
fighting, and cursing – i.e., his deviance or rebelliousness – coincided with the
death of his father? Perhaps the most significant aspect to uncovering the son's
rebelliousness is this event.

Letter-32 offers us an "ideal type" as a way to analyze the way "chronic stressors"
such as death contribute to the child's rebelliousness. The mother speaks of the
son, the youngest of four siblings, as being "loved dearly" and "indulged" by all
those around him. All those except his father that is, who despite often being
away on business, treated him sternly and would sometimes beat him "ruthlessly"
when the son did not listen (again we see a perfect storm brewing: the overindul-
gent mother and absent, strict, and violent father). After being beaten by the father
the son was "able to be especially obedient." Under this maternal "love" and
paternal "guidance" the son was considered a relatively *good* boy until year five
of primary school. At the age of eleven, the father died of a chronic illness. Not
long after the father's death the mother was called to a school meeting along with
the parents of three other children. The mothers were told that their sons had
become the classes' "headache" because they talked during class, did not hand in
homework, and had declining grades. Feeling faint, the mother could not believe
that the son could become like this.

The mother reasoned that his deviance was due to not receiving supervision
from a young age and so his "disobedient personality spread unchecked." In addition,
because his father was absent then he was no longer "afraid of anyone"; as though
the best medicine to prescribe for disobedience is producing a fear of authority.
Significantly, a despotic father in Letter-19 operated under a similar regime, with
him severely terrifying and beating the son because he believed that in a dishonest
society such as his people needed to be a "wolf that is not afraid of anything."
And a wolf he became, as the mother ended up years later begging Tao Hongkai
to somehow miraculously halt the son's slide into "evil ways." Now back-tracking
on her earlier statement, the mother in Letter-32 confesses that the scoldings and

beatings by the father did not really produce obedience, as he was always "unable to really do what he was asked to do." It seemed that the parents operated under two opposing regimes: the mother tried to love obedience into him, while the father tried to beat it into him. Neither approach worked.

The son began playing online at the internet bar with these three other "bad kids" until dark. The mother was afraid that he would "study badly" at the internet bar, and so she bought him a computer to use at home. Like a tiger he consequently "dominated" the computer everyday by chatting and playing games. After discovering he had caught hepatitis B the mother tried to get him to eat more and sleep earlier. But in a classic case of "*fan gan*" (rebelling against everything his mother wanted from him) he would sleep until very late, and "if you told him to eat this he wouldn't eat it. If you told him to not get angry he would get angry and smash things."[82]

While the mother was worried about his health, he would say himself that he did not want to live for long anyway. Understanding his devaluation of life it is perhaps not surprising that the mother discovered in his third year of middle school that he had been: cutting school; not listening at all when at school; and had not even opened his textbooks. In a classic case of attribution, this rejection of school the mother attributed to two teachers that he quite liked having left, therein "disrupting" his schoolwork.

The mother subsequently cheated him into going to live in Xiamen in order to "leave this environment" that was teaching him "how to do bad things in society." Considering that these friends had obviously become the central and most important part of his life – as they allowed him to avoid aloneness, isolation, and connect him with a world outside of himself – then it is not surprising that he refused to leave and did everything in his power to return once he had left. Despite all these problems the mother acknowledges *he has experienced a great deal*. Nevertheless, she believes that "he doesn't know what to do with himself" even though, like most of the other parents, she does not understand what he is thinking. His problems are made all the more confusing because the other three children are all considered obedient and so she is left to wonder "how can he be like this?" Her conclusion being that his "disobedient personality spreading unchecked." This despite the fact that being the youngest sibling he was "loved dearly" and "indulged" by all those around him.

In trying to make sense of this case, as an ideal type of other similar narratives, we should not merely link it back to the father's death but also link back to the way the father, like many of the fathers of "internet addicts," "ruthlessly" beat the son. In fact a growing body of research findings is indicating that a child who is subjected to corporal punishment by his/her parents subsequently displays disobedient and aggressive behavior themselves.[83] For example, researcher Catherine Taylor studied a mother's use of corporal punishment upon the 3-year-old child. Analyzing 2461 children across twenty cities in America, Taylor and her research team wanted to investigate the link between a 3-year-old child being physically punished and that same child 2 years later exhibiting aggressive behavior – even after controlling for the child's initial level of aggression along with other seemingly important maternal parenting risk factors and demographic features. Each of the confounding factors – i.e., neglect by the mother; violence or aggression between the parents; maternal stress and depression; the mother's use of alcohol and drugs; unwantedness of child during pregnancy – contributed to the children's aggressive behavior at age five; however, they could not explain all of the violent tendencies at that age. That is, a positive connection between corporal punishment and aggression remained strong even after these confounding factors had been accounted for. Basically the finding of the research is as follows: the more corporal punishment inflicted upon the child at age three the more aggressive behavior (approximately 50 percent) that same child displayed when he/she was 5 years old. In short, "the child learns to be aggressive by being treated directly with aggression."[84] While supposedly finding "statistical links" or "correlative predictors" in relation to human behavior makes research findings such as this study appear more "scientific," the "facts" more hard, and thus the findings more "true,"[85] nevertheless, we should merely be cognizant of the important picture drawn from this research. As the letters clearly indicate, there appears a strong tendency for *fan gan* (resistance/rebelliousness) to be evoked within the child when the child is beaten.[86] Additionally, in contrast to the children who were not hit in the study, those who were physically punished were more likely to demand immediate satisfaction of their wants and needs, to be defiant, get frustrated easily, have temper tantrums, and lash out physically against others.[87] Moreover, the study pointed out that children who had merely a "visiting" relationship with the father – i.e., a neglectful and absent father – were at risk for higher levels of aggression.

In addition to physical violence we can, I believe, add symbolic violence as a factor engendering *fan gan*. We can also factor in non-family members as contributing to the production of *fan gan*, such as teachers. For example, the son in Letter-4 with "very strong self-respect" was skipping class with his friends to go to the internet bar to play games. This was discovered by the teacher and instead of reprimanding the group the teacher apparently decided to only punish the son in order to "kill the chicken to scare the monkey" (i.e., to signal one person out for severe punishment as a warning to others). Feeling his self respect severely insulted he refused to go to school again. And after flunking out of school he did not go home and have his pride dented even further, so instead he ran off to the internet bar. Even taking into account the possibility that this situation provided him with an attribution in order to secure an escape from school ("the teacher left me with no choice but to quit"), nevertheless, the teacher's method of using him as an example to threaten others must be understood as playing a contributing factor in increasing the son's internet use. Therefore such research findings should be kept firmly in mind when we are searching for the "causes" for deviant behavior such as becoming the class "headache" or increased internet use. If the mother looked at the way the son was treated by his parents she may learn how he "could become like this." It is not simply that the child learns to be aggressive through having aggression rained down upon him (i.e., aggression = aggression) but more so that, as Fromm argued, *the individual and social conditions that make for suppression of life produce the passion for destruction.*

This chapter has focused upon conceptualizing a number of contributing factors leading to the production of the family war-machine and how the son "could become like this." In particular I have argued that intensive internet use cannot be reduced to the perceived failings of the (pathological) individual, but rather begins with filiarchical relations and reaches its apex during the individuation process, which is itself a search for freedom *from* primary ties and the freedom *to* become more autonomous and more in control of one's *own* lifeworld. The subsequent production of *fan gan*, or rebelliousness, of which online gaming is central, is the result of the fight over this search for freedom, wherein the parents, who as the psychic agency of society are trying to get the son to devote his whole existence to school-work, find themselves scolding, beating, and locking away the son as ways in which to arrest this process. This, inevitably, produces *fan gan* within the child and leads to increased deviance and internet use. In this way I have put forth the proposition that intensive internet use stems from a position of ontological insecurity due to the production of a tiger-mouse character structure and, at the same time, a thwarted or suppressed life. In the following chapter I extend this argument further with reference to the push and pull factors relating to internet use.

6   Push and pull factors

This chapter, as the name suggests, focuses upon the push and pull factors relating to intensive internet use. Like a coin, the internet – or its driving mechanisms – could be said to have two sides. One side contains push factors while the other contains pull factors, but both are magnetic in that they "attract" the person into its sphere of influence. That is, the internet serves particular functions for certain people. The push factors can be understood as stemming from what Fromm and Laing would call acts of self-preservation, and which can be understood as constituting part of the son's "mouseness." Basically, the retreat from normalcy and advance toward the freedom of the internet, the internet bar, and one's peers, is done partly in order to preserve one's autonomous self (separateness). This thwarting and suppression of the autonomous self is conceptualized using two main concepts: engulfment and depersonalization. Both of which can be said to "push" the son away from a normalcy they experience as emotionally stifling, and toward the internet which is experienced as liberating because it reinforces autonomy and individuality. The pull factors, on the other hand, principally stem from more intensive strivings – relatedness/transcendence/orientation and devotion – and can be understood as constituting part of the son's "tigerness." This is also the "devotion" to feelings of success, achievement, power, prestige, and domination – which the biomedical model conceptualizes as an "addiction" but which in reality is them attempting to adhere to society's dominant values and ethics within a socially devalued (cyber)space. Fromm notes that these strivings, what he calls "frames for orientation and devotion," are rooted in the same need from which religious and philosophical systems spring for they stem from the attempt to make sense of one's existence and place in the world.[1] That is why the internet bar is like a kind of monastery, because it is a space in which people can attend to that central paradox in their existence: the simultaneous seeking of closeness and of independence, or the striving for oneness with others and at the same time the preservation of one's uniqueness and particularity.[2] Thus the underlying premise of the push/pull mechanism is the following: "the nature of all life is to preserve and affirm its own existence."[3]

Letter-13 – turning the child into a grade-making machine

While parental death, divorce, absence, neglect, and symbolic and physical violence play important contributing factors toward the child's rebelliousness, the parents', and in particular the mother's, over-investment in the child's education must be given its due importance in pushing the son away from the family unit and school yard and toward cyberspace. Basically, what the parent considers to be "providing" for the child in terms of education may result, for the child, in a depersonalized experiential process of being "loved to death." Letter-13 provides us with an ideal type highlighting the way the parents turn the child into a *depersonalized* grade-making machine, and the son's subsequent reaction, or *fan gan*, to this *engulfing* "love":[4]

> I write this letter to you with a very heavy heart, I want to ask you to help solve my child's severe problem during his prime. As he is infatuated with computer games he is not studying properly, and his school grades have suffered a disastrous decline. None of the methods we have tried have had any effect, we are afraid that if this continues then it will destroy his life.
>
> 1) Introduction of Basic Circumstances
>
> 1. Xiao Liang is at a key middle school in Beijing where enrolment is according to primary school grades. (Middle and high school are continuous so there is no need to attend the high school exam.) The class has 48 students, with just 16 males, the others are all females.
>
> 2. His grades in primary school were really good. We did not push him too hard in his studies, and he was a really obedient child. He also took on the responsibility of class head. When he graduated from primary school he was elected one of Beijing's "three good" students, and so was smoothly admitted into this School. This made us feel very happy.
>
> 3. Due to the school being quite far away from home, then in middle school Xiao Liang was willing to board. In his first year of middle school he relied on himself to study hard, and both his grades and his behaviour were very good, and he was elected a "three good" student. Everything was normal. In the class the girls were eager to have better grades than the boys, and so the front ten were all girls.
>
> 4. Family relations were harmonious, although before we were quite strict on the child's discipline, and perhaps some problems existed with our methods, but we never exceeded unreasonable or excessive boundaries.
>
> 2) Abnormal situation begins
>
> 1. From November of 2004 an abnormal decline in grades began, and he went down to 20th in the class. It was here his physiology underwent a noticeable growth, his height increased very quickly, his voice became course, and he started to pay attention to fashion. It was here when two things happened.
>
> A) He shared a desk with the female class head. Once I took him travelling and his mobile phone accessory was lost, but Xiao Liang was the only one

who worryingly looked for it, yet he didn't say to us why, so I angrily criticized him. Later I figured out that this was certainly related to this girl.

B) In December we had a very formal talk with him. This was because the semester was about to end and his mid-semester exam results had declined, so we were hoping to get him to accelerate and firmly grasp his studies so that at the end of the semester his grades would be good. But he did not speak ideally, revealing some reactionary emotions, saying "The current education system is not good, teachers and parents just want to know about school grades." We emphasized to him that parents do not attach special importance to grades; rather we just want him to work hard and that to learn knowledge is good enough. He was not willing to listen to his parents, and said that he does not want us to interfere with matters relating to study. We essentially respected him, and did not control too much. The result was that at the end of semester his grades still declined.

2. During the winter vacation communication with Xiao Liang was so-so, and no big conflict emerged. But after the second semester of the second year of middle school there emerged a very big change.

A) While boarding at school he did not adhere to work and rest time regulations, and he started going outside the school by himself to relieve boredom. He did not study by himself at night, and his expression was very unhappy. He was unwilling to communicate with us, his temper was irritable, and he resisted against anyone.

B) Xiao Liang said that that he wanted to transfer schools. He did not want to board as there are too many controls and restrictions. We went about handling the procedure of suspending his boarding.

C) After attending day school we discovered that he was really infatuated with games. He would frequently go to internet bars, and twice he did not come home until at 2 am. Once he did not come home at all.

D) Because he was excessively infatuated with games, this has produced an aversion to study and he does not do homework, sleeps in class. After coming home he does not read books. After the mid-term exam his game playing became even more severe, we therefore tried to restrict him, but this was of no use. We also talked rationally with him, and reasonably arranged good study and game playing time – study for 2 hours, and play games for 2 hours. But he did not listen. Basically he has never read a book or done homework at home.

E) Due to excessive use of games, he only sleeps at 11–12 pm. The next day he doesn't pay attention to time and so dawdles about until he is late. You can try to reason with him until you are blue in the face but he won't listen. The teachers definitely give him pressure. He has been truant for three classes, and so has been criticized by the school.

3) We think the overall behavioural situation is:

1. Excessive infatuation with games and detest and rejects studying. He thinks there is a future in playing games (can attend Counter Strike gaming competitions and receive prize money). Sometimes even if he is at the internet bar playing games when he returns home he is unhappy. It seems as if it is like he has lost interest in life.

2. Has agitated emotions that fluctuate quite a lot. When playing games he gets annoyed with himself if he plays badly. When we communicate with him he uses words that are improper. He is able to immediately change emotions, and so can produce a rebellious psychology. He is not willing to communicate with his parents but communicates with other people ok.

3. An inferiority complex exists for sure. At primary school he was always in the top few of the class, after starting middle school, he cannot get within the top 15 in the class. He also doesn't have a special strong-point. His sole strong-point is his computer knowledge.

4) Some of the parental measures

1. Basically we have tried to patiently convince him to give priority to education, even to the extent of coaxing him. To the best of our abilities we have shown concern for him, and communicated with him. When we say little he groans a promise, but it won't actually result in action. When we say a lot he is really annoyed and goes silent. Occasionally, we sternly criticize him, and once I even hit him with my hand, but the effect was even worse.

2. We also tried to satisfy him materially, and to make him feel happier. For example, we bought him things that he likes such as brand sports shoes, clothes, a mobile phone, a bicycle. Before when he wanted these we weren't be so forthright in promising them, so we began one-by-one to satisfy him, but he didn't change. On the contrary, matters just got worse.

3. We also let his cousins live at our house so that through lots of contact with him they could communicate and guide him through playing and chatting, but the situation just got more rotten by the day.

4. We recently had a discussion with a teacher and asked for five days leave so that he could have time at home to adjust his mental attitude and work and rest; the effect wasn't great.

He is such an intelligent, progressive and good kid, how could he become like this? We will spare no effort in saving him, we cannot let him continue to degenerate like this. We have already exhausted all the tricks, we earnestly request you to help us save our child.[5]

Letter-13 – engulfment

Letter-13 is arranged into four parts. Part one ("basic circumstances") highlights how when he has getting good grades Xiao Liang was "good" and the parents were "very happy," and so this situation was considered "normal." Part two ("abnormal situation") summarizes his decline into *abnormality*, which starts with his grades and ends with excessive infatuation with games and aversion to school. Part three is the mother's pseudo-psychiatric diagnosis of the son's "overall behavior," in which his unhappiness, loss of interest in life, improper language, agitated and annoyed emotions – that fluctuate and change rapidly – are the result of an excessive infatuation with games, a detestation of school, and an inferiority complex (i.e., mouseness). Part four summarizes the parent's attempts, through certain "parental measures," to deal with the son's slide into abnormality by using a carrot (by trying to coax him back to school using persuasion and material rewards) and a stick (symbolic and physical violence through stern criticism). Let us first deal with what the mother called the son's "basic circumstances," for this reveals, I would argue, the pathology of normalcy that passes for the normal functioning of society.

It is revealing that what the mother considered to be "basic" and "normal" is a son whose "really good grades" allowed him to enter a "key middle school." And this coupled with him being a "really obedient child" resulted in him, twice, being elected a "three good" student.[6] In reality there is nothing "normal" about the "three good student" because the few, the so-called top of the class, who receive such a reward are awarded so not for their normality but rather their abnormality; in that they are abnormally good, disciplined, and obedient students. But for the child to "get ahead" they are required to accumulate such awards for being abnormally obedient. While the mother initially claims they did not push him too hard in his studies she then admits that they were "quite strict on the child's discipline," a method she now, upon reflection, believes created "some problems." While she believed their education toward the son "never exceeded unreasonable or excessive boundaries" there are enough revealing comments to suggest otherwise. For example, in a letter addressed to a person she is begging to help her son overcome "internet addiction" why would she write the following: "The girls were eager to have better grades than the boys, and so the front ten were all girls?" Likewise, when a parent wants to have a "very formal talk" with the son under the sole aim of getting him to "accelerate and firmly grasp his studies so that at the end of the semester his grades would be good," then what does that tell us about the parent's relation to the son's school grades and the conceptualization of the son as principally someone who should, above all else, be getting good grades?

When we look at the son's basic circumstances, according to the mother, we get a rather distorted picture of Xiao Liang. His most important elements, his foundation, are all about his schooling and his school grades. But what about him as a *person*? The only information offered about Xiao Liang as a person is in relation to schoolwork: he was really obedient, took on the responsibility as class head, and so was elected a "three good" student; he relied on himself to study hard at boarding school and so his grades and behavior were good. We could, on the other hand, ask: What about his spiritual health? His physical health? His psychological health? His hobbies? His passions? His relation to nature? His relation to his classmates, to his city, and to society? This letter, which is similar in focus to most of the letters, offers us a window in which to view where parents place their *value*. While this over-investment in school and school grades may be the mother expressing her "love" for the child, however, this is not necessarily love in a productive sense. Rather this kind of engulfing love has the potential effect of producing not love in return but rather resistance, rebellion, and even hate. For, as quoted earlier, the child may end up saying the following to his parents: "*All you – and my teachers – care about is school grades, school grades, and school grades. I hate you and I hate school.*"

R.D. Laing, in his studies of the dynamics of family relations wherein one member, usually a child, is said to be "mentally ill," discovered a common feature of the *inter*personal relations between parents and child. Laing bases his understanding of identity upon the following: "A firm sense of one's own autonomous identity is required that one may be related as one human being to another. Otherwise, any and every relationship threatens the individual with loss of identity."[7] And so if the individual cannot feel himself to be autonomous this means that he can experience neither his relatedness to, nor his separateness from, the other in the usual way. That is, the process of individuation, as outlined by Fromm, becomes suffocated. This lack of a sense of autonomy, according to Laing, implies that one feels as though one's being to be bound up in the other, or that, conversely, the other is bound up in oneself, in a way that transgresses the actual possibilities within the realm of human relatedness. For the person bound up, smothered or engulfed by the other, they feel they are in a position of "onto-logical dependency" to the other, which is the opposite of a sense of attachment and relatedness based upon genuine mutuality. Tied in this interpersonal knot, the individual experiences him/herself as a person who is constantly saving him/herself from an existential drowning by the most strenuous and desperate activity.[8] This engulfment, for Laing,

[I]s felt as a risk in being understood (thus grasped, comprehended), in being loved, or even simply in being seen. To be hated may be feared for other reasons, but to be hated as such is often less disturbing than to be destroyed, as it is felt, through being engulfed by love.[9]

This sense of being drowned or destroyed by engulfment is nicely captured by the son in Letter-26, a son who has a mother that focused on grades and a father who "strictly controlled" him, to the point of beating him severely and even locking him in the house. During the second year of middle school the son, in a classic example of the individuation process, started changing his behavior due to what the mother called an "emerging self-awareness." This self-awareness, or what we could call his unraveling of the engulfment knot, resulted in him going against his parents "will." Not only did he want to play outside where he had lots more freedom, but he also said, "I didn't come home to listen to your nagging; keep nagging and I will leave again."[10]

Laing also argued that in order to understand the development of psychoses then we must look into the *intra*personal "make up" of the individual, or what he called *primary ontological security.* For Laing an ontologically secure person will encounter all the social, ethical, spiritual, and biological hazards of life from a centrally firm sense of his or her own and other people's identity and reality. In contrast, and more importantly for the potential development of psychological problems, is the ontologically insecure person, who, as the term suggests, possesses a partial or even complete absence of a secure sense of an autonomous self, which in turn allows anxieties and danger to arise in relation to their own selfhood and the attempts to deal with such dangers and anxieties. As Laing says,

> We can say that in the individual whose own being is secure in this primary experiential sense, relatedness with others is potentially gratifying; whereas the ontologically insecure person is preoccupied with preserving rather than gratifying himself: the ordinary circumstances of living threaten his [or her] *low threshold* of security.[11]

And because one feels threatened by the actions of the other, say, for example, the obsession by the mother over the child's school grades, they seek out acts that will lead to self-preservation so as to "save" themselves from some kind of drowning-of-autonomous-self. It is in this sense that online gaming during the individuation process, when they are pressured to "accelerate" their schoolwork, can be thought of as a *remedy* – in saving one's autonomy and a search for freedom – as opposed to a kind of imported *poison* called "electronic opium." To reiterate my earlier statement: *socially problematic internet use is often the outcome of a thwarted life* (and not a disordered mind).

And so when Xiao Liang was "going outside the school by himself to relieve boredom" (and to seek excitement), it was not simply because he was "addicted" to the internet but partly because the internet can keep the engulfed person existentially alive. In this sense internet use can function as a counter-measure against the stress-tensions that contemporary Chinese society is generating during a process of a disorienting modernization.[12] As noted earlier, due to the specific conditions of China's modernity, in which citizens are partly condemned to individualization and so must constantly adapt to changing social conditions, then they are forced to find ever-new biographical and individual solutions to the social and structural contradictions in their existence. Specifically, deregulation and privatization – i.e., handing over the individual to State-managed market forces – has meant that individualization is like a kind of socio-political sentence in which individuals are congratulated when they succeed yet perhaps condemned as "addicts" when they rebel or fail.[13]

This social reality has been neatly captured by a large scale survey. A total of 629 history students at 33 universities throughout China were questioned on their attitudes, behavior, and belief systems. The findings, which were deemed too sensitive to be published in the mainstream press, reveal both the individualization *and* individuation processes taking place among the *children of the market* as they come of age in an increasingly consumer-based society. When asked about their belief system 72.2 percent of respondents significantly choose "individual strug- gle." In addition, more than 94 percent said they had been influenced by Western culture, while more than 61 percent said they identified with liberalism.[14] The belief that they must struggle individually in order to get through and advance in life is a reflection upon them being generally forced to seek individual solutions to social problems, while their belief in Western culture and liberalism (as associ- ated with capitalism and individualism) help us understand the individuation process taking place among Chinese youth today, and the subsequent individual struggle of youth for personal power and freedom. This is why we must juxta- pose to this individual struggle the results from another survey in which more than 50 percent of the 500 post-90s students surveyed said they worship "them- selves" more than any other role model or hero, while saying "happiness" was the most important thing in life.[15] It is thus no coincidence that the host of Hunan TV's popular dating show "Take Me Out" would say that if the show contributed something to the lives of the young contestants it was to hopefully help them to *love themselves more*.[16] The children of the market, who must ideally learn to market themselves as *products* on the market, are able to "worship" and "love" themselves more through the powerful feelings of personal satisfaction, achieve- ment, and "happiness," obtained while gaming, blogging, micro-blogging, etc.[17]

Most importantly, and one of the keys to understanding the family war- machine and the child's intensive internet use, is that the only way to unravel this cloak of "love" that engulfs them is through *detachment* and *isolation*. While the parent's existence is necessary for the child's survival, it is, nevertheless, also a potential threat to his/her existential survival.[18] In this sense, the "love" of some Chinese parents toward their (only)-child could be referred to as *deathly love*, in that driven by an attribution that states "no sacrifice is too great to give my child all the things I didn't have in order to insure his happiness," they deplete the child's sense of autonomy. The son, for his autonomy and individuality, rebels through *fan gan* by escaping the family nexus therein detaching himself from the "normal" functioning of society. Meanwhile, the military-style boot camp's self- interested goal is to exploit, for maximum economic gain, the parent's desperation and heart-break stemming from the child's retreat from school and subsequent advance in a new cyber-direction.

So the child's deviant behavior is not simply a rejection of school *per se*, but partly a response to engulfment by their parents *over* school. "Love" partly drives them into the individualized and socialized space of both the internet bar and the internet, for only here, as the center of *their* universe, can they feel autonomous and not threatened with the loss of individuality during the process of individua- tion. Indeed, this is where an autonomous identity can in fact be produced and claimed. Thus, engulfment can be understood as one of the push factors driving the son away, in an effort to preserve his being, from that which is suffocating him and so is experienced as a threat to his autonomous self.[19]

Tao Ran is actually well aware of the way parental engulfment is a very serious threat to the child's identity, for on the wall in the entrance hallway of his hospital he had pasted the following veiled threat to parents: "Overprotection will make your children disabled."[20] If it is parental overprotection or engulfment that is "disabling" the child, thus pushing him or her toward the internet and gaming, then how is attacking the child with medicine, psychotherapy, and military exercises going to attack or untangle this parental engulfment? Here, again, we see a contradiction between his theory and his practice.

While the mother in Letter-13 recognized "some problems" in her method – one problem we could call an excessive infatuation with school-grades – another mother was more cognizant of the way engulfment and the production of *fan gan* are two sides of the same coin. The mother in Letter-16 wrote: "Due to me excessively paying attention to his school grades, and having inappropriate educational methods, then this *aggravated his rebellious psychology*.[21] That is, engulfing love can be the catalyst driving them to advance in a new direction: autonomy and freedom from engulfment. But this is ultimately an untenable or negative freedom because the self feels safe only in hiding, and in being isolated from that which is experienced as a threat. And the best place for the child full of "rebellious psychology" to hide and isolate themselves from a deathly love is the internet, which is experienced as a safe haven for the children of the market. For as the son in Letter-20 said to his mother about engulfment: "I am most annoyed by people keeping track of me."[22] The father, who both neglected the son, yet, at the same time, took out his anger from, and hatred toward work on the son, blamed the son's deviant behavior on the mother for "spoiling" the child. And so, according to the father, the son's deviance is "retribution" for the mother spoiling him. In defense of the mother, however, we should note that the father using the son to *fa xie* (give vent to) his frustration and anger surely played an important part in the son's "retribution.'

To return back to Xiao Liang's "basic circumstances" we should therefore ask the following: how much of all his proud achievements and good behavior (being class head and a three good student) were expressions of his own will? The important question is not how good or how bad Xiao Liang was, but whether he developed a sense of being the origin of his own actions, of being the source from which his actions are generated, or, alternatively, whether the source of his actions came, not from within himself, but from within his mother (and father). It may have occurred at primary school that Xiao Liang perfected the required skills to become a three good student and that he did all that was expected of him, yet genuine self-action may never have become established to any real extent, and instead most action may have been in compliance and conformity with outside directives; directives functioning under a premise of being "quite strict on the child's discipline."[23] And so the child suddenly seeing *his* school grades decline may not experience it in the same dramatic fashion as the parents, because he never "really" believed in school grades to begin with, or at least did not over-invest his emotions in them – as his eventual rejection of school tends to indicate. Rather he was generally complying with the demands of his parents and teachers.

The mother and father, for their part, were willing to "spare no effort" in order to prevent Xiao Liang from "degenerating." Like many letters, there is a strong social-Darwinist thread running throughout Letter-13, for the mother sees competition as the way "forward" while to slip back is to "degenerate." Likewise, his "inferiority complex" is related to him becoming "weak" in competition with his (female) opponents. As Bakken has argued, there is a social-Darwinist streak running throughout the entire discourse on individual modernity in China, which is on clear display in the letters. The "survival of the fittest" doctrine is ever-present in the way competition over the child's position in the class and over school grades is defined as the striving for superiority over classmates, so that, for example, the top ten in Xiao Liang's class were all girls because they were more "eager" (i.e., more "hungry" for success). Likewise, desiring Xiao Liang to "accelerate" his studies, like a tiger chasing down prey, is seen by parents as a necessity in order for the *hurried* child to feel under sufficient pressure to strive harder. Everyone who is competing is expected to want to be superior in order to avoid losing out, and so these stress-producing feelings are meant to engender within students a desire to strive continuously.[24] Under this competitive pressure-cooker the slow and lazy (i.e., uninterested/bored) student will simply drown or "degenerate." However, these so-called inferior students experience existential stress through trying to keep up on the treadmill of this hurried hyperculture. Therefore, these drowning students who attempt to keep themselves existentially alive by gaming competitively online are in no way outside the reality of conventional Chinese modernity. In reality, online gaming is inside this modernization process because the marketplace value of competition is a central component in Chinese life whether one is in the classroom or in the internet bar. This can be clearly seen in the way Xiao Liang, like many "internet addicts," desired to attend Counter Strike gaming competitions to receive prize money through competing and (hopefully) winning. The problem for Xiao Liang was that he was competing in the wrong game.

Letter-13 – producing *fan gan*

If we look closely at part two of Letter-13, "abnormal situation begins," an interesting picture emerges. First, the mother writes that "abnormality" begins when there is an "abnormal decline" in his grades. That is, the threshold separating normal from abnormal – from the mother's perspective – lies not principally in the thoughts, speech or general behavior of Xiao Liang but rather in his grades and their decline to "20th in the class." Only then does she attempt to interpret his lifeworld against the backdrop of declining grades – and not vice versa. Then she basically describes the individuation process at work: a teenager going through significant physiological changes, which is accompanied by attraction to persons outside of himself and his primary ties, and a search for both conformity with peers and a desire to create an identity through the consumption of fashion. As Fromm argued, this quest for freedom and independence is part of the task of orienting and rooting himself to the world in order to find security in other ways than those which were characteristic of his preindividualistic existence.[25] And central to this process for Xiao Liang, and countless like him, is detaching himself from engulfment.

Perhaps most significantly of all, when having a very formal talk with him Xiao Liang expressed to his parents a "reactionary emotion." "The current education system is bad," reacted Xiao Liang, "because teachers and parents just want to know about school grades."[26] As if to drive home this search for freedom from engulfment he then tells his parents to stop interfering with matters relating to *his* schoolwork. Quite simply, by focusing almost obsessively on *his* school grades the parent's actions, in the eyes of the child, reduce him to a kind of grade-making machine, which is to *depersonalize* or "machinify" him. His reaction is to react – to *fan gan*. And despite attempting to placate Xiao Liang by trying to convince him that they do not engulf him in a straight-jacket made of school grades by arguing, contrary to facts, that it is "good enough" that he "works hard" and "learns knowledge," the mother, nevertheless, adds that he did not listen to his parents and *therefore* at the end of semester "his grades still declined." Like a bungee jump cord Xiao Liang's actions always bounce back onto a platform made of school grades.

Tao Hongkai, whose work he believes is as much centered around getting the parents to unwrap the cloak they have draped around their children as it is in getting the children to untie their "addiction" to the internet, offers in his courses and lectures to the parents his "three no's." He insists that parents say no to three emotionally driven disciplinary mechanisms when dealing with the child: "1) no control, 2) no worry, and 3) no fear."[27]

In order to enforce this message he accompanies this advice with a sentence he projects onto a large screen for them to reflect upon. It reads: "Its ok, let it go, everything will be just fine." When confronted with these "home truths" during Tao's lectures many parents do indeed let go of – *fa xie* – their pent up worry, fear, and anxiety over the child's success/failure by often crying uncontrollably. As a qualification, he then tells them that the more they employ these three no's the worse the situation will become. What he is essentially telling the parents is that there is a kind of "inverse reaction" (a *fan gan*) to the parent's engulfment, in that the now-teenage and resistant child is thinking "the more you control me the more I will resist you." And so when the parents use violence – whether symbolic violence through cursing or physical violence through beatings – in order to "teach" the child to stop going to the internet bar, the result is likely to be a child who runs off to the internet bar more angry and for longer periods of time. In short, the child learns to be aggressive by being treated directly with aggression.

In one session I observed, Tao Hongkai chastised the parents for constantly telling their child to "study hard, study hard." He followed this up by asking the children themselves if this educational measure actually works. Two quickly replied that no it does not, adding that in fact such pressure tends to have the opposite effect. Tao Hongkai then told the parents that their children do not want to be constantly criticized, controlled, and pressured about school and school grades. And so, according to his advice, the best method is to teach their children how to control themselves. Tao Hongkai basically sees his task as turning kids who he says are harming themselves (by playing "violent" video games) into kids who love and control themselves. This makes him somewhat of a Confucian master instilling self control into the young person by *convincing* them to be able to give up – for their parents, their education, their society, and their future – pleasure and desire for *unproductive leisure* and, instead, direct these feelings into pleasure and desire for *productive work*.[28] Otherwise, Tao Hongkai argues, the child will not have a "successful future" (read: get into university then find white-collar employment) for they will have no direction in life because they are not autonomous and independent enough – that is, not individual enough – to find their own *dao* (way; road). For example, while seemingly understanding the way Xiao Liang was playing online games at the internet bar as a way to search for happiness, the mother said "even" playing online did not appear to bring him out of his black hole and so it seemed to her that he had "lost interest in life." Perhaps it is more accurate to state that he had lost interest in *family and school life*, as not only did he express a desire to carve out a future life as a professional gamer but he also, despite being unwilling to communicate with his parents, communicated "ok" with other people. The problem was that Xiao Liang, during his *detachment* and *isolation* from the normal functioning of society (home and school), was funneling himself toward a one-way path: he was heading down *devaluation road*. That is, he was devaluing his future exchange value in relation to him being able to become a sellable commodity in the near future. Therefore his mother, justifiably, bemoaned the fact that this "excessive infatuation" with the computer had pigeon-holed him resulting in Xiao Liang's "sole strong-point" being his computer knowledge. This very real parental fear is premised on the fact that the saleability – or more worryingly un-saleability – of China's future labor-power is largely left to the private fears and worries of individual men and women living within (sometimes stem) nuclear families, who must now be acutely aware of their "market value" and how to sell themselves and their family members, using their individual abilities and *guanxi networks*, within a market where employers often have a strong preference for free-floating, flexible, unattached, multi-talented and ultimately disposable employees.[29]

What Tao Hongkai is arguing is that underpinning "internet addiction" is the engulfment of children by parents. Or what we could call in relation to serious cases the *creation of ontological dependency and the production of ontological insecurity*, which not only fails to make them autonomous subjects but, more problematically, thwarts them from developing socially appropriate self control mechanisms. And so when the son in Letter-28, whose mother "kept guard over him every day" says "Mum, I also want to study well, but I can't control myself," is it accurate to claim that his "failure" to control himself is *his* problem and his problem alone?[30] To prove his point that many parents are using excessive "love" in order to educate their child, Tao Hongkai often tells parents of one child who slept in the same bed with the mother until the age of twenty-one, asking them rhetorically "should you blame the kid, is this love?" Adding that, to him, this is a kind of "selfish love."[31] Coincidentally, listening to this particular lecture was a friend of Tao Hongkai's niece who had come in order to learn his method so that she could hopefully "save" her cousin from "internet addiction." On the second day of the trip she told me she was missing her mother terribly as her mother is like her best friend, adding that they even sleep in the same bed together. She was 17 years old at the time. It is this very entangled knot that Tao Hongkai has spent countless hours trying to untie. In short, many parents, under intense pressure from the normal functioning of society, are not producing autonomous subjects that are genuinely separate from their parents, and so behavior such as *excessive* internet use is itself partly the outcome of *excessive* love. Or as Fromm put it slightly differently: *domination* (of parents and other gamers) *and destruction* (of one's present and future) *is the outcome of a thwarted life.*

Material rewards and consuming love

In order to convince Xiao Liang to give priority to his education, the parents tried to use material rewards in order to "satisfy him, and to make him feel happier." Such a strategy or parental measure can be understood as contributing to both the tigerness within the child and as a pull factor drawing him into a world-of-consumption. Using a very similar strategy, Tao Ran, in an extremely unethical and unscientific use of medication, reportedly said: "We use these medicines to give them happiness, so they no longer need to go on the internet to be happy."[32] The strategy is to replace one form of consumption for another. While Tao Ran appears to be saying that happiness can be obtained by becoming dependent upon medication (i.e., replace one so-called addiction with another), Xiao Liang's parents seem to assume that rewarding their son with the latest fashions will work to buy him off by making him feel both satisfied and happier; and thus soften his rebellious psychology thereby hopefully obtaining his compliance.

First, instilling a materialistic reward-based value system upon him may indicate to him that people can be bought off with material rewards. Second, it is ironic that it is excessive consumption of online games that they are criticizing and punishing him for, yet, at the same time, they reward him for what they consider good behavior by offering him conspicuous consumption of the brands he "likes." So on the one hand they condemn his consumption, yet on the other hand they encourage it, thereby producing an array of mixed and contradictory messages – an entangled semiotic knot – by saying that they are both for and against conspicuous consumption.

On this point the exemplary example or ideal type of using material rewards in order to buy off the son is given in Letter-4. The brother writes that the son had "completely plunged into a crazy state, living a secluded life at home playing computer games."[33] Despite the son having a "sickly constitution" and being both "weak" and "frail" as a child, he was nevertheless said to have been "naturally endowed with intelligence" while also possessing a "natural gift for mathematics." He was initially praised for winning prizes at mathematics competitions, and there was great expectation (read: pressure) upon him to get into one of China's most prestigious universities. But then in the third year of middle school he started sneaking off to the internet bar to play *Counter Strike* (*CS*), slowly achieving the recognized status of "*CS* master" with dreams of becoming a professional player (and not a mathematician). In order to unplug his connection to *CS* and reconnect him to school, the parents used both the carrot and the stick. First they spoke "rationally" with him, and if this did not work then they would curse him, which simply made him angry. Two months before the most important event on the family calendar, the *gaokao* or college entrance examination, he escaped to the internet bar saying he did not want to sit the exam and instead wanted to "walk down his own path" and "choose his own future."[34]

In essence, he was searching for freedom and autonomy, and so his mastering of *CS* allowed him to orient and root himself to a new world and to find security in ways other than those which were characteristic of his preindividualistic existence, while, at the same time, giving him control and domination over his existence through perceived feelings of achievement and satisfaction. Subsequently his *gaokao* score was a disappointing 400, a mark which "astounded" everybody. Anxious for the child to have a bright future (*wang zi cheng long*) the parents persuaded him to retake the *gaokao*.[35] Upon promising to do so the parents borrowed 7000 yuan to buy a computer for the son. After re-sitting the *gaokao* he did not study hard because the family now had a computer at home, and so instead of doing his homework he would play games at home after school. In effect, the parents had bought the son the very device they claim is "poisoning" him as a material reward.

It is this very materialistic behavior that Tao Hongkai argues partly underpins both the parent's engulfing love and the child's own love of consuming online games. His critique of excessive materialism, wherein the parents use material goods and/or money to "bribe" the child into becoming a grade-making machine, is said to explain why "internet addiction" – itself a leisure activity which is part of a larger phenomenon we could call a *love-of-consumption* – is not only occurring in "problem" families exhibiting violence, divorce, death, poverty, etc, but is also prevalent in what appears to be "successful" families. That is, seemingly well-adjusted families who have money and a child who does well academically at school. His argument is that within families with the economic means to do so many parents – guided by the principle that "no sacrifice is too great to give my child all the things I didn't have" – are loving their children to death through excessive conspicuous consumption, therein producing young people who seek a *life-of-leisure* over a *life-of-work*. In his talks, which are repeatedly peppered with the same anecdotes, he uses a story to highlight this point.

Three children are asked who they love the most: 1) the first child says he loves his Dad the most as he has the most money; 2) the second child says she loves her Mum the most as her Mum buys her many things; and 3) the third child says he loves Grandma the most because he had bought him a new bag.

Tao then asks the parents rhetorically what is it that the child really loves, adding it is not principally the *person* themselves but rather the material goods that that person provides. He also asks if you can really blame the child for their love-of-things, as the parents use material goods for rewards for their children in order to "express their love." This is really to obtain their compliance to "study hard, study hard," but by being "loved" they are placed under an unsolicited obligation.[36] While chastising parents for using what we could call a *consuming love* in order to get their children to devote their existence to schoolwork, Tao Hongkai, however, downplays the fact that the parents themselves are part of the whole commercialization of Chinese society. From central government policies downwards, China is going through a consumer revolution, the beginning of which coincided with the birth, and subsequent socialization, of the post-80s children-of-the-market.[37] In effect, Tao Hongkai is attempting to contain this profound consumer revolution by convincing parents to implement the three no's (control/worry/fear) so as to use not counter-productive consuming and deathly love as parental socialization measures but rather love that is productive.

What is important, however, is the element of *choice*. For example, the parents were bought up in a world of severely limited choices (scarcity) while their children are increasingly encountering a world surrounded by excess choice (over supply) and an advertising machinery literally engulfing them with messages of *consume, baby, consume*.[38] The unleashing of parental consumer love is, itself, partly the effect of the CCP's own destructive political history, and so the desire to "give the child all the things I did not have" is surely an unintended consequence of the materially starved lifeworld of the *children of Mao*. As Farquhar has argued, the now grown-up children of Mao, living in a culture of excess, are gaining gratification and pleasure from indulging in the consumer-based pleasures that were either forbidden, unimaginable, or simply unavailable when they were young.[39] But for today's urban youth in particular, life is already electronically mediated wherein *social* life has become synonymous with *electronic* life and *consumer* life. For example, the results of a 2008 Asia-wide survey conducted by MTV found that China was the only country in the region where people claimed to have more friends online than off.[40] And so much of social life in the cities is now conducted through the *nowist* mediums of the internet and mobile phone that it is obvious to the young themselves that they do not really have a choice if they want to have a social life. As Renfei said, "the internet IS my world." And this penetration of the internet into the lifeworld of Chinese youth is happening at a very young age. According to a 2007 nationwide survey by Beijing-based *Answer Marketing Consulting Ltd*, nearly 40 percent of children aged 7–10 use the internet, while nearly 60 percent of those aged 11–13 are getting online.[41] That is, living a consumer-based social life electronically is almost a social necessity for China's urban youth. In many ways "social death" awaits those who have as yet failed to *turn on, boot up, and log in*.[42] As Huang He told Yang Yongxin just before he was subjected to electric-shock treatment: "I get online; at present how many young people don't actually get online?" *China Internet Network Information Center's* (CNNIC) biannual "Statistical Report on Internet Development in China" gives us a general answer to Huang He's rhetorical question.

First, it is important to note that in 2009, for example, 72.2 percent of internet users were living in cities and townships,[43] and that while the overall penetration rate of the internet throughout China was about 25 percent, in larger eastern urban centers and areas – Beijing, Shanghai, Tianjin, Guangdong, Zhejiang, Fujian – the penetration rate among the population ranges between 45 percent and 65 percent.[44]

In short, internet use has been a relatively urban phenomenon. Moreover, approximately 60 percent of the 380 million internet users in China at the end of 2009 were aged between 10 and 29, which basically means that about 228 million (the vast majority of which are living in urban areas) of the altogether 375 million or so aged between 10 and 29 years in China are getting online.[45] Likewise, in 2009 175 million, or 51.8 percent of all internet users, were teenagers, while 28.8 percent of this 380 million were students. In short, internet use has been a relatively youthful phenomenon (but this is changing fast as older people are migrating on mass to cyberspace). Acute penetration of the internet into the lifeworld of China's urban youth has been followed by the rapidly increasing penetration of internet accessible mobile phones. Mobile internet users increased from 117 million in December 2008 to 233 million in December of 2009.[46] Little wonder then that CNNIC's 24th Report points out that mobile internet use is not merely a useful portable electronic tool, but has become, more importantly, a symbol of fashion and an integral part of popular culture. After all, the ultimate goal of technology companies is to have their product transform from mere *use* into a daily *habit* (or what is sometimes called an "addiction").

Thus while parents are helping to instill into the child a love-of-consumption, the consumer-driven society they are all embedded into is, at the same time, doing all it can so as to make social life synonymous with both electronic life and consumer life.

The search to be somebody

Coupled with the production of a love-of-consumption is the way consuming online games attempt to satisfy the central component of tigerness: the desire to *be someone.* Incessant consumer activity among students, which is being funded by parents and grandparents, is partly driven by an individuation process within a consumer-based individualized society wherein people must first *recast themselves as commodities.*[47] If people like Xiao Liang are sought after (as a *"CS* master"), they are somebody, yet if they are not popular, they are simply nobody. Or as "Rachel" the wanna-be-famous character in the wildly popular American program *Glee* bluntly put it: "Nowadays being anonymous is worse than being poor."[48]

Interestingly, Swedish research company *Kairos Future* carried out a survey on the values of middle-class Chinese youth, and according to their data young middle-class Chinese youth are much more keen on becoming famous than their American or European counterparts. Likewise, such youth, who said their number one interest was surfing online, also told researchers that they are very concerned about fitting in, thinking it is important to "look good" and to be "in style." Moreover, 81 percent of participants said material possessions provide "meaning in life," while 60 percent said that certain brands are important for "expressing their identity"; a figure they claim is three times as high as comparative studies in Europe.[49] Yet beneath this search for respect, success, and fame, of which the "Super Girl" singing contest is the exemplary example, resides a desire to not dissolve into the grey, faceless mass of commodities that is the city. There is a collective dream of turning into a notable, noticed, respected, talked about and powerful commodity, a commodity that is able to stand out from the mass of tens of millions of other commodities, a commodity impossible to overlook, to deride, or to be dismissed.[50]

A good example of the desire to "worship" and love oneself through being someone is that of Huang He mentioned at the beginning. Huang He, recall, was bought to Yang Yongxin's clinic after he was drugged with sleeping pills by his parents. After receiving the now-banned electric-shock treatment we learn that while disappointed in real life he, nevertheless, had found dignity and honor in the internet world. Huang He said that "since my skills are relatively good then people on the internet called me *laoda* [big brother/Mr. Big/master]. Even though I was only 30 or 40 people's *laoda*, however, if you really compare the skills then it is above a few million people or a few tens of millions of people."[51] This important statement by Huang He, which is generally dismissed by those who are working against the tide of increasing internet-based social relations in China, informs us that the internet empowers young people like Huang He by providing them with a sense of self-perceived dignity, honor, self-confidence, respect, and power.

In this sense Huang He's love of gaming can be partly understood as an expectable response to not feeling respected in the "real" world, and not simply the result of some internal dysfunction, for through the display of his gaming skills he was able to obtain the respect of his fellow gamers. This aspect of the internet gaming experience is important for youth because these *existential trophies* are not available to them in a "real world" that places a premium upon academic-based success and achievement. And so online gaming, through the respect of fellow players, increased Huang He's self-confidence, self-esteem, and self-worth, just as mastering any academic or leisure pursuit provides. Therein Huang He, far from being the parasite opposed to "real" life the TV documentary made him out to be, is in fact attempting – albeit in a delegitimized space – to adhere to contemporary China's neo-liberal entrepreneur-based dominant social norm of *achieving individualized success* (i.e., "socialism with Chinese characteristics"). But parents, moral entrepreneurs, and medical crusaders believe that because this leisure activity, which is now a global professional sport, is taking place in an "unreal world" then these experiences, feelings, and emotions are themselves also not considered real.

And so in order to be someone, and thus socially alive, one must be online. And if one can do so looking stylish wearing the latest brand shoes and using the latest popular mobile phone then all the better for increasing one's (pop)cultural capital and perceived sense of meaning in life as a somebody. Under this system the parent's own choices are not simply of their own choosing, for in a system emphasizing consumption a child who is literally not up to play within the realms of fashion and popular culture is socially poor (i.e., abnormal). Filiarchy and filiarchical relations are, then, partly a logical outcome of this larger structural process of turning China into an urbanized consumer-based social system. Let us continue on this larger structural level so as to understand the family's relation to this consumer society and the way they are being forcibly nudged, and even deceived, to seek solutions to their problems in consumption.

Consumerism – happiness and satisfaction

> We must keep expanding domestic demand, especially consumption, and
> make sure we implement and improve policies to stimulate consumption.
>
> Premier Wen Jiabao[52]

While supplying the child with consumer goods that he "likes" – likes which
are themselves planned, created, and organized through the political process and
the market economy as ex-Premier Wen Jiabao's quotation informed us[53] – may
keep him or her socially alive this does not, however, offer any guarantee that it
will "satisfy him, and make him feel happier." The satisfaction of desire through
instant gratification and the assumed production of happiness actually runs contrary to the efficient functioning of a consumer-based society.

Zygmunt Bauman, in his analysis of the ways consumerism is becoming the
principal propelling and operating force of society, argues that the supreme value
of such a society – or more accurately the *promise* of consumerism – is the promise of a *happy life*. But not only does a consumerism promise happiness in *earthly
life*, which in China during the reform period has been expressed through the CCP
promising to deliver a "a well-off society" in exchange for power, authority, and
legitimacy,[54] but more specifically it promises *instant* and *perpetual* happiness in
the *here and now*. But while the "official transcripts" of a consumerist society – the
happy faces of celebrities standing next to the latest product to have reached
the market in the latest marketing campaign – associates happiness with the
gratification of desire, the actual functioning of the system itself, on the contrary,
does not reach for the satisfaction of desire but rather aims for an *ever-rising
volume and intensity of desires*.[55] Consumerism urges the consumer to look to
commodities for their satisfaction – e.g., Chinese consumer electronics firm
Skyworth using Taiwanese pop-star Jay Chou to sell their latest LED TVs under
the slogan "healthy wonderful life" – while, at the same time, urging the same
consumer to promptly use and speedily replace the very commodities that are
hoped to gratify them.

As Bauman succinctly put it: "New needs need new commodities; new commodities need new needs and desires."[56]

Far from being a machine patented to continually churn out an ever increasing
volume of happiness until the consumer is fully satisfied, consumerism is, on the
contrary, more like being on a "hedonic treadmill."[57] That is, the life of the consumer, during the production of their subjectivity, is a continual chase after an
ever allusive horizon: you run after a horizon called happiness and satisfaction
but the horizon moves as you run and so you never actually catch up with it.

In this way the precious resource "unobtainium" in the film *Avatar*, which the
US military-industrial machinery was extracting from the planet Pandora, can be
used as a term to understand the way the market continually functions so the consumer is forever non-satisfied, always left wanting more, for the newest and latest
fashion item – e.g., that Apple's newest invention is going to be the one to make
your life more "convenient" and "pleasurable." But fashion within the market

economy functions to quickly go "out" of fashion, and thus like the receding tide leaves one feeling slightly drained until the new tide of fashion rolls into the beach. So the premise of satisfaction or gratification in a consumer-led society is "unobtainium" because it is simply unobtainable. That is, one can never really obtain satisfaction and happiness through consumption.[58]

In a *China Daily* article called "Why are Chinese people so anxious?" analyzing why the *xiaokang* (well-off) society Deng Xiaoping promised has brought China's now materially well-off anxiety rather than happiness, the author captures the unobtainium trick of consumerism perfectly. First, the article points out that "ordinary Chinese" (i.e., those not yet fully "well-off") are anxious about personal relationships, housing, employment, and education.[59] Basically, economic stress conditions that have themselves created neologisms such as *Fangnu* (house slave), *Chenu* (car slave), and *Hainu* (children slave) to demonstrate the *pathology of normalcy* relating to having to "keep up" on the treadmill. Then the author points out the now well-off, who in theory should have transcended the economic anxiety relating to the high cost of housing and education, are even themselves anxious. "When they are affluent enough to purchase a flat, they want a villa," the author contends. "When they possess a car, they wish for a limousine. When they are millionaires, they dream about ten million yuan, but once they fulfill that, aren't they anxious about being billionaires?"[60]

It is precisely this *non*-satisfaction of desires, coupled with constantly renewed and reinforced "anxiety" that each successive attempt at reaching satisfaction has partly failed, that is the genuine cycle of the consumer-led economy. Quite simply, consumerism thrives as long as it can perpetually produce *non-satisfaction* in its members.[61] In this sense, the concluding summary of this article, wherein the anxiety pervading Chinese society is understood as an unavoidable process that the people in a transitional economy must experience while "developing," is greatly misguided. This yawning gap between promise and delivery, in that money and happiness are assumed to correlate, is not simply a transitional problem related to (under)development. On the contrary, to be constantly *dissatisfied*, *ungratified* and always wanting more is the necessary condition of a properly developed consumer-driven society; a society the CCP is trying its utmost to create. Understanding this helps us to partly understand why buying the latest brand products for Xiao Liang in the hope that this will "satisfy him and make him feel happier" ended up not solving the family war-machine. These material rewards for good behavior function to attempt to bring him back to a position he does not want to return to, which would take more than a new mobile phone to achieve.

Nevertheless, what begins as an effort to satisfy a perceived need must, in an ideal sense, ends up as a kind of obsession and compulsion, or what is known popularly as an addiction. As long as people are eagerly encouraged to seek solutions to problems (such as bribing your child with material rewards) and relief from pain, anxiety, and meaninglessness in shopping and consumption, then of course we are going to see consumer activities like online gaming congeal into a daily habit. In many ways online games are the perfect product for a consumer-led society because they are designed to continually leave a seemingly "happy" user ungratified with their non-perfect score. The mantra being: "next time I will get to that new level and acquire those new rewards." While the games themselves are designed to continually *suck in* the user, the internet bar owners are also doing all they can, usually through the market's enticing yet deceptive strategy of "the more you consume the cheaper it is," in order to prevent the consumer from leaving the building. It is in this sense that "internet addiction" can only be a product of China's reform and opening up policies. That is, were are dealing with a problem of development rather than with a problem of pathology

If the *search for happiness* is to go on, and on, and if the new promises to become *xiaokang* (well off) are to be continually alluring and enthralling, then promises already made must be cyclically broken, while hopes of fulfillment and satisfaction must be routinely frustrated. Each promise made, such that the new internet-accessible mobile phone will enhance your social life and happiness, must be at least exaggerated if not deceitful – i.e., the latest LED TV will not give you a "healthy wonderful life." Otherwise the zeal and intensity needed to keep the circulation of commodities going between coal mine, factory lines, shopping malls, and rubbish dumps may grind to a halt (and with it 8 percent annual GDP growth). In short, without a hedonic treadmill that keeps the consumer wanting to come back for more – through the production of non-satisfaction – consumer demand would run out of steam. It is the *excess* of the sum total of the promises made by companies, their marketing apparatuses, and CCP propaganda alike, that partly neutralizes the personal frustration and anxiety caused by the disjunction between promise and non-delivery (consumption and non-satisfaction) that allows the accumulation of frustrating experiences to stop short of draining confidence in the perceived effectiveness of the continual search-for-happiness.

What Bauman is arguing is that perpetual, prolonged, and daily consumption – actions which when applied to certain forms of behavior using a biomedical-based model are called "Shopaholism/ Nomophobia/Tanorexia/Internet Addiction"[62] – is not simply a kind of individual pathology, but is rather the behavior par excellence of a person living within a social system in which consumerism is the principal propelling and operating force of society. Consumer-based "addiction" (i.e., compulsive and repetitive productive activity) far from being an individual *deficiency* or *failure* is, in many ways, the supreme behavioral condition of consumerism. At the same time Bauman is also saying that the capacity of consumption to enhance human happiness is very limited, for consumerism actively promotes dissatisfaction, non-gratification, and insecurity; cyclical conditions that then themselves become the source of the ambivalent fear it promises to "cure" or nullify.[63]

Bauman is basically following Fromm's line of argument in that the process of consumption is essentially an alienating process. Fromm first points out that while we acquire goods with money, a process largely taken for granted, this process is, in reality, a very strange way of acquiring things. For while money represents labor and effort in an abstract form, it does not, however, necessarily represent *my* labor and *my* effort.[64] This is especially so for young people who are acquiring goods using money acquired through their parent's labor and effort in the form of a "reward" for their own valued labor and effort. Second,

Fromm asserts that while the act of consumption could or should be a productive and meaningful human experience, within a consumer-led society it is essentially premised upon the satisfaction of artificially stimulated fantasies that are planned, created, and organized through the market economy.[65] For example, while chatting to "Pheeb V" on QQ one afternoon about her life and work in Guangzhou she told me that Hong Kong is a "heaven for ladies" because it is a "shopping paradise," adding that she desired to travel to Holland to see the flowers because "all girls love flowers."

In addition, Fromm highlights an obvious yet often overlooked dimension in regard to the things we consume: we are engulfed by things whose origin, nature, and inner workings we know little about. We may know how to manipulate, use, and consume the technological devices and machines we rely on and replace with cyclical regularity, but we generally do not know on what principle they function except in the most vaguest and mystified way. In this sense we manipulate at the surface-level and consume things without any direct and concrete relatedness to the objects which we depend upon for our daily functioning. We are one-step-removed from the things which are meant to bring us happiness. But at the same time, company after company, through research and development, are expending the most excessive amounts of capital, energy and human resources to create new forms of pleasure and hopefully new "needs" or dependency in groups of consumers. This is the particular task of those working for online gaming companies, and so by creating artificially stimulated fantasies they hope to be able to create new needs in particular gaming cultures ("you need to check out this game, it is awesome"). And so the more dependent the consumer within that group feels in order to maintain membership then the more "successful" the result is for the company. The exemplary example being internet-accessible mobile phone companies, as such usage has become a "need" for tens of millions of youth who feel it is "necessary" to own such a device if they are to be socially and electronically alive.

In this sense, it is not so much the internet bar itself that is in direct war with school over the time and interest of the student, but more so the gaming companies. The internet bar is simply a social conduit between the producer and the consumer (as the monastery is a spiritual conduit between Earth and heaven). If young people like "Pheeb V" dared to articulate her concept of heaven we may surmise that she would envision the biggest department store in the world, displaying the latest brand products and gadgets, and herself having plenty of money with which to purchase them. She, who on Earth always plans to shop on her day off work but usually ends up sleeping because she is too exhausted, would wander, open-mouthed, in this paradise of commodities and technological devices, provided only that there are ever more and newer goods to consume.[66]

As surveys such the *Kairos Future's* survey cited earlier is indicating, Pheeb V is far from alone for this is the kind of consumer-dream for many Chinese youth today, a dream being fostered upon them by the twin processes of (globalized) State-lead market reforms and urbanization. Chinese urban residents are literally becoming boxed in by shopping malls, and so the cities are becoming dominated by two different kinds of architectural designs: the high-rise residential apartment and the commercial spaces. Add on to these processes the CCP's policy-driven drive to get the Chinese people to increase their consumption levels, and we have the creation of a consuming dream and love-for-consumption.

The subtlety of what we could call the semiotic architecture of the consumer society, in particular consumer product advertisements, was nicely captured during the *Focus Point* mentioned earlier where Tao Ran, Tao Hongkai, and other well-known public figures debated the legitimacy of the term "internet addiction." Just before the program shot to an advertisement break, Tao Ran said: "When there was no internet China was a gambling nation."[67] This comment was designed to show that there is a natural connection between gambling and gaming, and that in Chinese culture, and thus in Chinese people's "human nature," it is expected that some will be addicted to leisure pursuits whether it is gambling, gaming, opium, or alcohol. The viewer is then presented with an advertisement for rice wine. The following advertisement was also for another kind of expensive rice wine, while the third advertisement was by Samsung advertising their latest mobile phone (with Western actors). Ironically, these professionals are debating ways in which to best deal with a social problem called "internet addiction" (i.e., love-of-consumption), yet at the same time the program is bombarding viewers with images of alcohol and technology. Do they not see the contradiction involved and the way the market is playing an important part in producing this problem, which the show itself is implicated in?

With this structural shift from production to consumption we are likewise witnessing a shift in the relationship of a *person toward him/herself*. As Fromm said of American society during the 1950s–60s, this reorientation of the relationship to oneself involves a diminished orientation toward "hoarding" (e.g., saving income) and a subsequent increased *receptive* orientation, in which the purpose is to receive, to "drink in," to have something new to consume cyclically and so to live, as it were, with a continuously open mouth.[68] It is therefore noteworthy that the term for "tween" (those between approximately 10–13 years old) has been translated into Chinese as the "swallow generation."[69] In this sense online gaming is in no way a "deviant" act that is outside of social norms, for it is following the orders set down by the consumer society, and so like good consumers, young people – consumerism's target audience – should be ready and prepared at all times to receive, to "swallow," the latest games and other internet applications. So when Tao Hongkai says that internet addiction is not simply the child's fault (but more so the parent's and education system's), we should add that it is also consumerism's fault, for young people are not only in a battle with their parents but also with consumerism, which is spending vast amounts of resources in order to win their *heart and minds*.

Mo Zijin, an ex-chief creative officer in an advertisement company, captured the nature of the relationship between the consumer market and the family perfectly by likening a successful advertisement aimed at children to "a shining golden chain"; each ring of which has been crafted with careful planning and design. When the advertisement is beamed into the family via the television or internet, the chain "clicks tight and locks the children's hearts and their parents" purses."[70] Thus when we speak of the family war-machine between parents and child over the child's excessive consumption we must say that the consumer society is the third chain in this link.

Deathly love and productive love

Tao Hongkai is attempting to contain this profound consumer revolution by convincing parents to not use deathly love and consuming love as parental socialization measures, arguing that it results in the parents smothering their kids, thus producing dependent children who only love things. He says that if parents do not understand love then the child will not understand love. But what is meant by this notion of love?

Laing argues that genuine love, which is productive and not harmful to the construction of an autonomous identity, is based upon "understanding."[71] Laing says that what is important is knowing how a person is experiencing himself and the world. He argues that if one cannot understand the other, then one is hardly in a position to begin to love the other person in any effective way. That is, in an ideal world, young people like Xiao Liang should be able to say that he had a mother who loved him, *all of him*, and loved him just for being himself and not simply for what he could do (in an exam).[72]

Similarly, Fromm understands love, in an ideal sense, as a passionate affirmation of an "object."[73] Love for Fromm, however, is not simply an affect such as "falling in" love with someone or something such as the internet, but is an "active striving and inner relatedness, the aim of which is the happiness, growth, and freedom of its object."[74] As it is for Laing, Fromm argues that genuine love is rooted in productiveness and so what he calls *productive love* is, itself, rooted to or conditioned upon four particular elements: 1) care; 2) responsibility; 3) respect; and 4) knowledge.[75] Care and responsibility, so central to the productive parent–child relation, is for Fromm not simply based upon an affect or passion but rather signifies love as an *activity*. Love in this active sense therefore implies both care and responsibility for the other's physical existence but also, and more importantly, care and responsibility for the development and growth of *all* his/her human powers and potential. Productive love is, thus, a kind of phenomenological labor. In order to, as Laing says, love all of him, care and responsibility must be underpinned or driven by respect for, and knowledge of, the person whom one loves. Otherwise, Fromm argues, love may deteriorate into possessiveness and domination. Under such a condition, acts such as bribing the child with material goods in exchange for good grades and the expression of "natural" concern for the child may stem not from love *for* them, but rather from the love of domination and ownership he/she has *over* them. The child is therefore put into a kind of "golden cage" in which it can have everything – brand sports shoes, clothes, mobile phone, bicycle – provided the child does not want to leave the cage (and run off to the internet bar and play with "unreal" friends). That is, the parents may give the son everything they economically can as "no sacrifice is too great to give my child all the things I didn't have," except two things: the right to be free and independent. The potential result of this *dominating love* in which the child is placed under an unsolicited obligation of *goods-for-grades* is often, according to Fromm, a fear of love on the part of the child when he grows up because to him "love" implies being caught and blocked in his own quest for freedom.[76]

In addition, this respect for the person whom one loves is not, as the father in Letter-19 believes, based upon the production of fear so as to produce a "wolf that is not afraid of anything." But is, on the contrary, based upon the active ability of knowing how the beloved person is experiencing him/herself and the world, which implies being cognizant of his/her individuality and uniqueness.[77]

In order to really know the transforming child Tao Hongkai's colleague Fu Xueyu tells parents that they need to pay attention to the kinds of online games their children are playing.[78] Not in order to encourage them to play games but in order to educate themselves about what their child is actually doing online. In addition, teacher Fu also asks parents to try and experience the child's thoughts and to face, and hopefully solve, the child's problems together with the child. But she warns parents to not simply pretend to like everything the child likes, so that one ends up being like a friend to the child (as opposed to a parent), for this will simply continue engulfment. Amazingly, many parents simply do not know what their children are doing online, and so when I have asked a parent what games their children are playing, they have usually replied that they did not know. This is important, as it is through understanding what exactly the child is doing online that will help to see how they are feeling and what games and applications they are using to deal with their pressures. Chatting on QQ is not the same activity as playing *World of Warcraft*, just as playing *Perfect World* is not the same activity as watching a movie, for all are driven by differing existential and emotional needs.[79]

However, for the grade-obsessed parent "love" is a misdirected love and may produce more harm than good. Their love is not principally based upon understanding and accepting their child for who he/she is (i.e., productive love), but is a restricted and conditional love that tends to only function, in the eyes of the child at least, if it is closely connected to schoolwork and school grades.

Tao Hongkai, unknowingly echoing Laing and Fromm, attempts to get parents to realign this misdirected love by getting them to focus upon the Chinese character for "knowledge."[80] He separates the character into its component parts: know + understand. He talks about parents crying over their child's issues with school because they "love" the child so much. This crying, he says, comes about after they have scolded the child and then perhaps hit the child, which they do out of apparent love for the child. He tells the parents that knowledge, if used properly, can result in real quality education (*suzhi jiaoyu*); or what Fromm called productive love. In order to highlight their excessive misguided love, or love *out-of-balance*, he presents them with a power-point slide that reads:

家长对孩子的六大教育误区 (Six great misunderstandings in parental education towards the child)

1）重玩轻育 (heavy emphasis on education over play/leisure)

2）重养轻育 (heavy emphasis on education over nurturing)

3）重智轻德 (heavy emphasis on intelligence over morals)

4）过度关爱 (excessive love)

5）过度保护 (excessive protection)

6）过度期望 (excessive expectations)[81]

These parental measures, which are part of a larger *culture of excess* and *intensification-of-life* permeating contemporary China, basically encompass the central components of engulfing love: excessive and intensive attention toward a) education, b) information, c) protection, and d) expectations. But employing the term "engulfing love" is itself somewhat misleading because this engulfment is as much driven by the emotion fear as it is by a misdirected love. To understand how love and fear are two sides of the same coin we can cite an extreme case as a symbolic example.

In February of 2010 a picture circulated around the world causing moral indignation.[82] The picture shows a 2-year-old toddler chained to a lamp post outside a shopping center during a freezing Beijing winter day. While most were quick to condemn the father for being cruel and inhumane, an alternative picture slowly emerged that rationalized the father's actions. The son was apparently chained to a post not in order to prevent him from running away, as the motorcycle taxi rider father could not afford to pay for childcare, but rather to prevent others from abducting him.[83] The father claimed that his daughter was abducted from the same spot two weeks ago, while he was working and she was playing with her young brother. He had not seen her since.[84] A story that began about cruel parenting ended up highlighting a growing problem in China: the cruel abduction of young children by criminal gangs. Nevertheless, the father claims he chained up the boy out of *love* for the child because he *feared* losing him. In a symbolic way, "normal" parents are *chaining* their children to schoolwork out of love for the child and, at the same time, out of fear that the child's successful future may never be realized.

Depersonalization

Coupled to engulfment, and the other dominant push factor relating to the family war-machine, is the way this parental obsession with schoolwork produces what we can call depersonalization. Not only do some parents depersonalize their child by turning him/her into a grade-making machine, which is itself a potential producer of *fan gan*, but understanding depersonalization also helps us to understand the nature of this problem. In brief, depersonalization is underpinned or driven by the parents placing emphasis on exchange value over use value when evaluating the child's *qualities*. Instead of simply laying the blame of depersonalization at the feet of parents, however, we must understand that this process is itself a consequence of the rise of the market orientation character in which young people have to recast themselves as commodities – and parents have to do all in their power to have this come to fruition.

While the differing forms and intensity of engulfment described earlier can be understood as a socially and structurally-produced interpersonal process driven by an array of intrapersonal emotions, such as love and fear, aimed at preventing the often only-child from drowning academically within a hypercompetitive education system, this very process, at the same time, engenders on both sides another non-productive and emotionally harmful affect. Coupled with engulfment is the process of depersonalization that itself underpins the break down of communication between parent(s) and child.

One of the ways in which ontological insecurity arises is through depersonalization. According to the *WHO* depersonalization is: "A rare disorder in which the patient complains spontaneously that his or her mental activity, body, and surroundings are changed in their quality, so as to be unreal, remote, or automatized."[85] According to Laing, however, depersonalization is not simply an *intra*personal, or even rare, phenomenon, but is rather based upon *inter*personal relations functioning as a way of dealing with another person who, in their eyes has become, for example, too troublesome and/or disturbing. That is, a person no longer allows oneself to be responsive to the thoughts and feelings of the other, and as a result is prepared to treat him or her as though he or she had no feelings. By de-personalizing the other, by stripping them of *personal* feelings, one is, in effect, turning the other to stone.[86] This aspect of depersonalization we can observe when children turn their parents to stone by refusing to communicate with them about their schoolwork, their leisure activities, and their whole lifeworld in general.

For example, in Letter-8 the parents say that when "exasperated" with the child they sometimes beat him, the result of which was him hitting them back. In addition he had broken three doors while giving vent to (*fa xie*) his "dissatisfaction." While living at boarding school the son would sneak away to the internet bar. Upon discovering this, the parents told him to stop and "requested" he rectify his attitude by trying hard to correct his existing "deficiencies." In response, the son, like most of the sons, either did not say anything at all or would have a "temper tantrum." These two depersonalizing strategies – silence and violence – are ways in which the son can shut the door on the parents by building a great wall around himself. But we also see parents "closing down" the relationship with their children, acts which, in themselves, end up being one of the contributing factors relating to the son's deviance in general and online gaming in particular.

For example, Letter-11 describes the father, an apparently corrupt and gambling-loving education administrator, divorcing his second wife and marrying his third wife. Communication with the first wife, the "internet addict's" mother, had closed down completely. After problems with schooling, including the father using his professional connections to get someone else to sit the son's middle and high school diploma exams, the father then shut down communication with the son refusing not only to talk to him but also refusing to allow the son to live with the father. Basically the son went back to his father's house after the school semester ended and after arriving no one at home responded or spoke to him, and he was not offered food. This was understood as a way to get the son to leave. This depersonalization and paternal rejection, according to the mother, caused the son great pain and suffering. The son had subsequently taken up gambling online and idolized the opium den owning gangster from Republican-era Shanghai Du Yuesheng and his partner-in-crime Huang Jinrong, telling his mother one day: "Nowadays good people can't live."[87] This had left the mother feeling "psychotic" and "helpless" because she could not change the family, the school, and society that she said had all caused the son harm.

Or we can mention the son in Letter-17 whose now separated parents (both government employees) felt "annoyed" by the son's questions when he was growing up and so would just "carelessly reply" to him. In addition to this depersonalization, they were both very busy working and trying to advance their careers when the son was young and so they communicated very little with him. Since the son started gaming for five hours a day at university the parents attempted to communicate with him, but to no avail. "Now we want to talk to him," the mother said regretfully, "but he doesn't want to talk to us, this is our punishment [for depersonalizing and neglecting him]."[88] Likewise, we can refer back to the father in Letter-6 earlier who had "always been indifferent to the son's education," and after the parents divorced he extended this indifference to include the son's whole lifeworld by basically giving up on the son altogether. Should it then be unexpected to find that his personality became "very introverted" and he would often go out at night and not return home to the mother? How is a son who has been abandoned by his father meant to act? Not "normally," that is for sure.

The fact is depersonalization, or more accurately, partial depersonalization, is a universal phenomenon because most interpersonal relationships are based upon some degree of depersonalization.[89] In public space in China (which has also become the marketplace) partial depersonalization is ubiquitous and can be seen where people simply act like the other – usually someone attempting to market or sell something on the street – is simply invisible.

However, it is when depersonalization becomes a threat to one's self that existential dangers arise. For example, when a person experiences the other as deadening and impoverishing as they do not simply want to turn you into stone but, rather, into a grade-making machine. Instead of finding oneself enlivened and the sense of one's own being enhanced by the other, one may, on the other hand, experience the other as a threat to his or her capacity to act autonomously.[90] By turning their child into a grade-making machine, by depleting him of his personal aliveness, the child, in turn, experiences the parents as treating him like a piece of machinery because they want to reduce the child – impoverish him – to a kind of factory that spits out school grades. The child's "health" is often not based upon his happiness and satisfaction with *life*, but rather on whether he is studying hard or not; which, in turn, is the parent's threshold for their own perceived happiness.

Likewise, the mother in Letter-16 writes that in "teaching" the child to stop being "crazily enthralled" with Formula One racing she would use the carrot and stick method, which often resulted in her hitting the son during an argument. Unsurprisingly neither the carrot nor the stick had any positive effect. More importantly, the father was basically absent from the son's life as he had been working away from home for a long period of time. Significantly, the son would *"denounce the teachers' educational methods as improper and the education system as unreasonable."*[91] However, the mother simply put such comments down to "bickering unreasonably." What was reasonable for the mother was sending the son to a private school in another city so he could retake the third year of middle school. The mother subsequently praised the son because he obtained the top grade in his chemistry class, while each major subject grade "made clear progress." The mother's "heart was very gratified" because the son would come home every month and communicate with her on matters concerning teachers, and classmates, even taking the initiative to give an account of "every subject's exam grade." What made her believe that the son had become more "thoughtful" (i.e., had left his crazy enthrallment with F1 behind) was when he told her that before an exam he went with classmates to the toilet to read until late into the night. In essence, when the son showed a passion for F1 it was attributed to him being "crazily enthralled," yet when he began to study excessively, to the point of doing so inside a toilet, then this was attributed to his "thoughtfulness" and to him "making clear progress." In an ideal situation, which would make the mother's heart feel most gratified, would be her son becoming "addicted" to school and school grades. This would eliminate the son "bickering unreasonably" about the oppressive state of the education system and his mother's obsession with it.

In response to being turned into a grade-making machine the child's strategy may be to reject this person who is experienced as a threat to his self and his autonomy, therein robbing the person of their power to machinify him and so undercutting the risk to his aliveness. Adolescents who are rejecting school – killing it – and therein making their parents life a kind of living hell, is understandable only if we fully comprehend their relations to their parents, their school, their peers, and the world of consumerism in which they are embedded. Within the home we find an entangled knot of interpersonal problems, of which a misdirected love for, and fear of, the child's schooling looms ever-present. Increased internet use is partly a response and *reaction* to these interpersonal relations – important push factors. So if a child is depersonalizing their parents – ignoring them, arguing with them, destroying them, and going against them – it may be because they themselves feel depersonalized by the parents trying to *reduce* them to an *exchange value*. As Laing put it "the man who is frightened of his own subjectivity being swamped, impinged upon, or congealed by the other is frequently to be found attempting to swamp, to impinge upon, or to kill the other person's subjectivity."[92]

The resulting strategy may be to kill the thing the parents most desire – good school grades – and then continue, or even accelerate, the activity they fear the most – internet gaming. This then makes it primarily an issue of *rebellion* and not one of mental illness. This defensive strategy of rejecting both their parents and school comes *after* the offensive strategies of both school and parents. It is a *response* to a violent imposition upon him, wherein, as Renfei tells us, exam preparation is experienced as a kind of imprisonment. And so to claim his problem is because he is addicted to the internet fails to take into account the whole situational context that brought about the gaming, and in particular increased gaming, in the first place. Quite simply, excessive online gaming is not merely about the correlation between individual and technology (i.e., individual connects to internet = internet makes individual addicted/pathological), but more stems from the individual's *inter*personal relations to significant others and the structural conditions of his/her existence.

Depersonalization may be reflected through interpersonal relations but for understanding the engine of depersonalization I suggest we refer back to that important distinction between use value and exchange value. As mentioned, today's graduates must first recast themselves as commodities. That is, they must market themselves as products capable of catching attention and attracting demand and customers.[93] This transformed relationship to oneself, itself a product of China's economic transformation, has resulted in the emergence of the "marketing orientation."[94] Fromm invented the marketing orientation to indicate that people living within a consumer society experience themselves as a thing to be employed successfully on the market. Because his/her sense of value greatly depends on his/her success, one's sense of self does not principally stem from his/her activity as a loving and thinking individual, from his/her *human qualities* as a human *being*, but rather from his/her socio-economic role as a human *doing*.[95] Within this system a person's sense of their own value largely depends on factors extraneous to oneself, in particular on the fickle judgment of the market, which decides upon a person's exchange value as it decides about the value of commodities. Like all commodities that cannot be sold profitably on the market, he/she is considered worthless as far as his exchange value is concerned, despite the fact that his/her *use value* may be considerable. And so if there is no use for the qualities a person offers, then, as far as the market is concerned, he/she has none, and therefore becomes just as an un-saleable commodity (i.e., underemployed) and a "nobody."[96]

The child becoming an un-saleable commodity is the great fear of parents whose child loses interest in school, while, simultaneously, gaining interest in the internet and its multiple applications and pleasures. They are afraid that their child will not be able to be sold profitably on the market, that is, that they will have no exchange value because he/she (and not the family) has failed to make it to university. This is why Tao Hongkai's greatest exemplary model is the *failed* student, who, through self control and ambition, passes through the black-hole of excessive internet use and, to the great relief of parents, makes it to university.

Yet this transformation of consumers into commodities does not begin upon graduation, because upon graduation the market-oriented character must "hit the ground running." Rather, as shown earlier, this transformation often begins at kindergarten with acts such as mock graduation ceremonies, in which hurried children are being forced to play "miniature adults" before they are physically, psychologically, and/or socially prepared to do so. In this sense he must first be a success with passing school exams before he can sell himself on the market, and so if he fails in the exams, or in school more generally, then it is *his* failure – but the family's tragedy. Children and parents quickly learn that the most prized exchange value is the school grade in learning to become a commodity and market oriented. Conversely, through discipline and punishment, they learn what happens when one does not quantitatively measure up. "Because my school grades were no good," the "slow" son in Letter-24 lamented, "then this meet with corporal punishment from my parents and cursing abuse from my teachers." In short, what we are witnessing is the child who is evaluated not for his use value, his/her usefulness, beauty, character, etc, but, on the contrary, more so for his exchange value, that of school grades.

Specifically, the school grade, in particular the *gaokao* grade, is said to be an indicator of the future exchange value of the child, and so his/her use value is *secondary* to his exchange value (on the marketplace). And in this way of experiencing things sight of what goes on concretely is lost. For example, the child's concrete experience of school and life is *subsumed* under the weight of school grades. The child, for his/her part, experiences this as both the quantification and abstraction (i.e., depersonalization) of their lifeworld by their parents and school (and to a lesser extent society as a whole).

Through the letters we can observe how the parents valuate the "quality" of the child (*goodness* vs. *badness*) against the "quantity" of the school grading system, therein showing us that the war-machine within the family is partly one between quality (use value) and quantity (exchange value). For example, when the child is seen as a "good" boy because he got 93 percent in his exam, thus putting him 3rd in the class and 5th in his year, then we are no longer speaking of his certain human qualities but refer to him as an abstraction whose value is expressed in a quantitative figure. It is this distinction between use value and exchange value that can be said to underpin depersonalization.

This depersonalization, in turn, denies or partly *dissolves* the rich and concrete personal characteristics and qualities of the child, for the richness and concreteness of human life is expressed in the abstract formula of an educational function. The dissolution of a concrete or qualitative frame of reference in the process of living means that the child does not experience oneself – all of oneself – as the center of his/her world and so, in a way, becomes estranged from oneself. They may not be the principal creator of their own acts, rather their acts and their consequences may have largely become their parents and the education systems, who they have often obeyed because at home they receive material rewards for doing so and at school receives punishment for not doing so. As one student told Tao Ran and Tao Hongkai on the *Focus Point* program:

> Beginning from the start of primary school our parents have already told us that everything you do is for study and everything is for grades. No matter if you do things well everyone just wants to know what your grades are like, and if your grades are good then everything is ok.

Another student in the audience then added that parents have no way to communicate with their kids because parents are extremely busy at work and their own social pressure is great. And because of these socio-economic factors then, according to this student, parents just became concerned about the child's grades.

Under this sense of estrangement from one's concrete human qualities we can understand the powerful attraction of the internet. The people one encounters and socializes with in cyberspace is partly based upon a desire to overcome this dissolution of any concrete frame of reference in the process of living out of balance, for peers do not depersonalize them, rather they relate to them through an emphasis on the richness and concreteness of human qualities. This qualitative function is nicely captured by netizen Sun Lingsheng who said

> I love the internet because you have complete freedom to talk with people all over the world … online, what you think and feel is more important than who you are or where you're from. In the outside world, there are so many walls between people – class walls, cultural walls, and national walls. But the Web is like a ladder that helps us climb the walls, and maybe someday melt them.[97]

To counter this estrangement of not experiencing themselves as the center and creator of their world, because, for example, they have been forced to see their classmates as rivals and thus as threats, then they enter the *World of Warcraft* or the *Perfect World*. For it is here, and nowhere else, where they can experience themselves as the center – and master – of their world. That is, they are in the control tower rather than on the ground being controlled. This attraction to being a master of one's universe is seen in the way online games promote themselves. In order to attract new players the online game "*Wulin 2,*" for example, described their game in the following way: "It brings the players to the unpredictable world of *Wulin* where they can *do what ever they like*, while trying their best to *become a hero.*"[98] And so gaming, whereby the individual's own acts are ruled by him, or perceived to be ruled by him, must be partly understood as a remedy in which he attempts to overcome estrangement, that is, a life that is not his own.

Summary of push factors: unleashing the tiger and the mouse

Through filiarchy, engulfment and depersonalization we observe the son, as the center of the family nexus, being chained up in a deathly love wherein he is rewarded with material goods, authority, and power if he is willing to transform himself into a grade-making machine. From the parent's perspective it is hoped that giving the child everything they didn't have will, in this way, be enough of a sacrifice to ensure the child can successfully pass the college entrance exam (*gaokao*), make it to university and, finally, become a saleable commodity in the highly competitive marketplace. While sacrificing themselves in this way for their child's success they may, in practice, be actually creating a child who is a tiger at home and a mouse outside – i.e., an ontologically insecure person who desires to be a *laoda* (master) in cyberspace. The parents seem to assume that the child will *naturally* want to study ferociously by drinking in, or swallowing, schoolwork with a continuously open mouth in the *same way as everybody else*. But the parent's wishes are in competition with the consumer society which is doing its upmost, using a shining golden chain, to lock-in the hearts and minds of the children-of-the-market so as produce a me generation that is prepared to receive, to drink in, and to swallow the latest consumer fashions with cyclic regularity and intensity. The so-called internet addiction phenomenon pivots around this competition for the hearts and minds of this individualizing adolescent.

As the parents see the child drift over to the *dark side* of the internet, which is to see their tear-stained sacrifices sink down the drain, the best they can do to arrest this process is by scolding, beating, boarding up, or locking away the child. This unleashes both the tiger *and* the mouse within the child, who is prepared to fight to detach himself from having to swallow schoolwork, whose bitter taste he dislikes, in order that he can attach himself to a pleasurable activity where he can continuously drink in the sweet taste of success while being able to avoid the bitter taste of failure. In this sense, we could say the mouse stems from a feeling of being threatened by an engulfing and depersonalizing outside world, wherein they feel *their* autonomy is being thwarted, curtailed and suppressed by the constant pressures relating to school. The tiger, on the other hand, stems from a desire for a sense of power and domination over others, which has been fostered both within the filiarchal home and through the hyper-competitive education system and the consumer society, with the underlying mechanism being the struggle for freedom and independence. As Fromm informs us, these two energies – the withdrawal from the "normal" world and the desire for domination over others – are part of the same process. That is, the inflation of oneself through a desire for domination, expressed through intense and competitive online gaming, may itself be rooted in the insufferableness of individual failure and powerlessness – within a system that over-values individualized achievement. And so the ontologically insecure person can *escape* these feelings of failure, isolation, and powerlessness by attempting to dominate others or even oneself. A process which can be understood as an attempt to save oneself from being swallowed by a pathology of normalcy. To repeat again, *socially problematic internet use is often the outcome of a thwarted life*. Or to put it another way: intensive internet use cannot simply be reduced to the perceived failings of the individual because this negates the particular social and structural conditions from which such use stems.

Xiao Kang – becoming a *laoda*

While we have dealt extensively with the "push" factors relating to the migration toward cyberspace and intensive gaming in particular, we can use Xiao Kang's letter provided later as an ideal type in which to understand more completely the important "pull" factors underpinning intensive internet use. Through Xiao Kang's narrative we can observe the tigerness at work, which I have framed within the desire of becoming a *laoda* (big brother/master), as well as the very powerful pull factors at work within online games. As we will see, through gaming Xiao Kang was able to feel like a pseudo-hero, an existential experience which provided him with infinite pleasure and was centered around the *quest for excitement* Elias and Dunning said underpinned leisure activities. I have divided this letter into five parts as a way in which to analyze the process wherein online gaming – vis-à-vis his lifeworld – unleashed the tiger within him. Part One shows him *becoming estranged* from his lifeworld, which should be understood as the catalyst that, so to speak, let the tiger out of the cage. Part Two describes him *becoming intoxicated* with gaming, while Part Three shows him *becoming angry* after fighting with his parents over his exam failure, and so produced *fan gan* and contributed to him increasing and intensifying his gaming. Part Four highlights him, at least within his own eyes, *becoming an idol* to others through his gaming. And Part Five analyzes the apex of his tigerness wherein he and his fellow gamers experienced *becoming the world's savior*.

In short, Xiao Kang, a graduate from Jiaotong University in Xi'an, wrote to Tao Hongkai in order to tell his story of "conquering" his *enthrallment* to the internet.[99] Xiao Kang, who subsequently became a volunteer for Tao Hongkai, hoped to inspire those currently *indulged* in the virtual world of online games by stirring them to "conquer the internet and conquer themselves."

Part one – becoming estranged

Upon entering Jiaotong University I was full hope in the future, and had life planned out. A famous school and a famous major made my friends praise me endlessly. More so, my family thought I had already entered into a magnificent future. I did not have the slightest anxiety.

However, at university I encountered students from poor areas whose gaokao grade was 50–60 points higher than mine. Their diligence gave me a very big shock. Their assiduous study was something I did not even want to think about, for compared to them I was simply like the pampered son of the wealthy family. Listening to them made me feel unprecedented pressure. From this day on my competition was going to be with those who could put all their energy into studying. I could not be like them and put everything into my studies.

My worry came true. These classmates did not have any kind of life outside of school. Only after the light in the self-study room had gone out did you see them in the dorm. I would easily get fed up reading in the self-study room, and so I had no choice but to go outside campus for a walk by myself. Slowly I started to experience loneliness, and discovered that I had absolutely nothing to talk about with the classmates that surrounded me. I could not even find anyone to go hiking with in the weekend. In their eyes I had become a different species.

After exams I idled about, unable to find a higher purpose. I couldn't be like them and study hard every single day; that was just too tiring. In my eyes, they were wasting their life. They were just a group of simpletons that didn't understand life. My relationship with these classmates became distant, and so I became arrogant and frivolous. From then on I did not go into the self-study room and began cutting school.

In order to understand Xiao Kang's "enthrallment" in online games we need to first contextualize his social existence. What we see is Beijing-raised Xiao Kang becoming shocked and worried after learning first-hand the nature of his "competitors" at university, whom through hardship, industriousness, diligence, and fierce competition had managed to locate the route out of the village and into a prestigious university. The "unprecedented pressure" he felt in contrast to these incredibly driven students was underpinned by the quick realization that he could not compete with them. The fact that from the outset he conceptualizes them as competitors tells us much about the Xiao Kang's pre-university socialization. For example, as "Wang Gang" told a reporter while confined to Tao Ran's military hospital:

> Perhaps the problem is that the whole society gives us too much pressure. Pressure at home and school is too much. All our parents say is 'achieve, achieve, achieve.' My classmates and I don't have any brothers and sisters, and so I hope that we are able to become friends, but instead it is like we are rivals. Like this, there is only one place where you can escape these problems and make friends, and that place is the internet.[100]

Worse than not being able to compete with these rivals was Xiao Kang not being able to bond with them. While they, as a group, put everything into their studies Xiao Kang, however, desired to have what he called a "life." This meant going outside the campus for walks and hiking, activities he felt he had "no choice" but to do alone. As a result he experienced loneliness, which was further compounded by the perception that he could not communicate with these classmates/rivals as, in his eyes, they had absolutely nothing to talk about. While in their eyes they perceived him as being a different kind of species (the pampered son of a wealthy family). From the outset of his migration to Shanghai he is *estranged* from those closest to him, an estrangement made all the deeper by his initial positive sense of his place in the world and the bright future he perceived lay in front of him.

Following Laing, we can say that what is pertinent to understanding Xiao Kang's situation, and more importantly his participation and non-participation in it, is how a) he perceives and acts toward the others, b) how they perceive and act toward him, c) how he perceives them as perceiving him, and d) how they perceive him as perceiving them.[101] It is this situation that is central to Xiao Kang's narrative. In this way, his perception toward himself as being unable to find a "higher purpose" is in response to his perception of them of having this higher purpose (i.e., achieve, achieve, achieve), a force which allows them to "study hard every single day" together in the self-study room. His perception of them, once filtered through his deflating pride, becomes one of self-preservation in which he first depersonalizes them by thinking they are "wasting their life," and then, despite their *gaokao* grade being significantly higher than his, he taps into the common urban prejudice toward rural citizens by calling them "simpletons" who do not "understand life" (i.e., modern urban living). This self-preservation falsely inflates his arrogance while, at the same time, builds a kind of inter-personal moat between him and them thereby creating a relationship premised upon distance. He thus feels alone, estranged, and alienated. In short, being a tiger at home (the perceived pampered son of a wealthy family) had accelerated his transformation into a mouse in the real world.

Part two – becoming intoxicated

As for encouragement, I had my computer. Everyone marveled at this cher-ished thing, because this was the first time many had used a computer. In high school my family bought a computer, but that was for my older brother to use for study. Now this computer completely belonged to me, and because I didn't have other people's restrictions I could do on it any-thing I wanted. I proudly taught others how to use the computer, and from the expression in their eyes I could see envy, even to the point of jealously, and I felt an unparalleled satisfaction. Classmates were able to use my computer at any time. I was therefore very happy.

From the first day I was in possession of the computer I installed the latest games. Every day I was intoxicated with them, and I delighted in the games and never got tired of them. Through the games I was best at it was as if I had found the easiest kind of method for gaining respect. This, compared to study, was much easier and more relaxing. Every time I broke my own record I was able to experience the joy of achieving. Nearly every class-mate who returned from self-study would say: "did you reach the level"? How did you pass it?" I became the whole dorm's focus, and it seemed that every person was looking forward to hearing about my affairs, and I had to con-tinuously challenge a new record, for only then could I continue to obtain their recognition. My reputation as a good gamer got bigger and bigger, to the extent that students from other departments would come to my dorm and watch me play. I always took delight in telling them how to plan the character's death, how to design rational tactics, and how to acquire treasure in the game.

Only through understanding Xiao Kang's estrangement from those around him and his feelings of loneliness and isolation is it logical and rational that the computer quickly becomes a "cherished" object he utilizes for encouragement. His estrange-ment is narrowed by the sense of belonging he gains through *possessing* the computer, a possession that is heightened by the new-found realization that there are no paren-tal restrictions over his use of it. It is his and his alone, and he can do whatever he likes on it. In a more general sense, it is this new found freedom students gain from parental controls (whether at boarding school or university) that is an important contributing factor in excessive online gaming, for some of the engulfing knots are untied for the first time in their life. Their subsequent "enthrallment" is therefore partly in response to them being severely restricted (thwarted) from enjoying themselves prior to university. Through his ownership over and competence on the computer Xiao Kang's sense of aloneness evaporated as he became a *somebody* in the eyes of others. He felt "unparalleled satisfaction" from perceiving what he thought was envy and jealously toward his computer skills, while he also gained happiness from their appreciation toward him for teaching them important computer skills that the university was failing to do. As O'Conner and Rosenblood argued, the existential need for *affiliation* is generally believed to motivate individuals to seek out social contact.[102]

Xiao Kang found, in contrast to his difficulties in the real world, and study in particular, that obtaining a sense of respect through online gaming was both much easier and more relaxing. This is partly why online gaming is so dangerous to study and the education system, for it is simply much easier, more relaxing, and more pleasurable as it is premised upon continuous feelings of gratification in the *here* and *now*. Thus Xiao Kang was able to easily experience the "joy of achieving." However misleading and however transitory, this sense of achievement he experienced through online gaming he could not experience in relation to school. Can we therefore call a person who desires a sense of achievement mentally disordered, for is this not one of the values and goals of the education system – to produce winners and the feeling of being a winner? Can we blame youth, who are told that achieve, achieve, achieve is the ultimate goal, for seeking out this end?

Tao Ran's psychologist, Xu Leiting, has said "internet addicts" "*escape* to the virtual world to *seek* achievements, importance, and satisfaction, or a sense of belonging."[103] Not only does such a statement negate the possibility that the "internet addict" has an internal dysfunction, for there is nothing internally dysfunctional about seeking achievements, importance, satisfaction, and belonging as these are highly desirable social values. But this also negates the social context, for if a person is unable to find a sense of achievement, importance, satisfaction and belonging in the real world, then is it not rational that they would seek it in the virtual world? The problem lies in placing a value judgment on the "real world" while taking it for granted as something inherently good, yet, at the same time, devaluing the same process conducted online. Here, the so-called internet addict is condemned because they cut themselves off from the society-of-work and, instead, escape into what they believe is a world of simulacrum and fantasy. And while "attached" there they are thought to produce nothing real, and because they are being non-productive then they are said to be wasting their time.[104] But how can someone *escape* in order to *seek*, for escape means to go into hiding while to seek means to advance toward a stated goal? As already highlighted, they are not simply escaping by hiding or taking refuge; rather they are advancing in another direction.

Xiao Kang lapped up being the focus of other's attention (i.e., like being at home), which in turn drove him toward continuously challenging himself by beating his own record, for he perceived this fickle recognition and respect to be premised upon continuous success. In order to continue to *be someone* – remember that no one wanted to go anywhere with him before – he felt like he needed to continue to perform for his "fans." As his reputation grew bigger so too did his inflated sense of himself as a *laoda* and as someone individually special. In taking delight in showing others how to plan, strategize, and design rational and logic-based tactics he was not only doing applied science but he was also becoming more and more like the "simpletons" he used to despise. He was becoming a diligent, industrious, and fierce competitor. The problem was he was playing the wrong game.

Part three – becoming angry

> As the exam period got closer, and I was still intoxicated with the satisfaction that the games brought me. I failed three courses. I took this disappointment, irritability, and a depressive feeling back home with me. After my parents heard about my situation it was like the sky had fallen in, and they were completely unable to accept it. Everyday Dad wouldn't say anything, and closed himself off in his room and would not come out. Everyday Mum wagged her tongue off cursing me, and so there was not a moment of peace. I really could not understand their reaction. The child that they usually really trusted had failed in an exam just this one time, yet I had become a person without a single virtue. The whole holiday there was not one day of peace, I nearly did not want to go on living. The spring festival had yet not finished, and I left home and went back to Xi'an.

> In the spacious and deserted dormitory, I was even more attached to gaming, from morning to night I didn't leave the computer. It wasn't necessarily that the game had completely sucked me in, but rather leaving the game would result in me having to think about many matters, that included study, family, etc. I didn't dare to think about such things. Every time I thought about quarrels at home, I could not help but to want to throw things around.

Xiao Kang, like many others, mistakenly believed that he was intoxicated with the satisfaction that the game brought him. As is clear, it was not the satisfaction that the game gave him, but rather the sense of satisfaction that gaming brought him *in relation to* his classmates, which, in turn, changed their perception of him from someone virtually invisible to the center of their attention. He had become popular.

What we also see here is his gaming impacting directly upon his school grades. His exam failure quickly deflated this fragile and insecure sense-of-self, while his parents' excessive reaction to it merely further compounded his problems. In a classic case of depersonalization, his father chose to completely close himself off to Xiao Kang. If we ever see a case of a person wanting to escape reality, surely it is here in the father's response to Xiao Kang's exam grades. Xiao Kang, in trying to maintain a tenacious grasp on his lifeworld after entering university, attempted to take advantage of the computer to overcome his loneliness and estrangement. However, he was left mystified by what he perceived as an excessive overreaction on the part of his parents, which made him feel worthless and left life meaningless. His reaction was to *fan gan* (rebel) and head back to university early.

In contradistinction to Tao Ran's claim that virtual gaming leads to real-world violence, we see Xiao Kang using gaming in order to prevent real-world violence by giving vent to (*fa xie*) his anger and frustration online. It was not that he was simply escaping reality by gaming but rather he was using the internet in order to deal with reality. The question then becomes: why was he using this – and not something else – as a remedy to his socially-produced problems? That is, why is gaming one of the few weapons young people in China have in order to deal with the dangers of modernity? What does this tell us about contemporary Chinese society, and in particular the lack of any effective relief mechanisms available for young people during a time of rapid and disorienting social change?[105] As Bakken noted, the opening up and reform period is an inherently *destabilizing* process because it is caught between a failed Maoism and a hoped for but unrealized successful State-led capitalism.[106] Thus both lost equilibrium and lost control are experiences characteristic of the reforms due to the inherently transformative and contradictory nature of the reform policies. Within this transformation it should be expected that many individuals are going to have serious problems trying to "adapt" to an inherently destabilizing historical process, while others are going to go from one extreme to the other in their attempts at locating balance in a world inherently out-of-balance. Thus in part, online gamers can be framed within the space of lost equilibrium that has been created by the inherent contradictions and destabilizing transformations within the reform process. That is, Xiao Kang's behavior is both an outcome of, and response to, this process.

Part four – becoming an idol

After the semester started there were many students who wanted to buy computers, and so I naturally became their advisor. Very quickly half the dormitory had computers and we started to plan and prepare to organise a local area network. Therefore I specially studied information correlated with the internet, and so I studied MSCE (Microsoft Certified Systems Engineer). After successfully establishing the internet network, I now had even more choices of games to play. Because "infinite pleasure comes from the battle with others," I very quickly discovered the attraction to internet games when broadly compared with single player games, because in internet games people are mutually engaged with one another, and this mutual conjunction gives people a new kind of feeling. Within the games, every person can become a leading character, and the focus, and so they can also enjoy the victor's joy and happiness.

Through the internet I got into friendships with some classmates who, like me, played games everyday. Everyday we communicated with each other about what we had learned about games, and discussed any new tactics. In this circle, no one talk about matters relating to study, and no one unrealistically compared each other's grades. Likewise, it just happened that I became the shinning light of the group, to the extent that if player beat me just once he would go and publicize it. I had already become their goal, their idol … and the sole powerhouse.

In contrast to playing singularly, Xiao Kang discovers the way being "mutually engaged" with his peers gave him a "new kind of feeling." This is a crucially important observation in understanding the pull or attraction of online games. The attraction is not premised upon escaping reality, but rather upon the mutual conjunctions that people entangle themselves in, and the new kind of feelings that emanate from such interpersonal conjunctions. That is, online gaming is not inherently premised upon disconnection and desocialization but rather interpersonal connection, and thus is driven by friendship-making and socialization.[107] A key element in online gaming is not simply the pleasure of playing games, in and of themselves (for games are simply a tool to other means and not an end in themselves), but rather the "infinite pleasure that comes from the battle with others." Contrary to the opinion of anti-gaming crusaders these "others" are not some unreal virtual character, but rather real people, and often real friends. Many parents dismiss them as "real" friends, not principally because they are in cyberspace and thus not real, but because these friends are attributed as being a negative influence upon the child's schoolwork.

The other key element, and the main focus of Xiao Kang's narrative, is the way online gaming allows the individual to become the "leading character" and the "focus" (center of attention) so that the "victor's joy and happiness" can be experienced as *my* victory and *my* happiness. By feeling like a master of their universe they feel as though they are leading and thus in control. Existentially, this is one of the most powerful pull factors for young people, whether they are a "loser" or "winner" at the game-of-life, as it allows the loser to feel like a winner and the winner to continue to feel like a winner in a new whole realm, thus continuously encouraging them to extend and deepen their winning ways. And when they do lose, unlike in the game-of-life, there are little or no negative consequences. It is simply a matter of starting over again by pushing the restart button. This is partly how two hours immersed playing quickly becomes six. It is this "me worship" – or "*laoda* effect" – that is so attractive to those who gain no pleasure from school and home life, yet who are immersed in a social system that constantly reinforces the high social value of individual achievement and an individualized life. As Fromm said, these actions are part of their necessity to find ever-new solutions for the contradictions in their existence, and to find ever-higher forms of unity with their peers and with themselves.

Xiao Kang then talks about a deepened and intensified relation to the computer involving researching tactics and, through problem-solving, learning how to both operate and manipulate the game to his own benefit. In short, he was doing applied science, for as literacy expert James Gee noted, commercial video games are basically problem-solving spaces.[108] As Fromm pointed out, most people do not understand the nature and inner workings of the objects they consume, but what Xiao Kang was doing was attempting, by applying the methods of logic and science, to understand the inner functioning of the game so as to be able to manipulate his environment. Is not the highest value of education to have a student who can take a platform and learn how to operate and then manipulate it in order to produce something new? Is this not the basis of science?

Not only did he attempt to manipulate the technological aspects of his leisure activity but, at the same time, he was actively trying to *advance* his knowledge by listening and learning through the experience of others. Being part of this inner circle – as opposed to being an isolated wolf hiking alone in the woods – Xiao Kang and his friends were both solidifying their friendships and increasing their socialization skills, for far from online gaming resulting in the shrinking of their world it, on the contrary, had expanded their social world. How could anything compete with the pleasure this brought him, for it was based upon him obtaining power and domination over others? Like Huang He mentioned earlier, he felt like a *laoda*.

But as far as the education system and the so-called normal functioning of society is concerned, this inner circle was both revolutionary and dangerous, for they were not discussing matters related to study, by, for example, devoting their time to "unrealistically comparing each other's grades." What was considered deviant to the education system was, for them, part of the attraction, for this allowed them to get away from the burden of school grades – a breathing space and breath of fresh air. The problem as far as their relationship to the normal functioning of society was concerned was not the qualitative premise of this activity, but the quantitative degree to which they took it.

As he points out, the education system could not compete with the way in which he felt like the "sole powerhouse" in the game and the "shining light" within the group. As people like Foucault have shown, the education system has both normalizing (you are like everyone else) and individualizing (I am like no one else) functions, and because of these twin processes there is only a very small number in each class who are able to become the sole powerhouse in a particular activity (i.e., the top in the class).[109] But online games offer pseudo-heroism to a large number of competitors, for every victory is a potential feeling of individual power and powerful individuality.

Part five – becoming the world's savior

> In the second year the university had put the internet in every dorm and every student could apply to open an IP address. At Tsinghua University they established a *Starcraft* server under the name Smith, and so we encountered an opponent even stronger than us, which was as though we had found an even higher purpose than ourselves, the excitement was endless, and so I was even more indulged in online gaming.

> Even though every battle team member's school report cards were bad no one talked about study, as everyone had the same thirst for getting away from the real world. It was as if one was a character in the game, and we were both the hero in charge of the important task of saving the world. Once in a while when we returned to the real world, emptiness and feelings

of loneliness appeared, but they were able to vanish without a trace during competition. It was like we were chasing a life time career, but we never thought whether this "career" was real or not. Everyone was fantasizing that one day the "devil" would fall into the world and oneself would be mankind's sole hope.

Here, Xiao Kang informs us of the central role the university is playing in creating the technical possibility for students to be able to *frequently* and *repeatedly* reproduce the act of online gaming, even when alone.[110] For those like Tao Ran who argue that the internet has some kind of inherent addictive quality in that "so long as they can get access to a computer there will be addiction,"[111] the actions of the university then becomes akin to Shanghai gangster Du Yuesheng opening an opium den in every dormitory. More accurately, through the university's active encouragement of installing the internet in every dormitory, so that students can develop a "scientific outlook on development," Xiao Kang and his circle were able to encounter an "opponent even stronger than us," which both reinforced their in-group qualities while providing them with "an even higher purpose than ourselves." Xiao Kang had found that higher purpose (achieve, achieve, achieve) that the "simpletons," in his eyes, already possessed. Through finding this higher purpose – just as newly converted Christians in China believe they have found a higher purpose in Jesus Christ, God, and a "secure" doctrinal ideology – the internet had opened up their world thus allowing them to overcome *the need to avoid aloneness, and the need to avoid isolation by being related to the world outside oneself.*[112] It is in this sense his gaming is premised upon "devotion" and not "addiction.'

Xiao Kang also writes that those in the circle all had the same "thirst for getting away from the real world." But when we analyze their actual behavior, and the values driving their behavior, we see that what they thirst for is that which is actually highly valued in the real world: friendship (relatedness); belonging (rootedness); success (transcendence); attention; respect; appreciation; prized individual abilities and skills, etc. That is, they were seeking feelings of self-importance. For in a consumer-driven society if a person is sought after, they are somebody, yet if they are not popular, they are simply nobody.

Yet the realness of this real world is itself called into question by him describing a "lost feeling" and loneliness growing more distinct and intense, with the internet becoming the only place where he could obtain "disengagement" from it. We must ask why is the so-called real world such a lonely and desolate place? What Xiao Kang is saying is that it was not the games themselves that were sucking him into a void, but rather his reluctance to reenter the lonely real world where he felt lost and which had, in relation to the excitement of online gaming, become even more lonely and desolate. Can we blame a person for desiring to seek a safer and warmer environment? And does accusing him of simply wanting to escape reality amount to a productive conceptualization of his whole lifeworld? Is not his experience really a critique of this real world, in which almost from the beginning of university life his inner being was like a deserted island? Instead of simply demonizing video games and the internet, is not a more important task, one of improving the world outside gaming so that it is at least as attractive a place to be as cyberspace?

Finally Xiao Kang, in seeing his school grades suffer greatly, had in effect turned full circle and was again feeling empty, lonely, and inferior. In this way, it cannot simply be deduced that online gaming had *caused* these feelings to manifest themselves, for not only did he express a range of extremely positive emotions in relation to gaming (infinite pleasure; endless excitement), but these feelings are the same set of emotions he felt *before* starting to game. If anything his gaming had not, despite his initial feelings and thoughts to the contrary, allowed him to save and conquer himself. Rather, because there was no value attached to gaming as far as the university was concerned then the more he gamed the more problems he created for himself – both materially in relation to schoolwork and existentially in relation to him feeling like a failure vis-à-vis the normal functioning of society. His problem, as he said, was that he *could not wake up to the reality*. That is, he was not doing what he knew all along he *should* have been doing, and what his parents and the university *expected* him to have been doing. This is why the thing he feared most of all was hearing others talk about matters related to study, for this was the reality he knew he had to wake up to. In understanding this weight of reality we must understand the way any given society tends to form the character-structure of its members in such a way as to *make them desire to do what they have to do in order to fulfill their social function*.[113] The "internet addicts" are rebels because they *refuse* to do what they have to do in order to fulfill their social function, but then, paradoxically, seek the same values prized within the so-called real world. If he was a professional gamer or a "gold farmer" then he would not have such intrapersonal conflicts, for it was not his gaming per se that was so problematic, but rather the whole social context in which his gaming took place that continuously rammed home the fact he was *playing* when he should have been *working*.

7 *DSM-IV* – Internet Addiction Disorder

In light of the social context explained throughout the text, now let us look at the Young-Tao model through the prism of the *DSM-IV*'s own definition of a mental disorder. In the following pages I will again highlight the contradictions between Tao Ran's explanatory theory and his method in actual practice. Or to be more specific, by negating the social context he consistently goes against his own theory. As we have seen repeatedly, on the one hand he points to the social context surrounding intensive gaming, but because he has imprisoned his perspective within the strict confines of the biomedical model he then goes against his own empirical observations. Ironically, he consistently admits that the family is a war-machine and that the causes of internet addiction reside not within the disordered mind of some pathological individual but within this war-machine; however, he then washes this away. What we have seen, and will see again, is that instead of arguing that intensive gaming is a mental disorder he is, on the contrary, actually arguing that it is *not* a mental disorder.

We must begin by asking the following: is it valid to claim that the declining school grades, gaming, lying, stealing, fighting, cursing, talking, smoking, drinking, and other forms of rebellious, "abnormal," or norm-violating behavior stemming from the actions of the "internet addict" are caused by a mental disorder called "internet addiction?"[1] Or alternatively is it more accurate, when we take fully into account the actual social conditions within the families presented here as empirical evidence, to agree with the mother in Letter-32 who said her son *has experienced a great deal*?

One central task of both sociology and psychology – in the search for legitimacy, authority, and appropriate solutions to real-world problems – is to distinguish between mental disorders and a) normal reactions to stressful environments/situations/relationships and b) signs of existential distress such as feelings of alienation, aloneness, isolation, anxiety, melancholy, resistance, and anger. As noted, we need to contextualize norm-violating behavior such as increased internet use after one or more of the following situations occur: a) the death of a parent; b) parental divorce; c) a child subjected to acts of violence, absence, and neglect by one or both parents; d) feelings of intense pressure due to examinations and schoolwork; and e) feelings of depersonalization and engulfment due to parental pressure and over-investment functioning under the pretext of "love." Under such conditions is it more appropriate to conceptualize their reactions as normal – and not abnormal – responses to their stress environments? In offering an account of *a person* we cannot forget that each person, whether child or adult, is always acting upon others and always being acted upon by others, for no one acts or experiences in a social vacuum. As mentioned at the outset, this person who is described as an "internet addict" *is not the only actor in their world.*[2]

Another essential distinction to be made when persons in positions of authority are labeling the actions of people in a socially powerless position as stemming from a psychological "addiction" is the distinction between mental disorders and social deviance. Deviations from social norms, such as refusing to do schoolwork and demanding to play online, generally arise *not* because of internal pathologies but because of a range of other factors, including:

a) *Conflicting cultural norms* (i.e., desiring play/consumption over work/ production).
b) *Conformity to the standards of subcultures* (i.e., peer pressure to play games for "who is not playing games these days," means to *not* play games becomes "abnormal').
c) *A lack of adequate social control* (i.e., because of engulfment or "loving the child to death" parents have not instilled appropriate ways of acting in the child, and have also lost control over the child by, for example, allowing the son to play online all through the night and letting him sleep during the day).[3]

Tao Ran, in addition to claiming six hours of daily internet use that harms social functioning defines "internet addiction," also claims that all "internet addicts" have behavioral and psychological problems. The psychiatric symptoms of which include severe feelings of maladjustment, pessimism, and despondency; dread of social contact; pessimism toward schoolwork; being down in spirits; loss of interest in doing things; and reduced feelings of happiness.[4] As Tao Ran has argued: "The Internet Addiction Disorder can lead to autism, self-contempt, confrontation with family members and other mental or psychological problems."[5] What is clear is that a "confrontation with family members" is not a mental or psychological problem. Likewise, Wu and Zhang have argued that prolonged use of the internet has a negative influence upon brain development by, for example, partly decreasing intellectual capacity, causing a disorder in vegetative nerves and hormone levels, and reducing immunity which leads to headaches, anxiety, or even death.[6]

The diagnostic psychiatry model that Tao Ran employs uses symptoms to classify discrete psychiatric disorders, and the basic assumption of such a diagnostic framework is that the presence of enough particular manifest symptoms, generally regardless of the social condition from which the particular symptoms arise from, indicates an underlying disease such as "internet addiction." As mentioned, Horwitz reminds us that the classifications of distinct disorders that underpin diagnostic psychiatry are useful when two broad criteria are met:

1) That each constellation of symptoms is actually a valid mental disorder.
2) That using manifest symptoms to distinguish diseases aids in establishing distinct causes, prognoses, and treatments for each condition.[7]

With reference to the empirical data presented here let us repeat this proposition: does the so-called "Internet Addiction Disorder" meet these two broad criteria? That is, is the constellation of symptoms identified to "diagnose" a certain form of internet use actually a *valid* mental disorder called "internet addiction," and is using these symptoms to distinguish "internet addiction" from "internet use" aiding us in establishing distinct causes, prognoses, and treatments for this condition?

DSM-IV – expectable response to stress condition

The assumption – which we see in the Young-Tao model – that the presence of enough manifest symptoms indicates an underlying mental disorder called "internet addiction" is especially problematic when psychological and psychosomatic symptoms are *themselves* products of a stressful and taxing social environment, for such a model mistakenly equates *expectable responses to stress conditions* with a mental disorder. This is simply because no sharp demarcation is made between those who are under stress and those who are not. The *DSM-IV*, the authoritative text internationally accepted within psychiatry as the definer of what does, and just as importantly, does not, constitute a "mental disorder" is very clear on this point. As mentioned, the *DSM-IV* states that for a clinically significant behavioral or psychological syndrome, or pattern that occurs in an individual, to be classified as a mental disorder the syndrome or pattern under consideration: "Must *not* be merely an expectable and culturally sanctioned response to a particular event, for example, the death of a loved one."[8]

This is why bereaved people do not suffer from the mental disorder called "depression," because people are *naturally* depressed after the death of a family member or the divorce of one's parents. It is therefore *expected* that young people who lose their father are going to act for a period of time in abnormal and norm-violating ways, such as, for example, increased internet usage; severe feelings of maladjustment, pessimism, and despondency; dread of social contact; pessimism toward schoolwork; being down in spirits; loss of interest in doing things; and reduced feelings of happiness. This is because they are confronted with acute and chronic stressors and so cannot be expected to act normally.[9] Thus it is misguided to claim their increased time spent at the internet bar with friends is simply because they are suffering from a mental disorder called "internet addiction" because by negating the situational context we are unable to say whether their behavior is an expected or unexpected response to an acute and/or chronic stressor.

As pointed out earlier, Tao Ran himself admits, in direct contradiction to his diagnostic-based psychiatric model, that the so-called "internet addicts" that he claims suffer from a mental disorder have come from stress environments and have encountered acute and chronic stressors. As he has said: "Every child in this rehab center has a sad or miserable history, because their parents didn't treat them justly."[10] Likewise, on the TV show *Focus Point* Tao Ran said the following: "The kids that come to our base, 58 percent have been cursed and beaten by their parents."[11] Perhaps most significant of all, Tao Ran told a journalist that the family ranked as the first cause of internet addiction. "Parents who are violent toward their children and families where relationships are not good drive children to seek consolation from the Internet," Tao Ran was reported as saying.[12] In addition he has stressed the important role the father plays in the family, adding that from among the "internet addiction sufferers" confined to his military hospital "95 percent were boys who lacked the love of a father."[13] What Tao Ran is saying, in negation of the biomedical model of mental disorder he presents, is that "internet addiction" *is* an expectable response to a stress condition. Instead of arguing that intensive gaming is a mental disorder he is, on the contrary, arguing that it is not a mental disorder.

If he thinks that the family unit, and in particular parental violence, is the main cause of what he mistakenly calls "internet addiction disorder" then why does he force them to take unspecified types of medication, undertake pseudo-psychoanalytic treatment, and subject them to military-style exercises? Surely it should be the violent parent(s), first and foremost, who should be the ones forced to change? Moreover, he has also said that "under heavy pressure in life or work, some adults hope to escape reality or release their emotions in cyberspace."[14] Again, he is saying that internet use is simply an expectable response to a stressful environment, for the desire to "release" heavy life pressure is considered something that a "healthy" and "normal" person does and should do.

This is one of the fundamental malfunctions of Tao Ran's model as he attributes all the self-perceived "symptoms" of the "internet addict" – anxiety, irritability, pessimism, anger, low-self-esteem, inattentiveness, apathy, etc – as being caused by "internet addiction." Yet at the same time he actually acknowledges the taxing and stressful social environments these young people are embedded into, thereby negating the biomedical model on which he bases his theory. Thus while acknowledging the "sickness" of the social environment the person is embedded in, he, nevertheless, continues (and in contradistinction to the *DSM-IV*) to focus upon the perceived biomedical "sickness" of the individual. This is because in trying to appear "scientific," and thus adhering to the CCP's dominant ideology of "scientific outlook on development," Tao Ran, in actual practice, conceptualizes his so-called patients as a physical-chemical system or *organism*, and not principally as *persons-related-to-persons*. In trying to appear "objective" and "medical" Tao Ran depersonalizes those under his command by turning a person into a diseased organism, and as Laing has noted, when a person is seen as an organism and not as a person then there is no longer any central place for this person's desires, hopes, fears, despair, and anger (i.e., their agency). Rather, such a person must be drained of their intra-and-interpersonal social condition, or depersonalized, before he can become an "object of scientific study."[15] And through this medicalization of the internet user the subject is turned into a medicalized organism as this is seen as the first step in "curing" their "sickness." This scientific and medicalized depersonalization is nicely captured in what Tao Ran said on *Focus Point* when asked by the host if he uses medication on those brought to his hospital, normally against their will, by their parents:

> At the same time as having internet addiction 22% of internet addicts also have other diseases.[16] For example, attention deficit and hyperactivity disorder, of which 4% of patients also have an accompanying 'conduct impediment,' while 2% have an accompanying 'personality impediment.' We use medicine to treat all his comorbidity problems. We take his comorbidity problems and treat them, for only then can you rectify his internet addiction.[17]

He is arguing that "internet addiction" can only be cured if you first cure attention deficit hyperactivity disorder and personality disorders, because "internet addiction" is in some way an "outgrowth" of the young person's comorbidity problems. But if 22+4+2 percent (28 percent) have these additional (comorbidity) disorders then what about the other 72 percent, do they not then require medication? In any case, seen as a medicalized organism the internet user cannot be anything else but a complex of things, of *its*, and the processes that ultimately comprise an organism are *it*-processes, such as time spent playing, various accompanying "impediments," or physiological symptoms like "anxiety," "pessimism," and "irritability."[18] However, in order to understand the internet user and their internet use we need to understand them as a person that is a) in relation with other persons, b) in certain relations with themselves, and c) in a multitude of relations that are non-human (technological) and structural (political/economic). Their social condition, and the unexpected or expected responses to such a condition, must be brought to the forefront if a biomedical-based concept called "internet addiction" is to be valid. Basically, one must articulate what the other's lifeworld is and his/her way of *being* in it.[19]

The fact is a large part of the symptoms Tao Ran attributes to internet addiction or accompanying "impediment" or "disease" results from *before* they entered into an intense relationship with the internet, as well as from the entirety of relationships surrounding their internet use. This is because the internet sometimes functions as a remedy, or weapon, they utilize in order to deal with *existing* stressful social conditions. Another important failure resulting from simply confining himself to the "objectively" observable behavior of the person before him is related to their present circumstances of finding themselves inside Tao Ran's hospital. For after being cheated and deceived by their parents (thus draining the relationship of trust) and then being subjected, against their will and best wishes, to Tao Ran's militarized and medicalized regime then it is *expected* that they would be angry, irritable, anxious, pessimistic, and inattentive. For as Fromm says, any threat against a person's vital emotional and material interests creates anxiety.[20] These feelings brought about by suddenly finding themselves confronted with Tao Ran's regime are conceptualized, and "scientifically" legitimized by him, through labeling them as "withdrawal reactions" such as depression, irritability, impulsive behavior, and destructive actions, and so are consequently seen as part of their "psychological problems." Because of these manifest symptoms Tao Ran argues that, therefore, psychotherapy or behavioral intervention cannot be carried out smoothly at this stage because "compliance is not high."[21] In order to obtain compliance he administers drugs that can gradually make their mood more "balanced."[22] In short, he forces them to take medication in order to make them *docile* so that he can then attempt to alter their "rebellious psychology" through pseudo-psychotherapy. Thereby hopefully bringing about a "good mental state" in which they are willing, through soft and hard coercive and disciplinary measures, to return back to normality.[23]

Nevertheless, one of the major shortcomings of "diagnosing" people who are deceived into going to Tao Ran's medicalized military-style boot camp is that it is not simply the so-called internet addict him/herself who is exhibiting signs of distress or suffering, but also his/her parents, which is why it is them, and not the supposed "addict" themselves, who is seeking treatment for their child. As we have seen, the letters, which are painful to read, demonstrate quite clearly how distressed the parents genuinely are. For example, the mother in Letter-7 offers an ideal type: "I am in an utterly helpless situation, all day I wash my face with my tears, and feel that living is not as good as dying, while every day I am thinking about the heavy mood that has secretly ferried away the day." Likewise, parental distress is on ubiquitous display at any of Tao Hongkai's talks. For example, one mother attending his course in Beijing carried around with her an intense look of worry that had been carved into her face from excessive anxiety over her son not wanting to go to school and only wanting to play online games. Confessing that she worries too much, she said that, nevertheless, all the worry over her son had made her hair turn grey and had aged her prematurely. This worry was amplified by the fact that the son ran away from the course after seeing the words "internet addiction" written on the side of the building. Not only was the son resisting being labeled as a person with a mental disorder, but he was also reacting to his mother's strategy, for she had tricked her son into coming to Beijing, telling him that she is sick and so needed to seek medical treatment.

How can the son accept his mother's concern when she is using deception in order to get him to do something against his will? This deception breaks down the already fragile trust between them, which is essential if they are to maintain a positive and healthy relationship. This distraught mother, who had tied herself into a tight existential knot, then subsequently cried all throughout the first day of the four-day course. Since the course partly functions for the parents in a similar way that online games function for their child, in that it allows parents a therapeutic and spiritual-like space to *fa xie* (give vent to) their repressed feelings, then she looked a lot more relaxed on day two and even more at ease on day three. This despite the fact that the son was himself roaming the streets of Beijing alone. But Tao Hongkai insists that in order to change the child one needs to first change the parents. One of the reasons why parents need to deceive their children into seeking treatment is that the child does not consider themselves to be "mentally disordered" or "diseased." This partly explains why when they see the concept "internet addiction" written on the wall of the boot camp they often flee, for they think it is their parents, and not them, who are "sick." For presumably only a person in distress would willingly label their own child as suffering from a mental disorder that does not legitimately exist.

And since the internet sometimes functions as a remedy or weapon they utilize in order to deal with existing stressful social conditions, then when a son stops communicating with his parents after they scold and violently beat him for refusing to do his schoolwork, and chooses instead to play online, then such behavior can be understood as partly an expectable response to a stress condition. Or when the son runs back to the internet bar after his father beats him or locks him in his room, that is, likewise, an expectable response to a stressful condition, and not merely a sign that he is unable to control his internet use because he is suffering from a psychological problem called "internet addiction." Xiao Kang's migration to the internet and online games can also be seen as an expectable response to him feeling like an outcast, or "different species" as he thought it, and having no classmates to socialize with on the weekends because they were all studying excessively. Moreover, Xiao Wang's attraction to the internet is also partly an expectable response to being discriminated against for being overweight, as online he was able to overcome this stressful condition through the "faceless" mechanism of the internet. And so too was Huang He's love of online gaming an expectable response to not feeling respected in the "real" world, for through the display of his gaming skills he was able to obtain the respect of his fellow gamers. Likewise, the teenage girl's online behavior that resulted in her being sent to the boot camp in Jinan was an expectable response to stressful social conditions, because she desired to communicate her innermost feelings to another person yet was denied this avenue in the "real" world and so sought it out on QQ.

In reality, all these actions, which their parents and Tao Ran would say were symptoms of their "internet addiction," were in many ways their expectable responses to stressful social conditions, or what could be called *living in a world out-of-balance*. Tao Ran is correct to point out that one of the main attractions of seeking out the internet as a remedy is because "they believe the virtual world is beautiful and fair."[24] But, at the same time, he is mistaken to then say: "In the real world, they become depressed, upset, and restless – they are very unhappy."[25] This is because this tells us nothing about the conditions making them feel depressed, upset, restless, and unhappy, rather it just presents them as weaklings who cannot "adjust" to the normal functioning of society.

The *DSM-IV* is clear in that "distress that emerges from social conditions is neither a mental disorder nor a distinct disease condition."[26] The problem is that many parents do not detect their child's distress, for there seems to be an assumption that their kids are – despite the fact that they are caught in the eye of a social transformation perhaps no society has ever passed through – somehow made of steel, which is surely a result of a general lack of awareness about psychological health in China. A revealing example of this lack of awareness about the coping mechanisms of Chinese youth is the speed with which the State Council ordered all schools in Jiegu to reopen within two weeks of the devastating earthquake that struck Qinghai province on April 14, 2010. Just four days following the earthquake the (mostly Tibetan) students were forced back to attend classes in makeshift tents lacking books and stationary, this despite the fact that these cold, hungry, devastated, and mourning children, some of whom had just lost both parents and many of whom had lost friends and classmates, were themselves sleeping in tents or outdoors in sub-zero temperatures. But in a paternalistically governed *nowist* society obsessed with education should we be too surprised to hear Deputy Education Minister Lu Xin tell local headmasters to "*resume classes with all speed?*" Local secondary school principal Baima Ngacyang appropriately summarized the reality of treating blank-face grieving students as blank-faced grade-making machines: "I don't think anything from their textbooks is suitable to teach in such circumstances."[27]

The reality is that many students are under a lot of stress and distress, and so some partly use the internet and internet games as a mechanism to deal with this stress, while some take this leisure pursuit to socially unacceptable levels of intensity. More importantly, why do many of the "internet addicts', according to the letters sent to Tao Hongkai, come from broken homes and problematic families that have experienced traumatic events (divorce/illness/death/violence/absence/neglect)? To then call their gaming that exceeds acceptable levels as a mental disorder is both misguided and problematic, for it assumes that the problem lies in the relation between child and internet and so they are unable to see the socially produced distress that envelopes the family and that resides outside of the internet. That is, blaming the child for using the internet too much to the detriment of their schoolwork fails to understand the problems the child is having with school, school-relations, school-work, and family life. The mistake is to see the internet as the cause of the problem rather than as an effect of other, much more serious, causes. In short, effect is mistaken for cause.

DSM-IV – internal dysfunction

In addition to the behavior under consideration not simply being an expectable response to a stress condition, the *DSM-IV* adds that the following criterion must *also* be met in order for certain kinds of behavior to be classified as a mental disorder:

> Whatever its original cause, it must currently be considered a manifestation of a behavioral, psychological, or biological dysfunction in the individual. Neither deviant behaviour (e.g. political, religious, or sexual) nor conflicts that are primarily between the individual and society [i.e., the war-machine between parent and only-child over school and play] are mental disorders unless the deviance or conflict is *a symptom of a dysfunction in the individual*.[28]

Thus according to the American Psychiatric Association's *DSM-IV* a mental disorder – that is not simply an expectable response to a stress condition – must also be shown to have originated from a dysfunction *in* the individual, and, therefore, it must be proven that there is something wrong with the *internal functioning* of a person. Importantly, an internal dysfunction exists only when an internal mechanism – such as cognition, thinking, perception, motivation, emotion, memory, or language – is *unable* to perform its natural function, and not simply when it *does not* perform this function. These functions, according to Horwitz, "are not social constructions but properties of the human species that have arisen through natural selection. People with internal dysfunctions have some psychological system that is incapable of performing within normal limits."[29]

Thus, only symptoms that stem from internal dysfunctions, and are not an expectable response to a stress condition, reflect mental disorders.[30] According to this criterion a "disobedient personality spreading unchecked," for example, is *not* the result of an internal dysfunction but is rather a social construction made by a distraught mother as a way of making sense of her world and of her role in it. Likewise, just because a young person in Tao Ran's hospital is not paying attention, is not concentrating, does not look happy or seems irritable, this does not at all signify that they are unable to do pay attention, concentrate, be happy and non-irritable. Instead of suffering from what he calls "attention deficit and hyperactivity disorder," it is just as likely that they do not want to perform these functions for the simple reason that they do not like being cheated, deceived, tortured, held against their will, force-fed unspecified drugs and ordered to undergo quasi-military training. These "symptoms" are more likely the expectable reactions to forced confinement by a person who has committed no crime and who believes does not suffer from any kind of mental disorder. Therefore just what, exactly, are the internal dysfunctions that are universal qualities of the human species that sets the "internet addict" apart from the rest of the population? These cannot be emotional and/or behavioral qualities such as pessimism, low self-esteem, pleasure seeking, etc, for they are *not* internal dysfunctions but rather the contextual affects of the relation between a whole range of external factors such as relations between the individual and the computer; the internet; friends; classmates; parents; school; city; society; social policy; capital, etc.

Indeed, one of the strongest threads running through the letters is the parent's emphasis on highlighting how *functional* the child was prior to his problems. And so they described the son using words such as: normal, intelligent, good-natured, lively, obedient, kind-hearted, outstanding, enterprising, progressive. Even taking into account the parent's attributions, that is, the way they frame the narrative in order to emphasis that the child – and by implication their parenting – was generally "good" until an external factor called the internet descended upon the family like a thief in the night, we must come to the conclusion that it is very difficult to prove (as a diagnostic-based "internet addiction" model must) that their socially inappropriate internet use stems from an internal dysfunction. And as Horwitz clearly states: "If nothing is wrong with people's internal functioning, they are not mentally disordered."[31]

However, another thread running through the letters is the way a number of parents referred to the child having an "introverted personality." But a so-called personality "trait" such as being introverted, which is a socially-ascribed idiosyncratic form of behavior, is not at all the same thing as an internal dysfunction. An internal dysfunction indicates something is wrong with the *capacity* of an internal mechanism to function as it is designed to function, and not that an individual has made *bad* choices in how to behave or is criticized by others for not behaving how they would like them to behave. An internal dysfunction renders a person *incapable* of being able to conform to social norms and so their norm-violating actions are involuntary. Thus criticizing your child for being "introverted," even though he may have legitimate reasons for being so, does not necessarily render him incapable of conforming to social norms thereby making his deviance involuntary.[32] Rather, terms like "introverted personality" operate as judgment markers to indicate a social and biological *failure* of adjustment, but which in practice imply a certain standard of behavior to which the person cannot seemingly measure up.[33] In reality, by choosing to play on the internet over studying, the son, from the perspective of both social norms and future prospects, could be said to have simply made poor choices in how to behave. For it is this "poor" behavior that parents principally want changed.

The parents are not primarily concerned about the "mental and spiritual health" of the child, for if they were they would not want the child to study seven days a week, including holidays. That is, they would not be trying to turn the child into a grade-making machine. Rather all they really desire is that he/she chooses to leave the internet bar and return back to school, and thus back to the so-called "normal" functioning of a hyperculture-of-excess. They are also not asking people like Tao Hongkai, who is an educator, that they want internal dysfunctions changed into internal functions, because they already generally believe that the son has a "good nature." Rather they simply beg him to *convince* or *persuade* the son to stop behaving badly and start behaving in line with present social norms. Quite simply, the parents are not as concerned about the effect internet use is having upon the psychological wellbeing of the child as they are about the effect this internet use is having upon the *gaokao* exam.

DSM-IV – deviance and Skinner's box

It is this very focus on deviant behavior that constitutes the third, and final, part of the definition of a "mental disorder" set out in the *DSM-IV*. The *DSM-IV* is very clear in stating that neither deviant behavior (e.g., political, religious, or sexual) nor conflicts that are primarily between the individual and society are mental disorders, unless they stem from an internal dysfunction that is not an expectable response to a stress condition. That is, mental disorders, such as "internet addiction," must be distinguished from inappropriateness as defined by social norms (deviant behavior) as well as from expectable responses to stressful environments. This is because the inappropriateness of behavior is not sufficient, in and of itself, to indicate the existence of a mental disorder. To be deviant and to be disordered are two very different conditions arising from two very different explanatory models. So, for example, "heavy drinking need not indicate alcoholism, nor is career criminality equivalent to antisocial personality disorder. These would *only* be mental disorders if it were clear that they stemmed from internal dysfunctions that render alcoholics or sociopaths unable to control their conduct."[34] Or, alternatively, when is heavy internet use hedonistic/inappropriate/deviant and when is it a sign of an internal dysfunction?

Where is the boundary, line, or threshold used to separate socially inappropriate or deviant internet use and internet use stemming from a mental disorder? If the threshold is six hours or more per day then how does this indicate a sign of internal dysfunction? Measuring time spent doing an activity is in no way related to proving an internal dysfunction, rather it is simply a socially ascribed value judgment upon what is considered appropriate and inappropriate forms of usage. For example, the professional gamer or gold farmer who plays online games for eight hours a day, which is considered an appropriate length of time in order to earn a salary or practice for a major competition,[35] does not exhibit an internal dysfunction, rather such "productive" persons are considered to be "making progress." According to the *DSM-IV*, then, prolonged and daily internet use does not indicate the conduct is caused by "internet addiction" unless this use stems from internal dysfunctions that render the internet user unable to control their conduct (conduct which, in addition, is not an expectable response to a stress condition).

We could say that being "unable to control their conduct" means making a clear distinction between *having* to do something and *wanting* to do something. This is to say we must be very clear about action being voluntary or involuntary. Do internet users have a *choice* or do they not? It cannot simply be inferred that a person who keeps performing the same act over and over again *has* to, by necessity, do it; or that they cannot stop doing it.

The diagnostic-based model's approach to this distinction between voluntary actions (wanting to) and involuntary actions (having to) is, according to Booth Davies, generally underpinned by the operant psychology of B.F. Skinner. Skinner's model which underpins the biomedical-based explanation for addiction is centered upon behavior being controlled by external environmental factors, or as Booth Davies simply summarizes it: "Behaviour seems to be something that happens *to* people, rather than being done *by* them. In a similar way, "addiction" is not conceptualized as something that people do, so much as something that happens to them."[36] This model can be thought of when the arbitrary distinction is made between the amateur gamer who plays for leisure and the gold farmer who plays for work, in that "addiction" happens to the amateur gamer while for the gold farmer "productive work" is done by them. The amateur gamer is seen as a passive *player* while the gold farmer is seen as an active *worker*, this despite the fact that the two are engaged in the exact same activity.

Booth Davies highlights the way the addiction concept operates in the same fashion as the famous "Skinner-box."[37] A Skinner box basically contains one or more levers which an animal, usually a rat, can press one or more stimulus lights and one or more places in which reinforcers like food can be delivered. The idea, using Pavlov's notion of conditioned reflexes, is to "scientifically investigate" the stimulus-response reactions of animals, and by association humans, to various situations. So, for example, the finding that a rat dosed on a stimulant of some kind will work continuously to get further doses of the stimulant becomes the basis for claiming that the rat "has to" press the lever because it is "addicted', rather than it "wants to" because it "likes it." The implication is that stimulation of part of the brain, which is followed by a bout of incessant lever pressing, leads to the assumption that the owner of the brain has no say in the matter, and so the brain's own reasons, motives, intentions, and will have little or even no part to play in the activity. Once it has been established that a "drug" has a measurable pharmacological effect upon someone,[38] then it is assumed that *therefore* that person has no further decision-making capacity because the pharmacology of drug action is assumed to compel the behavior irrespective of, or even against, the person's own will.[39]

This perspective, which envisions the user as a kind of slave to the stimulant, was expressed by Tao Ran when he said *their souls are gone to the online world.*[40] But as Booth Davies argues, conceptualizing the relationship between rat and stimulant in terms of external pharmacological influences washes over the more powerful relation – the interaction of interpersonal *and* intrapersonal factors – and so hinders, rather than helps, our understanding of why people take stimulants. As he concluded,

> Incessant lever pressing by a rat cannot be taken to indicate that it 'has to'; since by implication this means that less-constant activity is voluntary; that is, a lower rate of response indicates that the rat presses the lever even though it doesn't 'have to'.[41]

In relation to "internet addiction" this is to claim that the person who uses the internet for less than four hours per day, a daily rate Tao Ran has defined as a person being "cured" of internet addiction, does so because he *wants to*, while the person who plays for more than six hours does so because he *has to*. Before discharging "patients" from his hospital Tao Ran wants them to be sensible and have strict time control over their internet use. Therefore if they want their "addiction" to dissipate then their use should not exceed four hours a day, while continuous usage should not exceed one hour, which should include a rest period of 5–10 minutes.[42] Thus he presents a very confusing threshold, because if six hours expresses "addiction," while four hours expresses being "cured" of this addiction, then what does the time between four and six hours express? For example, if a young man leaves his hospital "cured" and then proceeds to spend five hours per day online then how can be said to have "relapsed" because he has not exceeded the original six hour threshold used to define addiction? Likewise, this conceptualization is the equivalent of saying, for example: six standard drinks per day means a man is addicted to alcohol while reducing his consumption to four standard drinks per day means he is cured of his alcoholism. How can a mere 33 percent reduction define the threshold between addiction and cure? Nevertheless, Tao Ran then offers us the real underlying reason for his method. He says that after being discharged the internet user should, in the face of the complex information network of the internet world, remind oneself at all times what is the actual *purpose* of the use.[43] That is, they must possess a clear ability to distinguish between use that has a purpose (i.e., usage related to study/work) and use that has no purpose (i.e., usage for leisure). In short, they must be able to make the distinction between exchange value and use value.

Or, alternatively, we could say that the person who uses the internet for 10 hours per day at work does so "voluntarily," while the same person who uses the internet for six hours per day for non-work-related purposes does so "involuntarily." The conditioned-reflex model suggests that people become "addicted" to drugs because some mechanism over which they have no control forces them to do so. It implies ultimately that the reasons for using a drug, or now computer game, lie at a level beyond personal knowledge or control because, for example, the "child" is an unripe fruit who lacks the cognitive abilities to resist the bright lights of the internet. For as manager Chen wrote in Letter-1 about the internet: "It is devouring young people's frail mind and body." This particular conceptualization is common among the medical and psychiatric professions in China.

An example is the volunteers who were sent from Qinghai Normal University to offer medical and psychiatric assistance to the mostly Tibetan victims of the devastating April 2010 Jiegu earthquake in Qinghai province. The day after the earthquake volunteers told *China Daily* that some patients were *still* in fear and a few *even* yelled and started crying in their sleep.[44] Liu Lingping, director of the hospital's intensive care unit, attributed these manifest symptoms to their "psychology" being "very weak."[45] The fact is there is nothing weak about a person expressing fear and shedding tears the day after a horrific and tragic event such as a deadly earthquake. Rather, these expressions are simply expectable responses to such an event. That is, they were acting normally under the present social conditions.

This general conceptualization of essentially the "weak" and "vulnerable" child also implies that the user does not have any valuable and valid reasons of his/her own – e.g., that he/she hates going to school and would much prefer to leave. And so while some claim that their child is "unable" to stop playing online games, this in no way proves that he is playing because he cannot control himself, rather he may simply prefer playing to non-playing (i.e., it is more fun, and provides him with a sense of achievement he is unable to find in the "real" world). A good example is Xiao Kang, who was able to stop gaming after slowly tiring of playing and gaining the support, and most importantly trust, of a friend. And thus overnight he put down his mouse and picked up the school books without any kind of physiological "withdrawal symptoms."

And so attributing their son's rebellious and norm-violating behavior to "internet addiction" implies that the son uses the internet because some mechanism over which he has little control forces him to do so, and his subsequent behavioral change is a function of the internet and not of the internet user. It is not taken seriously that the son may have his own reasons that are worth mentioning, for improper internet use is seen as a function of outside forces, and not of the person concerned.[46] This conceptualization of "internet addicts" as naïve "unripe fruit" being subverted by others ('bad friends who don't study') or as a consequence of personal weakness ('introverted personality') and the inability to resist outside pressures ('lacks self control') has arisen because this is the picture both the parents and people like Tao Ran *want to have* – as it serves functions for them both. As Booth Davies summaries this addiction-model function: "Addiction is therefore a conceptual Skinner box, into which drug users are put when they get into trouble."[47] For parents this picture that the child's behavior is not his own to control diverts their own complicity in the production of the deviant child. While for moral entrepreneurs and medical crusaders like Tao Ran and Yang Yongxin, it legitimizes their "intervention" and "treatment" for they present themselves as the science-based professional who has the scientific and medical tools in which to wrestle the dreaded internet addiction from the clutches of the "weak" child. They then use military-style discipline in order to make the child "strong" so that he/she can resist, like the Great Wall, the perceived addictive temptations of the internet. But this explanation overlooks some very basic truths, such as the fact that internet use and gaming is desirable and so they may do so because they *like it*, rather than simply because they are forced into it by outside forces.[48]

Understanding that internet use is desirable directs us to the underlying concern by authority figures, whether they are inside the home, the school, or government departments: *desire is dangerous*. Desire is dangerous simply because it is revolutionary. It is revolutionary in the sense that it can undermine and disrupt the established order of a society, which in the case of internet use is the disrupting, and thus undermining, of the educational order. To skip school for the internet bar is to openly and defiantly declare that I prefer the latter over the former. For it is school, and not online gaming, that they are actually forced into by an outside pressure.[49] Because a desire such as to play online games threatens the established order of society it is then vitally important for society to repress this desire, and even to establish something much more efficient than repression, so that repression, exploitation, hierarchy, and servitude are themselves desired.[50] The "internet addict," in their rejection of school and thus the normal functioning of society, is refusing to play this particular game of desiring their own repression within a pathology of normalcy; rather, they have chosen the search for freedom over conformity. And in order to repress this desire for freedom, society's authority figures need a tool in which to attack and rein in this threat. The internet addiction disorder concept serves this function.

But the internet addiction disorder concept is full of holes. When we look into these holes then it becomes clear that beneath the mask of a diagnostic-based psychiatric model resides the real face. As Thomas Scheff pointed out in the 1960s, "mental disorder" is often a category that observers use to explain norm-violating behavior that they cannot explain by any other culturally accepted or understood category.[51] While Scheff argued psychiatric symptoms are violations of social norms rather than intra-psychic disturbances of individuals, Horwitz, however, shows that while many of the "mental disorders" within the *DSM-IV* do not conform to the *DSM-IV*'s own definition, nevertheless, there are still a number of valid mental disorders that demonstrate internal dysfunctions or intrapsychic disturbances (e.g., schizophrenia and bipolar disorder). "Internet addiction," however, is not one of them.

The empirical data are clear that when the internet user's social condition and lifeworld are taken into account then their internet use does not adhere to the three critical requirements set out by the *DSM-IV*, namely, "1) mental disorders are internal dysfunctions, 2) mental disorders are not expectable responses to particular events, 3) mental disorders must be distinguished from deviant behaviour."[52]

Rather, "internet addiction" is a label that is used not to indicate some kind of intra-psychic disturbance or some underlying mental disease, for as the letters clearly show, according to the parent the child was a "good boy" when he was young, it was only when he came into contact with the internet and some "bad" friends that things turned bad. Likewise, as Tao Hongkai likes to point out, there are "internet addicts" from "good" homes who are considered to be "excellent" and "healthy" students. Moreover, the parents identify a problem not when the child exhibits some kind of intra-psychic disturbance, but rather when his internet use begins to negatively affect his/her school grades. And this may vary from family to family. The benchmark is not the mind and its breakdown, but rather school-grades and their decline.

Thus the so-called "Internet Addiction Disorder" does not meet the two broad criteria; that is, the constellation of symptoms identified to "diagnose" a certain form of internet use does not signify a *valid* mental disorder called "internet addiction." And so using these symptoms to distinguish "internet addiction" from "internet use" does not aid us in establishing distinct causes, prognoses, and treatments for this condition. In fact, quite the opposite, for it leads us further away from understanding the social reality of intensive internet use in contemporary China.

Conclusion: log off

Internet use as a partial answer to existential needs

> Sometimes I wish I had a brother or sister to share my doubts and fears with,
>
> And I wish I had a brother or sister to together ensure our parents' well-being …
>
> And yet on that very sense I feel alone … One is indeed the loneliest number.[1]

Since the concept "internet addiction disorder" is not a valid mental disorder as defined by the *DSM-IV*, then we need to shift the explanatory goal posts in order to make a more appropriate and accurate assessment. I propose that we follow Horwitz's model in helping us understand the underlying mechanisms driving intensive internet use. Horwitz argues that the primary reasons for the emergence of symptoms of distress, which diagnostic psychiatry often mistakenly defines as mental disorders, are the following:

1) *Social phenomena such as acute and chronic stressors* (i.e., parental divorce; death in the family; family violence; parental neglect; external pressure upon school-work).
2) *The strength and quality of social ties* (i.e., high level of distrust; lack of communication; engulfment and depersonalization by parents; lack of social support; absent parent).
3) *The degree of dominance and subordination in relationships* (i.e., being turned into a grade-making machine; filiarchal relations; becoming a tiger/mouse).[2]

I propose when trying to understand the psychology around internet usage to follow Fromm by basing our analysis upon Chinese youth's material, mental, and spiritual needs stemming from the *actual* social conditions of their existence.[3] When we do so we learn that it is the specific conditions of China's modernity, in particular its pathology of normalcy that passes for the normal functioning of society, that forces citizens to find ever-new consumer-based biographical and individual solutions to the social and structural contradictions in their existence. For as Fromm says of "man': "The necessity to find ever-new solutions for the contradictions in his existence, to find ever-higher forms of unity with nature, his fellowmen and himself, is the source of all psychic forces which motivate man, of all his passions, affects and anxieties."[4]

In this way we must therefore ask what role does the internet play in the life of China's youth in helping them find ever-higher forms of unity with nature (i.e., the game *Perfect World*), with their fellow citizens (i.e., relations of "equality" on QQ), and with themselves (i.e., where they can feel good about themselves, and where they can vent out their frustrations). Conversely, we must also ask: are the particular conditions of young people's real-world existence providing for their material, mental, and spiritual needs? That is, is a life of study in a large, and often polluted, segmented, commercialized, atomized, and consumer-driven city fulfilling their needs (and wants)? As Gao Wenbin, a researcher with the Psychology Institute of the Chinese Academy of Sciences, said: "Most children in China are the only ones in their families. They are told only to study hard, but no one really cares about their needs." This is why for him the major contributing factors underpinning excessive internet use is lack of family care, a lack of companions, and a lack of real-life games.[5] Likewise, Professor Yang Xiong argues youth today tend to be more isolated from the community than in the past. For example, those living in new residential complexes are worried about letting their children play outside because they do not consider it safe. The result is often an only-child forced to spend more time at home watching TV or playing on the computer.[6]

While most of today's urban youths have their physiological needs satisfied such satisfactions do not, in any way, solve their *human problems*, for their needs are not those rooted in their body, but are rather rooted in the very peculiarity of their incredibly complex social existence.[7] We may say Chinese youth's *passion* for the internet is partly an attempt to answer their existential needs, and even in certain cases, an attempt to avoid being crushed by life. "I have so many problems," 17-year-old Pang told *China Daily*, "and I have no way to solve them so I get online."[8] Is it accurate to say that Pang gets online simply to escape his many problems, or that getting online is itself an attempt, a last resort even, in finding a solution? This is why "attacking" the intensive gamers body with scientific instruments like electric-shock treatment and medicines is not going to rid them of their "infliction," for their problems are not rooted in their body (and so cannot be extracted from their body), but rather are rooted in their social existence – e.g., their relation to the school system and schoolwork; their relation to their parents (primarily vis-à-vis schoolwork); their relation to social values; their relation to their market-oriented city or town; their relation to the larger culture of excess; their relation – or lack thereof – to peers; their relation – or lack thereof – to spirituality; their relations of mistrust to strangers and even friends; their relation to technology and globalization, etc.

For example, and following on from the fathers who try to turn their son into a "wolf" (or tiger), a Shanghai-based newspaper, the *Xinwen Wubao*, conducted a survey and 90 percent of respondents said that being trusting and honest with strangers would, in most cases, result in a bad situation. Couple this with public signs in cities such as Wuhan that read: "Police Warning: Please do not answer any questions that a stranger asks you. Please beware of frauds," then who can blame youth for looking for alternatives to the so-called normal functioning of society?[9] Intensive internet usage must be understood from this interpersonal position, for the massive and quick embrace of the internet by China's youth is partly the result of a (spiritual) search for answers to their existence and stems from their desire to adhere to dominant social values (i.e., feelings of achievement and success). Unfortunately this is an existence which the "real" world does not necessarily give them the answer to, nor does a satisfactory job in providing them with the tools in which to seek and obtain such answers. This is because the CCP has focused excessively on satisfying their material hunger and not in trying to nourish, so to speak, their souls. Deposed Chongqing's Party Chief Bo Xilai seemingly understood this serious disjunction between material and spiritual security for he said: "Today's youth do not lack food or clothing, yet they need more spiritual nourishment."[10] Internet use is partly a remedy in the sense that it is a strategy to avoid drowning, which is being brought about by excessive schoolwork and a general sense of estrangement. For as "Dong', Tao Ran's ex-patient reportedly said: "My classmates study fifteen hours a day."[11] At which point another of Tao Ran's ex-patient's quickly added: "School is corrupted."[12]

The question we should therefore be asking is: has contemporary Chinese society provided spiritual solutions to the existential problems faced by young people who have grown up in a period of excessive capitalism and materialism? At least their parents had Maoism as a quasi-religious system to provide potential solutions to existential problems, but can neo-liberal State capitalism be utilized by the individual in order to seek solutions to existential problems? As Fromm and Bauman have taught us, obtaining happiness through consumption is ultimately a futile solution. Does not the rapid and excessive rise of Christianity, that has accompanied the same rapid and excessive rise of internet use, tell us that people – in a time of spiritual starvation – desire to seek solutions to their existential problems? For example, in a documentary about the impact of China's rapid social transformation upon the life-world of its citizens, a man with an internet tailoring business commented: "I found that the bible and Christ have all the answers I have been searching for. After being baptized I no longer feel lonely."[13] He believes that contemporary Chinese society is "dirty" and that "China is a country with no beliefs, and there are no role models. All the models are materialistic [and so] being a Christian seems to put a filter on my face and I can breathe through the filter every day." Likewise, the documentary also showed a hotel owner who has observed many of his friends "searching for a sense of spiritual belonging."[14] Similarly, a college student in the US, who was part of a study wherein 200 students were asked to give up all media for one day to observe "signs of withdrawal" from being detached from the internet and their mobile phone said that texting and instant messaging her friends gives her a "constant feeling of comfort."[15] "When I did not have those two luxuries," she continued, "I felt quite alone and secluded from my life."[16] Tao Ran, in a classic example of paternalism, has said that "internet addicts" cannot adjust to school and society, "so they try to escape their difficulties and avoid problems. They lack self-confidence and often don't have the courage to continue their lives."[17] Not only does Tao Ran wash over the pathology of normalcy that is the so-called normal functioning of school and society, but, in addition, he does not seemingly understand that far from escaping their difficulties and avoiding their real-world problems they are, on the contrary, using the virtual world in order to seek answers and solutions to their social and existential problems.

In this sense we must make an existential and structural connection to the mass migration to the internet, and in particular the desire to play so-called violent video games, and the spate of school stabbings that have occurred in China between March and May of 2010. At least six separate deadly stabbing attacks on kindergarten and primary school children understandably caused widespread concern over school safety and prompted analysts to explore deeper social implications beyond the CCP's political strategy of trying to reduce the killings to a few mentally disordered individuals. While Zhou Xiaozheng of Beijing's Renmin University overlaid a simplistic biomedical interpretation upon the killings by claiming the killers had "contracted a social psychological infectious disease" that then expressed itself in a desire to take revenge on society,[18] a more material understanding demonstrates more empirical sense. For example, one killer (Zheng Minsheng) had been jobless since June of 2009, another (Chen Kangbing) had been jobless since 2006, while yet another (Xu Yuyuan) had not found stable work since 2001, and so they are the kind of people whom are regarded as a *nobody* in a materialistic society.[19] In the search for social factors underlying these killings of innocent children, people put forth the possibility that these middle-aged men were seeking "revenge" on society because there are no social pressure valves, including the judicial system and civil society, where they can vent their growing anger against widespread social injustice. While one of the killers had a history of "mental illness" three others had a history of petitioning the government offices to address grievances without result. "Individuals took revenge against the whole of society," argued Geng Shen, an educator at the Beijing Academy of Educational Sciences, "because they cannot adapt to the fast social development and transformation, and their psychological needs are not taken good care of." Thus innocent children have become the most vulnerable victims of those seeking to release their anger and vent frustrations in a society that has inadequate effective relief mechanisms.

Others have pointed to the widening social chasm in which the gap between rich and poor is increasing rapidly and where the CCP has an excess monopoly on power over natural and social resources, which they violate with impunity as they do civil, human, and religious rights. Thus some writers argue that the CCP must realize that mainstream religions can provide much-needed spiritual comfort and guidance to tens of millions of people disillusioned by the rapid social changes sweeping China and its citizens.[20] This is because, as psychiatrist Lan Feng, pointed out, "The pressures of business and getting ahead in the new economy had altered the "balance" in Chinese society."[21] Do not all the actions of these killers adhere to Fromm's maxim that *domination and destruction is the*

184 *Conclusion: log off*

outcome of a thwarted life? Moreover, as I have argued, individuals are forced to seek biographical consumer-based solutions to social problems brought about from living in a world-out-balance. Understanding this, one understands the important function online games provide in allowing frustrated and angry youths (*fenqing*) to *fa xie* (give vent to) such feelings. That is, it partly provides for their psychological needs stemming from their social existence.

In this way we are not referring to a sick individual but rather a *sick* society that is not able to nourish the needs of the individual. As highlighted earlier, a "sane society," according to Fromm, would promote individual development and democratic self-expression within the context of an active and vibrant communal life. To do this, however, individual communities, cities, and society as a whole, must find ways to address certain universal human needs, including needs for 1) relatedness, 2) transcendence, 3) rootedness, 4) a sense of identity and 5) a framework of orientation and devotion. Has the CCP created a society to address these needs? To the extent that these existential needs go begging, or are inadequately met, states Fromm, the majority of people who adapt effectively to prevailing cultural norms and expectations partake in a "pathology of normalcy" which passes for health, but is really a kind of pseudo-sanity. Fromm also points out that the pathology of normalcy is embedded in the prevailing "social character." So that what is considered "normal" in contemporary China, that is, the "normal" market-oriented social character of the child who does little else but study from morning until night, is in fact really "pathological" because the whole social structure – that is, the relation between individual and society – is severely out-of-balance.

In the wake of this tragic spate of school stabbings, concerned citizens have been questioning the sanity of their social system. "*China is sick,*" well-known journalist and blogger Zhang Wen wrote echoing Fromm. For Zhang, China's pathology of normalcy – its sickness – consists of the following characteristics:

a) Life is getting faster, stress and pressure are building up, and the future is unclear.
b) People are worried about themselves and their own families, all the while gradually losing compassion towards others.
c) A one-sided emphasis on economic development has led millions on a single-minded quest for wealth and so the law of the jungle has entered into people's hearts.
d) The weak are food for the strong, and fairness and justice are in short supply.
e) Social classes are dividing and dissolving into opposition.
f) Relationships are mostly based on acquiring personal benefits and people no longer believe in traditions of mutual help and friendship.
g) Moral quality has degenerated because the ideas of Confucius, Mencius and Zhuangzi have been damaged almost beyond repair.
h) Popular expectations are outpacing changes in the social system, and in their confusion people have no faith to comfort them.

Zhang concludes by saying: "China is currently in a void." [22] What he is saying is that contemporary Chinese society has moved dramatically away from Fromm's conception of a sane society. Thus Zhang Wen is describing a social structure in which

1) There has been the break-down of *relatedness* between persons due to a single-minded quest for wealth and power.

2) Individuals find it difficult to *transcend* the separateness and aloneness of their individual existence.

3) Where people cannot experience *rootedness* because the hurried nature of the treadmill they are on is moving so fast.

4) Where *a sense of identity* has to be pieced together by fragments because of traditional moral and spiritual universes have been eroded by 'socialism' and market forces.

5) Where one is taught to *orient* and *devote* themselves to what Zhang Wen calls a law of the jungle ethic in which competing ferociously has become a necessity and normal part of living.

Only by understanding the *pathological* nature of the so-called normal functioning of contemporary society does the mass migration to the internet in general, and online games in particular, begin to make sense. Since it is the pathology of normalcy that is leaving them potentially separate, rootless, frustrated, fragmented, confused, and uncomfortable, then a (cyber)space which seemingly offers relatedness to others, the transcendence of aloneness and separateness, a sense of rootedness, orientation, comfort, and even spiritual nourishment is going to become *intensely* sought after. When we hear of an "addiction" to the internet, what we should really be asking is: why are millions of young people so *devoted* to this technological device? Let us now re-boot the discourse and begin from here.

Notes

Introduction: turn on

1 Taken from the documentary *"War with the Internet Demon"* (战网魔), which aired on the State-run CCTV-12 extolling the virtues of using electric-shock treatment to "cure" internet addiction. Go to: http://v.youku.com/v_show/id_XOD k3MT kwMDQ=.html.

2 The concept "lifeworld" is not used in the sense of an internal subjective viewpoint, but rather: a) in the way in which the world is experienced and lived (Husserl's being in the world), and b) as living with one another in the world ("living together"), and c) living within social structures and institutions ("living socially"). Thus we could say: lifeworld = intra-/inter- /extra-personal relations and lived human experience.

3 Letter written by an "internet addict" to his parents. The letter was then sent to Mr. Tao Hongkai by the mother, wherein I was given access to it. After being translated, the letter was edited slightly, but the main contents and argument presented by the son have not been altered or distorted in any way. Like all the names in the letters that follow, the young man was given a pseudonym.

4 Laing, R.D. *Self and Others* (London: Tavistock Publications, 1969, 82).

5 Ibid.

6 "Boy, 10, chained at home," *South China Morning Post*, July 20, 2010, A6.

7 The clip can be viewed at the following site: http://www.tudou.com/programs/view/ DuEm9G5QA Hg/.

8 现实中太多不公平的事情.

9 Ding Gang, "Lost Souls Falling Through Fast Social Change," *Global Times*, September 10, 2009, 9.

10 Filiarchy can de defined as children making family choices and decisions, as opposed to matriarchal-centered or patriarchal-centered decision-making mechanisms.

11 Fromm, Erich, *The Fear of Freedom* (London: Routledge & Kegan Paul, 1942, 158).

12 Derrida, Jacques, "The Rhetoric of Drugs." *High Culture: Reflections on Addiction and Modernity*. In: Anna Alexander and Mark S. Roberts, (eds.) (Albany: State University of New York Press, 2003, 19–43).

13 Beck, Ulrich, and Elisabeth Beck-Gernsheim, *Individualization: Institutionalized Individualism and Its Social and Political Consequences* (London: Sage, 2002, xxii).

14 Hewett, Duncan, *Getting Rich First: Life in a Changing China* (London: Chatto & Windus, 2007, 227).

15 Tai Zixue, *The Internet in China: Cyberspace and Civil Society* (New York: Routledge, 2006, 287).

16 See Yang Guobin, *The Power of the Internet in China: Citizens Activism Online* (New York: Columbia University Press, 2009).

1 Log in

1 Jia, Zhangke. 2005. "The World of Jia Zhangke. An Interview by Patrica R.S. Batto." In: *China Perspectives,* No. 60, (July–August), 46–50.

2 Ibid.

3 Connell, Robert W. *Masculinities* (Berkely, Los Angeles: University of California Press, 1995).

4 Burawoy, Michael. *The Politics of Production: Factory Regimes Under Capitalism and Socialism* (London: Verso, 1985).

5 I met Renfei when working for a private school teaching English in the city of Dalian, 2004–2005. Renfei was born in 1983 in the city of Anshan, but has been living in Dalian since 2002.

6 Turkle, Sherry *Life on the Screen: Identity in the Age of the Internet* (London: Weidenfeld & Nicolson, 1996).

7 Colebrook, Claire. *Gilles Deleuze* (London; New York: Routledge, 2002).

8 We were living in Renfei's now ex-girlfriend's mother's apartment, which because it was surrounded by three universities had a large concentration of internet bars.

9 This song is aptly titled "free to fly" (*ziyou feixiang*自由飞翔) by the group Phoenix Legend (*fenghuang chuanqi* 凤凰传奇). The fact is the frontier is one of the dominant metaphors for describing cyberspace, which is, as Tim Jordan remarked, to take a form of communication and conceive of it as space. *Perfect World* is the utopian frontier. See; Jordan, Tim, *Cyberpower: The Culture and Politics of Cyberspace and the Internet* (London; New York: Routledge, 1999, 176).

10 QQ was the most popular free instant messaging computer program in Mainland China. In addition to the chat program, QQ had also developed many sub-features including games, virtual pets, ringtone downloads, etc.

11 Kipnis, Andrew B. 2011. *Governing Educational Desire: Culture, Politics and Schooling in China*. University of Chicago Press: Chicago.

12 Fia Curley, *Detox Clinic Opening for Video Addicts* (http://www.breitbart.com/article.php?id=D8I489R80&show _article=1 – Accessed on June 3, 2008).

13 Maguire, Paddy, "Compulsive Gamers not 'Addicts'," BBC News, November 25, 2008 (http://news.bbc.co.uk/1/hi/ technology/7746471.stm – accessed November 26, 2008).

14 Adams, Jonathan, "In an Increasingly Wired China, Rehab for Internet Addicts," *The Christian Science Monitor*, January 6, 2009 (http://www.csmonitor.com/2009/0106/p01s03-woap.html – accessed January 7, 2009).

15 "Internet Addiction, Should it be Regarded as a Mental Disorder?" *Focus Point* (Anhui TV).

16 Zan Jiefang, "Hooked on Cyberspace. Chinese Psychologists Outline Criteria for Internet Addiction," *Beijing Review*, December 16, 2008 (http://www.bjreview.com.cn/health/txt/200812/16/content_170181.htm – accessed December 22, 2008).

17 Fia Curley, *Detox Clinic Opening for Video Addicts* (http://www.breitbart.com/article.php?id=D8I489R80&show _article=1 – Accessed on June 3, 2008).

18 望子成龙.

19 教子成龙. See the following clip on video sharing site *Tudou* for his general theory and method: http://www.tudou.com/ programs/view/DuEm9G5QAHg/

20 I was one of three foreigners accompanying Tao Hongkai. One was a graduate student from Oxford also writing on internet addiction. The other was an American law student who was interested in the topic and in helping both Tao Hongkai and the families involved.

21 Virilio, Paul, and Sylvère Lotringer. *Pure War*, Translated by Mark Poizzotti (New York: Semiotext(e), 1983, 82).

22 See, Macartney, Jane, "In God They Trust," *Post Magazine*, [date unknown] 2009, 14–17.

23 Lucrative in the sense that while I was there the base had 70 students paying approximately 6,500 yuan per person per month. That equates to 455,000 yuan gross income for that month. 800 had already passed through the base altogether since opening in 2007, and so a conservative estimate (6,500 × 800) tells us that it has received in excess of 5 million yuan in about two years of operating.

24 The answer, I believe, is because it deflects attention away from structural problems created by the Party-State, thus "hiding" the problem within individual minds.

25 Callinicos, Alex. *The Revolutionary Ideas of Karl Marx* (London: Bookmarks, 1983, 92).

26 Ibid, 114.

27 天下父母.

28 现生产，后生活. From; Mao Zedong, *Quotations from Mao Tse-Tung* (Peking: Foreign Languages Press, 1967).

29 For example, after one-and-a-half months the students can write a letter to their parents, at two months they are allowed to ring them on the phone, and at two-and-a-half months they can see them in person.

30 Chan, Anita, "The culture of Survival: Lives of Migrant Workers through the Prism of Private Letters." In: Perry Link, Richard P. Madsen, and Paul G. Pickowicz, (eds.), *Popular China: Unofficial Culture in a Globalizing Society* (Lanham: Rowman & Littlefield Publishers, 2002, 164).

31 If anything, the level of anxiousness and desperation may often be heightened for effect in order to grab Tao Hongkai's attention. But this is merely a matter of degree. Coming face-to-face with such parents gives a clear picture of their very real feelings of desperation and despondency.

32 Laing, R.D. *The Divided Self: An Existential Study of Sanity and Madness* (Harmondsworth: Penguin Books, 1965).

33 Horwitz, Allan V., *Creating Mental Illness* (Chicago; London: University of Chicago Press, 2002, 18). They are mistakenly classified as a mental disorder because deviant behavior stemming from chronic stressors are often an expectable response to a stress condition and/or conflicts that are primarily between the individual and society and so do not adhere to the *DSM-IV*'s definition of a mental disorder.

34 Kleinman, Arthur, *The Illness Narrative: Suffering, Healing, & the Human Condition* (New York: Basic Books, 1988, 49).

35 Chan, Anita, "The Culture of Survival: Lives of Migrant Workers through the Prism of Private Letters." In: *Popular China: Unofficial Culture in a Globalizing Society* 2002, 164.

2   The Internet Addiction Disorder

1 Electronic opium or electronic heroin is a commonly used term to derisively describe young people's attraction to digital media, in particular the internet. The underlying message is that, like the opium imported by the British into China in the nineteenth century, the 'West' is now bombarding Chinese citizens with online games which "enslave" youth. One mother even reportedly described the popular Taiwanese TV drama "*Meteor Garden*" as electronic heroin, claiming it had made her daughter become "weird" and "crazy" (Hewett, Duncan, *Getting Rich First: Life in a Changing China*. 2007, 161). We must understand this term not for its pseudo-attempt to link internet use to biomedical addiction, but rather to moral conduct. The term is not in the service of medicine or psychiatry but instead to social control and the policing of moral boundaries.

2 Tao Ran, *et al. Analysis and Intervention of Internet Addiction* (Shanghai: Shanghai People's Publishers, 2007, 165).

3 Cha, Ariana Eunjung, "In China, Stern Treatment for Young Internet 'Addicts'," *Washington Post* (http://www.washingtonpost.com/wp-dyn/content/article/2007/02/21/AR2007022102094_3.html – accessed November 13th, 2008).

4 Taken from, Virilio, Paul, and Sylvère Lotringer. *Pure War*. Translated by Mark Poizzotti (New York: Semiotext (e), 1983, 82).
5 Sun Zi, *The Art of War* (Beijing: Foreign Languages Press, 2007, 9).
6 As Robin Munro has extensively documented, addiction treatment centers throughout China such as Tao Ran's have a very dark history in persecuting political and social deviants under the guise of "addiction." See, Munro, Robin, *Dangerous Minds: Political Psychiatry Today and Its Origin in the Mao Era* (New York: Human Rights Watch; Hilversum, The Netherlands: Geneva Initiative on Psychiatry, 2002, 161).
7 Cha, Ariana Eunjung, "In China, Stern Treatment for Young Internet 'Addicts'," *Washington Post* (http://www.washing tonpost.com/wp-dyn/content/article/2007/02/21/AR2007022102094_3.html – accessed November 13th, 2008).
8 Ibid.
9 Reuters, "Game Over for China's Net Addicts," *China Daily*, December 3, 2007 (http://www.chinadaily.com.cn/china/2007-03/12/content_825231.htm – accessed Dec 16, 2008).
10 Lin-Liu, Jennifer, "China's e-Junkies Head for Rehab," *IEEE Spectrum*, February, 2006 (http://ieeexplore.ieee.org/stamp/stamp.jsp?arnumber=1584358&isnumber=33435 – accessed June 12, 2008). One does wonder, however, of the internet bar owner's role in this hibernation, and how the patient paid for six months of internet use at probably 1 yuan per hour (theoretically 4,368 yuan), and of how he sustained himself nutritionally.
11 For the case of Hu Ange, see "Man Poisons His Family Over Game Addiction," *BBGSITE@com*, November 17, 2008 (http://news.bbgsite.com/content/2008-11-16/20081116082600795.shtml – accessed December 23, 2008).
12 A copy of this TV show was given to me in disc form by Tao Hongkai, who was a fellow panelist on the show.
13 "Teenager Sells Family Car to Fuel Internet Addiction," *China Daily*, January 12, 2009, 5.
14 Reuters, "Online Addict Dies After Marathon Session," *Reuters*, February 28, 2007 (http://www.reuters.com/article/ idUSPEK26772020070228 – accessed March 4, 2008).
15 Ji Beibei, "'High-Pressure' Huawei Sets Up In-House Health Center," *Global Times*, June 19, 2009, 5.
16 Liu Xin, Alice, "Internet Addict Swallows Steel Saw Blade," *Danwei.org*, January 9, 2009 (http://www. danwei.org/– accessed January 9, 2009). Original article, 郝涛, 贾儒, "网瘾男子吞下钢锯条 术后仍念叨网游词语," 北京晨报, January 9, 2009 (http://news.xinhuanet.com/internet/2009-01/06/content_10607845.htm – accessed January 9, 2009).
17 See Lai Chloe, "Foxconn Deaths Spur Boycott of New iPhone," *South China Morning Post*, May 25, 2010, 2.
18 "China Statistics and Related Data Information Links," *China Today* (http://www.chinatoday.com/data/data.htm – accessed November 4, 2009).
19 Xinhua, "Road Accidents Kill Over 15,000 in the First Quarter," China Daily, May 4, 2009 (http://www.chinadaily.com.cn/china/2009-04/05/content_7650094.htm– accessed November 4, 2009).
20 Cohen, Stanley, *Folk Devils and Moral Panics: The Creation of the Mods and Rockers* (Oxford: Blackwell Publishers, 1987).
21 The numbers of traffic accidents and deaths on the road is annually published by the main police journal (*gongan yanjiu*).
22 Taken from Anhui TV's *Focus Point* – 焦点.
23 Tao Ran, and many others, often flip-flop between the differing terms mental disorder – *jingshen bing* 精神病 – and mental disease – *jingshen jibing* 精神疾病.
24 See Adams, Jonathan, "In an Increasingly Wired China, Rehab for Internet Addicts," *The Christian Science Monitor*, January 6, 2009 (http://www.csmonitor.com/2009/0106/p01s03-woap.html – accessed January 7, 2009).

25 Tao Ran, *et al. Analysis and Intervention of Internet Addiction* (Shanghai: Shanghai People's Publishers, 2007, 165).

26 Wu Zengqiang and Zhang Jianguo, *Prevention and Intervention of Adolescent Internet Addiction* (Shanghai: Shanghai Education Publishers, 2008, 14). 吴增强,张建国, "青少年网络成瘾:预防与干预" (上海: 上海教育出版社, 2007, 5).

27 Ibid, 6.

28 "China's Hu vows to 'purify' Internet," *OpenNet Initiative* (http://opennet.net/blog/2007/02/chinas-hu-vows-purify-internet-reuters – accessed January 29, 2010).

29 This documentary was originally made for a TV station in Henan, yet before airing it they let Tao Hongkai, who also briefly appeared on the program, to view it. Being opposed to *Tao Ran's* biomedical method and what he considers harsh and cruel treatment of Tao Ran's patients, Tao Hongkai told them that they should not air this as it is a terrible portrayal of the way authority figures are treating Chinese youth and so the TV channel will be heavily criticized. So it was never aired.

30 Tao Ran, *et al. Analysis and Intervention of Internet Addiction* (Shanghai: Shanghai People's Publishers, 2007). Tao Ran, Ying Li, Yue Shaodong, and Hao Xianghong. *Wang Luo Cheng Yin Tan Xi Yu Gan Yu Zhu* (Shanghai Shi: Shanghai Ren Min Chu Ban she). 陶然等，网络成瘾探析与干预 （上海市: 上海人民出版社, 2007, 165）.

31 See, http://www.psychologistanywhereanytime.com/famous_psychologist_and_psychologists/psychologist _famous_r_d_lang.htm – accessed October 8, 2009).

32 Griffiths, Mark D. "Video Games and Health: Video Gaming is Safe for Most Players and Can be Useful in Health Care," *British Medical Journal*, 331, (7509), 2005, 122–123.

33 Told to me during a personal conversation with Tao Hongkai. However, Tao Hongkai also retold this story, to Tao Ran directly, on the *Focus Point* program mentioned earlier.

34 Ibid. Moreover, I was told by an educator in Beijing – who works with families dealing with problems around internet use – that she had heard recently of two cases where the son who had been sent to a Tao Ran-style clinic attacked the father with a knife after he returned home.

35 We should not be too surprised to learn of Tao Ran's methods, as psychiatric hospitals in China – the infamous *Ankang* facilities – are known for using such torture-based methods upon deviants. For example, Robin Munro has shown an almost identical method of "treatment" handed out to *falun gong* practitioners. Detained practitioners have repeatedly reported being drugged with various unknown kinds of medication, tied with ropes to hospital beds or put under other forms of physical restraint, kept in dark hospital rooms for long periods, subjected to electro-convulsive therapy or painful forms of electrical acupuncture treatment, denied adequate food and water and forced to write confessional statements renouncing their belief in *falun gong* as a precondition of their eventual release. Munro, Robin, *Dangerous Minds: Political Psychiatry Today and Its Origin in the Mao Era*, 2002, 161.

36 He told me this while we were filming a TV show with *Tao Hongkai* in Wuhan.

37 On Anhui TV's *Focus Point* program (*Jiao Dian* 焦点). Italics added.

38 Grüsser, Sabine M., Ralk Thalemann, and Mark D. Griffiths, "Excessive Computer Game Playing: Evidence for Addiction and Aggression?" *CyberPsychology & Behavior*, Vol. 10, (2), 2007, 290–292.

39 Kutner, Lawrence, and Cherly K. Olsen, *Grand Theft Childhood: The Surprising Truth About Video Games and What Parents Can Do* (New York: Simon & Schuster, 2008, 102).

40 This figure is reported to have come from Shang Xiuyun, a Beijing judge who specializes in juvenile crime, which was cited in a paper by Liu Guiming, deputy secretary-general of the Chinese Society of Juvenile Delinquency Research. See "Juvenile Crime on Rise in China," *The Sunday Times*, December 6, 2007 (http://

www.asiaone.com/News/AsiaOne+News/Asia/Story/A1Story20071206-39928.html – accessed May 21, 2009).

41 Ibid. Incomplete social management is a veiled reference to the failures of the Party-State after retreating from the private lives of individuals and families and basically turning them over to the market.

42 According to Howard Becker, a moral entrepreneur, who is generally a person who seeks to influence others to enforce and/or create a norm, may be driven by factors such as genuine altruism or selfishness (or even both simultaneously). See, Becker, Howard, *Outsiders: Studies in the Sociology of Deviance* (New York: The Free Press of Glencoe, Inc, 1973, 147–153).

43 Conrad, Peter, and Joseph W. Schneider, *Deviance and Medicalization: From Badness to Sickness* (Philadelphia: Temple University Press, 1992). For moral entrepreneur see, Becker, Howard S. *Outsiders: Studies in the Sociology of Deviance* (New York: The Free Press of Glencoe, Inc, 1973).

44 Conrad, Peter, and Joseph W. Schneider, *Deviance and Medicalization: From Badness to Sickness*, 1992.

45 Ibid.

46 Jiang, Jessie, "Inside China's Fight Against Internet Addiction," *Time*, January 8, 2009 (http://www.time.com/time/world/article/0,8599,1874380,00.html – accessed January 18, 2009).

47 Ibid.

48 Kong, Linmeng, "Expert: Internet Addiction, Is It a Kind of Mental Illness?" [专家：网络成瘾，是不是一种精神疾病] *Ifengwo.com*, November 17, 2008 (http://www.ifengwo.com/xinwenzhongxin/hulianwang /200811/1719362.html#digg1 – accessed January 12, 2009). Italics added for emphasis.

49 Ibid.

50 Chappell, Darren, Virginia Eatough, Mark N. O. Davies and Mark Griffiths, "*EverQuest*-It's Just a Computer Game Right? An Interpretative Phenomenological Analysis of Online Gaming Addiction," *International Journal of Mental Health and Addiction*, Volume 4, (3), 2006, 205–216.

51 Reuters, "Game Over for China's Net Addicts,' *China Daily*, December 3, 2007 (http://www.chinadaily.com.cn/china/2007-03/12/content_825231.htm – accessed December 16, 2008).

52 Jenks, Chris, *Transgression* (London: Routledge, 2003, 25).

53 Tao Ran, Huang Xiu-qin, Yao Sumin, *et al.* "Analysis on the Epidemiology of 607 Inpatients with Internet Addiction Disorder," *China Journal of Epidemiology*, May, 2007, Vol. 28, (5), 519.

54 Adams, Jonathan, "In an Increasingly Wired China, Rehab for Internet Addicts," *The Christian Science Monitor*, January 6, 2009 (http://www.csmonitor.com/2009/0106/p01s03-woap.html – accessed January 7, 2009).

55 Virilio, Paul, and Sylvère Lotringer. *Pure War*, 1983, 82.

56 Castells, Manuel, *The Information Age: Economy, Society and Culture Volume II The Power of Identity* (Oxford: Blackwell Publishers, 1997, 125).

57 Virilio, Paul, and Sylvère Lotringer. *Pure War*, 1983, 99.

58 Tai Zixue, *The Internet in China: Cyberspace and Civil Society*, 2006, 170.

59 Virilio, Paul, *The Lost Dimension*. Translated by Daniel Moshenberg (New York: Semiotext(e), 1991, 15).

60 Kong, Linmeng, "Expert: Internet Addiction, Is It a Kind of Mental Illness?" (专家：网络成瘾，是不是一种精神疾病) *Ifengwo.com*, November 17, 2008 (http://www.ifengwo.com/xinwenzhongxin/hulianwang/200811/1719362.html#digg1 – accessed January 12, 2009).

61 Liu, Irene Jay, and Fox Yi Hui, "At Foxconn, Success and Tragedy Linked," *South China Morning Post*, June 1, 2010, 1.

62 Ibid.

63 Vause, John, "Inside China Factory Hit by Suicides," *CNN*, June 1, 2010 (http://edition. cnn.com/2010/WORLD/asiapc f/06/01/china.foxconn.inside.factory/index.html?hpt=C2 – accessed June 2, 2010).

64 Funk, McKenzie, "I Was a Chinese Internet Addict," *Harper's Magazine*, March 2007, Vol. 314 (1882), 65.

65 Taken from the infamous sign above the main gate at the Auschwitz concentration camp.

66 Elias, Norbert, and Eric Dunning, "The Quest for Excitement in Leisure." In; Elias, Norbert, and Eric Dunning, *Quest for Excitement: Sport and Leisure in the Civilizing Process* (Oxford: Blackwell, 1986, 67).

67 Fromm, Erich, *The Sane Society* (New York: Holt, Rinehart and Winston, 1955, 144).

68 Davis, Rowenna, "Game Overload," *South China Morning Post*, March 11, 2009, C1.

69 As one gold farmer put it: "The working conditions are hard. We don't get weekends off and I only have one day free a month." Ibid.

70 Said a professional gamer at the national finals of the World Cyber Games in Shanghai in August of 2009.

71 Sun Uking, "Chinese Society Mobilized for Gaokao Battle," *China Daily*, June 4, 2010 (http://www.chinadaily.com.cn/china/2010-06/04/content_9935778.htm – accessed June 5, 2010). See also; LaFraniere, Sharon, "China College Entry Test Is an Obsession," *The New York Times*, June 12, 2009 (http://www.nytimes.com/2009/06/13/world/ asia/13exam.html?ref=global-home – accessed June 13, 2009).

72 Tao Ran, Huang Xiuqin, Wang Jinan, Zhang Huimin, Zhang Ying, and Li Mengchen, "Proposed Diagnostic Criteria for Internet Addiction," *Addiction*, Vol. 105 (3), 2010, 556–564. Bold type added for emphasis.

73 Ibid.

74 Young, Kimberly S. *Caught in the Net: How to Recognize the Signs of Internet Addiction – And a Winning Strategy for Recovery* (New York: John Wiley& Sons, Inc, 1998, 4).

75 Ibid, 23.

76 Ibid, 21.

77 Ibid, 44.

78 Ibid, 9–10.

79 Cover, Rob, "Gaming (Ad)diction: Discourse, Identity, Time and Play in the Production of the Gamer Addiction Myth," *Game Studies*, Vol. 6, (1), 2006 (http://gamestudies. org/0601/articles/cover – accessed February 25, 2008).

80 Young, Kimberly S. *Caught in the Net: How to Recognize the Signs of Internet Addiction – And a Winning Strategy for Recovery*, 1998, 4.

81 Ibid, 13.

82 Ibid, 23, 13, 61 (respectively).

83 Ibid, 8.

84 Ibid, 32. Italics added.

85 Ibid, 4. I have altered the order of the question slightly so as to fit Tao Ran's list.

86 Ibid, 5. Italics added.

87 These response rates, which they reduced to calling merely "symptoms," are as follows: Symptom 1: 96.4 percent; Symptom 2: 95.5 percent; Symptom 3: 86.4 percent; Symptom 4: 83.6 percent; Symptom 5: 82.7 percent; Symptom 6: 82.7 percent; Symptom 7: 72.7 percent; Symptom 8: 48.2 percent. Altogether they average 81 percent, basically identical to Young.

88 Young, Kimberly S. *Caught in the Net: How to Recognize the Signs of Internet Addiction – And a Winning Strategy for Recovery*, 1998, 16.

3 Critiques of the Internet Addiction Disorder model

1 Wood, Richard T. A. "Problems With the Concept of Video Game "Addiction": Some Case Study Examples," *International Journal of Mental Health and Addiction*, Vol. 6, (2), 2008, 169–78.

2 Kong, Linmeng, "Expert: Internet Addiction, Is It a Kind of Mental Illness?" (专家：网络成瘾，是不是一种精神疾病) *Ifengwo.com*, November 17, 2008 (http://www.ifengwo.com/xinwenzhongxin/hulian wang /200811/17-19362.html#digg1 – accessed January 12, 2009).
3 Ibid.
4 See http://www.searo.who.int/en/Section1174/Section1199/Section1567/Section1827_8056.htm – accessed October 13, 2009).
5 See http://apps.who.int/classifications/apps/icd/icd10online/ – accessed October 13, 2009).
6 Golub, Alex, and Kate Lingley, "'Just Like in the Qing Empire': Internet Addiction, MMOGs, and Moral Crisis in Contemporary China," *Games and Culture*, Vol. 3, (1), 2008, 59–74.
7 Ibid, 64. For original see, Tian Bingxin, "Zhang Chunliang: Damned Internet Games," *Southcn.com*, January 2, 2005 (http://www.southcn.com/nfsq/ywhc/tbxst/shentan/200510260380.htm – accessed June 4, 2010).
8 Ibid.
9 Kohn, Livia, *Daoism Handbook* (Boston; Leiden: Brill, 2004, 825).
10 Kirkland, Russell, *Taoism: The Enduring Tradition* (New York: Routledge, 2004, 60).
11 Sun, Hualin, *Internet Policy and Use: A Field Study of Internet Cafes in China.* (PhD Thesis, The Florida State University. E-thesis. 2004, 102).
12 Ibid, 103.
13 Ibid.
14 See, Walter, Glenn D. *The Addiction Concept: Working Hypothesis or self-fulfilling Prophesy?* (Boston: Allyn & Bacon, 1999).
15 "Troubled Teen Survives Jump to Expose Boot Camp," *YNET.com*, June 7, 2008 (http://bjtoday.ynet.com/article.jsp? oid=21243835&pageno=4 – accessed April 28, 2009).
16 Dan Chongshan, "The Death of the Internet Addict Youth Deng Senshen, *Southern Metropolis Weekly*, August 14, 2009. English translation by *EastSouthWestNorth* (http://www.zonaeuropa.com/20090826_ 1.htm – accessed August 26, 2009).
17 Zygmunt Bauman (*Consuming Life*, 2007) uses the Stephen Bertman coined term "nowist culture" as a way to grasp the nature of the liquid modern phenomenon of consumerism, in particular, the way consumerism has enacted a *renegotiation of the meaning of time* in the sense that social behavior has become centered around the (power of) now and upon instant gratification (see Bertman, *Hyperculture: The Human Cost of Speed*, 1998). I would argue that this nowist culture is important not only for understanding the "causes" of excessive or intensive internet use among Chinese youth but also for understanding the parent's conceptualization of reducing and/or eliminating the child's use of the internet for pleasure and fun by seeking the service-based quick-fix solutions offered by the boot camps.
18 Stewart, Christopher S. "Obsessed With the Internet: A Tale From China," *Wired*, January 13, 2010 (http://www.wired.com/magazine/2010/01/ff_internetaddiction/all/1 – accessed May 31, 2010).
19 The term *biopsychosocial* comes from medical anthropologist Arthur Kleinman (see *The Illness Narrative: Suffering, Healing, & the Human Condition*, 1988, 6) who directs us to conceive of illness as a conjunction between body, self, and society, and so the production of illness is for Kleinman a dialectic between cardiovascular processes, psychological states, and environmental situations. The term "biopsychosocial" is an appropriate term in which to frame "inappropriate" internet usage for the activity involves body, self, and society, or the interrelation between them. That is, it is connected to the most acute physiological processes of the body and the macro processes of government policy, State ideology, market principles, urbanization, etc.
20 See, Charlton, John P. "A Factor-Analytic Investigation of Computer 'Addiction' and Engagement," *British Journal of Psychology*, 93, (3) 2002, 329–344. And, Charlton, John P.,

and Danforth, Ian D. W. "Distinguishing Addiction and High Engagement in the Context of Online Game Playing," *Computers in Human Behavior, 23*(3), 2007, 1531–1548.

21 In contrast, Wood says the "core" criteria relating to measuring addiction are often around issues of conflict, withdrawal symptoms, and relapse.

22 See, Wood, Richard T. A., and Griffiths, Mark D. "A Qualitative Investigation of Problem Gambling as an Escape-Based Coping Strategy." *Psychology and Psychotherapy: Theory, Research and Practise,* 80 (1), 2007, 107–125.

23 Turner, Nigel E. "A Comment on 'Problems with the Concept of Video Game *Addiction*: Some Case Study Examples'," *International Journal of Mental Health and Addiction*, Vol. 6, (2), 2008, 186–190.

24 Chappell, Darren, Virginia Eatough, Mark N. O. Davies and Mark Griffiths, "*EverQuest*-It's Just a Computer Game Right? An Interpretative Phenomenological Analysis of Online Gaming Addiction," *International Journal of Mental Health and Addiction*, Volume 4, (3), 2006, 205–216.

25 Blaszczynski, Alex, "Commentary: A Response to "Problems with the Concept of Video Game "Addiction": Some Case Study Examples," *International Journal of Mental Health and Addiction*, Vol. 6, (2), 2008, 179–181.

26 Laing, R.D. *The Politics of Experience, and, The Bird of Paradise* (Harmondsworth: Penguin, 1967).

27 Hofmann, Albert, *LSD: My Problem Child: Reflections on Sacred Drugs* (Los Angeles: J.P. Tarcher, 1983, 17–18).

28 Chappell, Darren, Virginia Eatough, Mark N. O. Davies and Mark Griffiths, "*EverQuest*—It's Just a Computer Game Right? An Interpretative Phenomenological Analysis of Online Gaming Addiction," *International Journal of Mental Health and Addiction*, Volume 4, (3), 2006, 205–216.

29 Cover, Rob, "Gaming (Ad)diction: Discourse, Identity, Time and Play in the Production of the Gamer Addiction Myth," *Game Studies*, Vol. 6, (1), 2006 (http://gamestudies. org/0601/articles/cover – accessed February 25, 2008).

30 Ng, Brian D. and Peter Wiemer-Hastings, "Addiction to the Internet and Online Gaming," *CyberPsychology & Behavior*, 8, (2), 2005, 110–113.

31 Kong, Linmeng, "Expert: Internet Addiction, Is It a Kind of Mental Illness?" [专家：网络成瘾，是不是一种精神疾病] *Ifengwo.com*, November 17, 2008 (http://www. ifengwo.com/xinwenzhongxin/hulian wang /200811/1719362. html#digg1 – accessed January 12, 2009).

32 Grüsser, Sabine M., Ralk Thalemann, and Mark D. Griffiths, "Excessive Computer Game Playing: Evidence for Addiction and Aggression?" *CyberPsychology & Behavior*, Vol. 10, (2), 2007, 290–292.

33 See, Sveningsson, Malin, "Cyberlove: Creating Romantic Relationships on the Net," In: Fornäs, Johan, Kajsa Klein, Martina Ladendorf, Jenny Sundén, and Malin Sveningsson, (eds.), *Digital Borderlands: Cultural Studies of Identity and Interactivity on the Internet* (New York: Peter Lang Publishers, 2002, 33).

34 See; Griffiths, Mark D, "Video Games and Health," *British Medical Journal,* 331, 2005, 122–123.

35 Griffiths, Mark D. "Videogame Addiction: Fact or Fiction?" In: Willoughby, Teena, and Eileen Wood, (eds.), *Children's Learning in a Digital World* (Oxford: Blackwell Publishing. 2007, 85–103). See also, Griffiths, Mark D. "Video Games and Health: Video Gaming is Safe for Most Players and Can Be Useful in Health Care," *British Medical Journal*, 331, (7509), 2005, 122–123.

36 Chappell, Darren, Virginia Eatough, Mark N. O. Davies and Mark Griffiths, "*EverQuest*—It's Just a Computer Game Right? An Interpretative Phenomenological Analysis of Online Gaming Addiction," *International Journal of Mental Health and Addiction*, Volume 4, (3), 2006, 205–216.

37 Matthew D. Shane, Barbara J. Pettitt, Craig B. Morgenthal and C. Daniel Smith, "Should Surgical Novices Trade Their Retractors for Joysticks? Videogame Experience

Decreases the Time Needed to Acquire Surgical Skills," *Sugrical Endoscopy*, Vol. 22 (5), 2008, 1294–1297.

38 Small, Gary W., Teena D Moody, Prabba Siddarth, Susan Y Bookheimer, "Your Brain on Google: Patterns of Cerebral Activation during Internet Searching," *The American Journal of Geriatric Psychiatry*, Vol. 17 (2), 116–127.

39 Musgrove, Mike, "Video Game Technology Gives Veterans New Lease on Life," *The Washington Post*, November 21, 2008 (http://www.washingtonpost.com/ wpdyn/content/article/2008/11/20/AR2008 11200 3731.html – accessed November 23, 2008).

40 Lott, Tim, "My Virtual Support Network," *The Guardian*, May 12, 2009 (http://www. guardian.co.uk/lifeandstyle /2009/may/12/cbt-nhs-beating-blues-computer – accessed May 12, 2009).

41 Mander, Toine (Rapporteur), "Report: On the Protection of Consumers, in Particular Minors, in Respect of the Use of Video Games," *European Parliament*, February 16, 2009 (http://www.europarl.europa.eu/sides/getDoc.do? language=EN&reference=A6-0051/2009 – accessed April 9, 2009).

42 Wood, Richard T. A., Griffiths, Mark D., and Parke, Adrian. "Experiences of Time Loss Among Videogame Players: An Empirical Study," *Cyberpsychology and Behavior,* 10, (1), 2007, 38–44.

43 Wood, Richard T. A. "Problems with the Concept of Video Game "Addiction": Some Case Study Examples," *International Journal of Mental Health and Addiction*, Vol. 6, (2), 2008, 171.

44 Cole, Helena, and Mark D. Griffiths, "Social Interactions in Massively Multiplayer Online Role-Playing Gamers, *CyberPsychology & Behavior*, Vol. 10, (4), 2007, 575–583.

45 Griffiths, Mark. D. "Videogame Addiction: Further Thoughts and Observations," *International Journal of Mental Health and Addiction*, Vol. 6, (2), 2008, 179–181.

46 Grusser, S. M., R. Thalemann, U. Albrecht, and C. N. Thalemann. 2005. "Excessive Computer Usage in Adolescents—A Psychometric Evaluation," *Wiener Klinische Wochenschrift,* 117, (5–6), 188–195.

47 Wood, Richard T. A., Griffiths, Mark D., & Parke, Adrian. "Experiences of Time Loss Among Videogame Players: An Empirical Study," *Cyberpsychology and Behavior,* 10, (1), 2007, 38–44.

48 Wood, Richard T. A., and Griffiths, Mark D. "A Qualitative Investigation of Problem Gambling as an Escape-Based Coping Strategy." *Psychology and Psychotherapy: Theory, Research and Practise,* 80 (1), 2007, 107–125.

49 See also; Griffiths, Mark D. *Adolescent Gambling*. (London: Routledge, 1995).

50 Skinner, Burrhus F. *Science and Human Behaviour* (New York: Free Press, 1953). Skinner's main principle can be understood as thus: "We tend to repeat behavior that is rewarded." Wallace, Patricia, *The Psychology of the Internet* (Cambridge: Cambridge University Press, 1999, 182).

51 Wood, Richard T. A. "A Response to Blaszczynski, Griffiths and Turners' Comments on the Paper "Problems with the Concept of Video Game "Addiction": Some Case Study Examples"," *International Journal of Mental Health and Addiction*, Vol. 6, (2), 2008, 179–181.

52 Kong, Linmeng, "Expert: Internet Addiction, Is It a Kind of Mental Illness?" [专家：网络成瘾，是不是一种精神疾病] *Ifengwo.com*, November 17, 2008 (http://www. ifengwo.com/xinwenzhongxin/hulian wang/200811/17-19362.html#digg1 – accessed January 12, 2009).

53 "Clinic Expert Defends His Internet-Addiction Claim in Face of Criticism," *China Economic Net*, November 26, 2008 (http://en.ce.cn/National/Local/200811/26/ t20081126_17506423.shtml – accessed December 23, 2008).

54 Cole, Helena, and Mark D. Griffiths, "Social Interactions in Massively Multiplayer Online Role-Playing Gamers, *CyberPsychology & Behavior*, Vol. 10, (4), 2007, 575–583.

55 In: *The Normal and the Pathological*. Translated by Carolyn R. Fawcett in collaboration with Robert S. Cohen, with an introduction by Michel Foucault (New York: Zone Books, 1989, 88).
56 Wakefield, Jerome C. "Disorder as Harmful Dysfunction: A Conceptual Critique of DSM-III – R's Definition of Mental Disorder," *Psychological Review*, Vol. 99, (2), 1992, 232–247.
57 Ibid.
58 Horwitz, Allan V., *Creating Mental Illness*, 2002, 20.
59 Ibid, 72.
60 Ibid, 73–74.
61 Ibid, 74.
62 Ibid, 11.
63 American Psychiatric Association, *Diagnostic and Statistical Manual of Mental Disorders: DSM-IV* (Washington, DC : American Psychiatric Association, 1994, xxi–xxii). Italics added.
64 Ibid.
65 Ibid.
66 Funk, McKenzie, "I Was a Chinese Internet Addict," *Harper's Magazine*, March 2007, Vol. 314 (1882), 65.
67 Ibid.

4 The humanistic intensive internet use model

1 Tai Zixue, *The Internet in China: Cyberspace and Civil Society*, 2006, 97.
2 Zan Jiefang, "Hooked on Cyberspace. Chinese Psychologists Outline Criteria for Internet Addiction," *Beijing Review*, December 16, 2008 (http://www.bjreview.com.cn/health/txt/200812/16/content_170 181.htm – accessed December 22, 2008).
3 Ibid.
4 Grüsser, S.M., Ralk Thalemann, and Mark D. Griffiths, "Excessive Computer Game Playing: Evidence for Addiction and Aggression?" *CyberPsychology & Behavior*, Vol. 10, (2), 2007, 290–292.
5 Conrad, Peter, and Joseph W. Schneider, *Deviance and Medicalization: From Badness to Sickness*, 1992. For moral entrepreneur, see Becker, Howard S. *Outsiders: Studies in the Sociology of Deviance*, 1973.
6 "War: Retreat of the 20,000," *Time*, December 18, 1950 (http://www.time.com/time/magazine/article/0,9171, 858986,00.html – accessed February 22, 2010).
7 Cover, Rob, "Gaming (Ad)diction: Discourse, Identity, Time and Play in the Production of the Gamer Addiction Myth," *Game Studies*, Vol. 6, (1), 2006 (http://gamestudies.org/0601/articles/cover – accessed February 25, 2008).
8 Fornäs, Johan, Kajsa Klein, Martina Ladendorf, Jenny Sundén, and Malin Sveningsson. "Into Digital Borderlands." In: Fornäs, Johan, Kajsa Klein, Martina Ladendorf, Jenny Sundén, and Malin Sveningsson, (eds.), *Digital Borderlands: Cultural Studies of Identity and Interactivity on the Internet* (New York: Peter Lang Publishers, 2002, 33).
9 Ng, Brian D. and Peter Wiemer-Hastings, "Addiction to the Internet and Online Gaming," *CyberPsychology & Behavior*, 8, (2), 2005, 110–113.
10 Ibid, 111.
11 Elias, Norbert, "Introduction." In: Elias, Norbert, and Eric Dunning, *Quest for Excitement: Sport and Leisure in the Civilizing Process*, 1986.
12 Associated Press, "Is No 3 Lama Prepared to Take the Reins?" *South China Morning Post*, March 13, 2009, A4).
13 Elias, Norbert, and Eric Dunning, "The Quest for Excitement in Leisure." In: Elias, Norbert, and Eric Dunning, *Quest for Excitement: Sport and Leisure in the Civilizing Process*, 1986, 67.

14 Maté, Gabor, *Scattered: How Attention Deficit Disorder Originates and What You Can Do About It* (New York: Plume, 2000, 24).

15 To view the cover art go to: http://www.evesound.com/images/cover-pink-floyd-the-division-bell.jpg

16 Jones, Steve, "Postscript: Academia and Internet Research." In: Fornäs, Johan, Kajsa Klein, Martina Ladendorf, Jenny Sundén, and Malin Sveningsson, (eds.), *Digital Borderlands: Cultural Studies of Identity and Interactivity on the Internet* (New York: Peter Lang Publishers, 2002, 33).

17 Elias, Norbert, "Introduction." In: Elias, Norbert, and Eric Dunning, *Quest for Excitement: Sport and Leisure in the Civilizing Process*, 1986, 66.

18 "To get rich is glorious" has been attributed (without evidence) to Deng Xiaoping's famous 1992 Southern Tour which helped to unleash a wave of personal entrepreneurship that continues to drive China's economy today.

19 Thompson, Clive, "How Video Games Blind Us With Science," *Wired*, August 8, 2009 (http://www.wired.com/gaming/gamingreviews/commentary/games/2008/09/games-frontiers_0908 – accessed August 12, 2009).

20 Steinkuehler, Constance, and Sean Duncan. "Scientific Habit of Minds in Virtual Worlds," *Journal of Science Education and Technology*, Vol. 17, (6), 2008, 530–543.

21 Ibid.

22 Tai Zixue, *The Internet in China: Cyberspace and Civil Society*, 2006, 120.

23 Xinhua, "China's First Law on Online Games Takes Effect, *China Daily*, August 1, 2010 (http://www.chinadaily.com.cn/china/2010-08/01/content_11077080.htm – accessed August 1, 2010).

24 Elias, Norbert, "Introduction." In: Elias, Norbert, and Eric Dunning, *Quest for Excitement: Sport and Leisure in the Civilizing Process*, 1986, 46.

25 Ibid, 50.

26 Elias, Norbert, and Eric Dunning, "The Quest for Excitement in Leisure." In: Elias, Norbert, and Eric Dunning, *Quest for Excitement: Sport and Leisure in the Civilizing Process*, 1986, 78.

27 The game takes place in 2065, where a computer named KAOS threatens to take over and destroy the world. The player's mission is to enter KAOS using a fighter plane and destroy it, thus both saving the world and becoming a hero.

28 Derrida, Jacques, *Dissemination*. Translated and Introduction by Barbara Johnson (London: Athlone Press, 1981, 125).

29 *Xin ling ji tang* – 心灵鸡汤.

30 *Du bu ji tang* – 毒补鸡汤.

31 Bremmer, Jan N. "Scapegoat Rituals in Ancient Greece," *Harvard Studies in Classical Philology*, Vol. 87, 1983, 299–320.

32 Huhtamo, Erkki, "Slots of Fun, Slots of Trouble: An Archaeology of Arcade Gaming." In: Joost Raessens, and Jeffery Goldstein, (eds.), *Handbook of Computer Game Studies* (Cambridge, Massachusetts: MIT Press, 2005).

33 Zimmerman, Eric, "Game Design and Meaningful Play." In: Joost Raessens, and Jeffery Goldstein, (eds.), *Handbook of Computer Game Studies* (Cambridge, Massachusetts: MIT Press, 2005).

34 Fromm, Erich, *The Sane Society*, 1955.

35 Zhang Jiawei, "China's Middle Class Under Great Pressure," *China Daily*, April 22, 2010 (http://www.chinadaily. com.cn/china/2010-04/22/content_9762269.htm – accessed April 22, 2010).

36 Beck, Ulrich, and Elisabeth Beck-Gernsheim, *Individualization: Institutionalized Individualism and Its Social and Political Consequences*, 2002, xxii.

37 Yi ge ren de zhandou. 一个人的战斗.

38 Fromm, Erich, *The Sane Society*, 1955, 65. "Orientation and devotion" simply means the quest for meaning and the attempt – by taking up a particular system of

thought – to make sense of one's own existence. Fromm, Erich, *Man for Himself: An Inquiry Into the Psychology of Ethics* (Greenwich, Connecticut: Fawcett Publications, 1947, 56).

39 Fromm, Erich, *The Sane Society*, 1955.
40 "As China Transitions, Beware Suicide Risk," *Global Times*, September 10, 2009, 8.
41 Ding Gang, "Lost Souls Falling Through Fast Social Change," *Global Times*, September 10, 2009, 9.
42 "As China Transitions, Beware Suicide Risk," *Global Times*, September 10, 2009, 8. Italics added.
43 Ding Gang, "Lost Souls Falling Through Fast Social Change," *Global Times*, September 10, 2009, 9.
44 Macartney, Jane, "In God They Trust," *Post Magazine*, [date unknown] 2009, 14–17.
45 Cochrane, Johanne, Hanhui Chen, Katherine M. Conigrave and Wei Hao, "Alcohol Use in China," *Alcohol & Alcoholism*, Vol. 38, (6), 2003, 537–542.
46 Jiang He, Gu Dongfeng, Chen Jing, Wu Kigui, "Premature Deaths Attributable to Blood Pressure in China: A Prospective Cohort Study," *The Lancet*, November 21–27, Vol. 374, (9703), 2009, 1765–1772.
47 Yang Wenying, Lu Juming, Weng Jianping, Jia Weiping, Linong Ji, Jianzhong Xiao, *et al.* "Prevalence of Diabetes among Men and Women in China," *The New England Journal of Medicine*, Vol. 362, (12), March 25, 2010, 1090–1101.
48 Lau Mimi, "Infertility Levels Raise Alarm on the Mainland," *South China Morning Post*, October 7, 2009, 4.
49 See, Rofel, Lisa, *Desiring China* (Durham: Duke University Press, 2007).
50 Associated Press, "Good Times Blamed for Resurgence of Syphilis," *South China Morning Post*, November 5, 2009, 7. For an exemplary example of a corrupt government official 'obsessed' with sex, drinking, and money, see the personal diary of disgraced *Guangxi's* Tobacco Bureau Chief Han Feng: "The Diary of Tobacco Bureau Chief," *EastSouthWestNorth* (http://www.zonaeuropa.com/2010030 2_1.htm – accessed March 5, 2010).
51 Watts, Jonathan, "China's 'Cancer Villages' Reveal Dark Side of Economic Boom," *The Guardian*, June 7, 2010 (http://www.guardian.co.uk/environment/2010/jun/07/china-cancer-villages-industrial-pollution – accessed June 7, 2010).
52 Bertman, Stephen, *Hyperculture: The Human Cost of Speed*, 1998, 75–76.
53 Fromm, Erich, *The Sane Society*, 1955.
54 Ibid, 24.
55 Ibid, 27.
56 Fromm, Erich, *The Fear of Freedom*, 1942, 158.
57 Ibid, 120.
58 The *danwei* was a socialist system guaranteeing job allocation. Workers were bound to their work unit for life, while each *danwei* created their own housing, schools, shops, services, etc. It was also multi-tiered hierarchy linking each individual with the Communist Party infrastructure. Thus while based on social inclusion it was also premised upon political suppression and repression.
59 The iron rice bowl, or "job for every worker," was a socialist welfare system securing employment and social welfare (yet, one which suppressed desire for a better material life). Whereas both the danwei and the iron rice bowl were based upon the ideology of socialist inclusion (and political repression), today we see a raw and often brutal capitalism engendering exclusion.
60 Fromm, Erich, *The Fear of Freedom*, 1942, 86.
61 As Zygmunt Bauman argued, individualization "consists in transforming human 'identity' from a 'given' into a 'task' – and charging the actors with the responsibility for performing that task and for the consequences (also the side-effects) of their performance." "Foreword by Zygmunt Bauman, Individually, Together," In: Beck, Ulrich, and Elisabeth

Beck-Gernsheim, *Individualization: Institutionalized Individualism and Its Social and Political Consequences*, 2002, xv.

62 Being "at sea" is the outcome of the individualization process, for Beck defined this process, which is part of post-industrial modernity (what Bauman called "liquid modernity"), wherein the individual has been "disembedded" from the social structure but without subsequently being "reembedded." Beck, Ulrich, and Elisabeth Beck-Gernsheim, *Individualization: Institutionalized Individualism and Its Social and Political Consequences*, 2002, xxii.

63 Ibid.

64 Xu Shenglan, "Bonus Inspires Independence," *Global Times*, September 10, 2009, 6.

65 Ibid.

66 Hewett, Duncan, *Getting Rich First: Life in a Changing China*, 2007, 166.

67 Ibid.

68 McNeal, James, and Kara Chan, *Advertising to Children in China* (Hong Kong: The Chinese University Press, 2004).

69 Ibid, 8.

70 Chan, Anita. *Children of Mao: Personality Development and Political Activism in the Red Guard Generation* (London: Macmillan, 1985).

71 总希望儿子，有回心转意的时候，会好好读书的.

72 Fromm, Erich, *The Sane Society*, 1955, 137–138.

73 Bauman, Zygmunt, *Consuming Life*, 2007, 6.

74 Fromm, Erich, *The Sane Society*, 1955, 137–138.

75 For example, consumerism is asking the subject to be an autonomous consuming individual, yet at the same time, this consumer is also being asked to conform to a social order where he/she must listen to what authority figures say and so must follow the collective rules and norms. See, Kleinman, Arthur, *The Illness Narrative: Suffering, Healing, & the Human Condition*, 1988, 99.

76 Leary, Timothy, *The Politics of Ecstasy* (Berkeley: Ronin Publishing, 1998).

77 Ibid.

78 Coltrane, Scott and Randall Collins, *Sociology of Marriage and the Family* (Belmont, California: Wadsworth/ Thomson Learning, 2001).

79 See; Munro, Robin, *Dangerous Minds: Political Psychiatry Today and Its Origin in the Mao Era*, 2002.

5 The family war-machine and the search for freedom

1 Letter-1. All the letters have been edited in some way so as to simply keep to the main argument.

2 Wu Zengqiang and Zhang Jianguo, *Prevention and Intervention of Adolescent Internet Addiction* (Shanghai: Shanghai Education Publishers, 2008, 14). 吴增强,张建国, "青少年网络成瘾:预防与干预" (上海: 上海教育出版社, 2007, 20).

3 Weber, Max, *The Methodology of the Social Sciences*. Translated and edited by Edward A. Shils and Henry A. Finch (New York: Free Press, 1949, 89–105).

4 Bauman, Zygmunt, *Consuming Life*, 2007, 27.

5 Letter-6. Italics added for emphasis.

6 *Wan shangyin*玩上瘾.

7 Huizhinga, Johan, *Homo Ludens: A Study of the Play-Element in Culture* (Boston: Beacon Press, 1955).

8 Tao Ran, *et al. Analysis and Intervention of Internet Addiction* (Shanghai: Shanghai People's Publishers, 2007). Tao Ran, Ying Li, Yue Shaodong, and Hao Xianghong. *Wang Luo Cheng Yin Tan Xi Yu Gan Yu Zhu* (Shanghai Shi: Shanghai Ren Min Chu Ban she). 陶然等, 网络成瘾探析与干预 (上海市: 上海人民出版社, 2007, 165）.

9 Huizhinga, Johan, *Homo Ludens: A Study of the Play-Element in Culture*, 1955.

10 Letter-1.

11 Letter-12.
12 Letter-13. *San hao xuesheng* 三好学生. Good in 1) study, 2) attitude, and 3) health.
13 Letter-13.
14 Letter-25.
15 Letter-30.
16 Letter-28
17 A political-economic example of China's culture of excess, wherein overcapacity or over-supply of goods is itself tied to the CCP's policy of maintaining excessive economic growth rates, is the way local governments just add capacity because they are often judged by how much economic growth they are generating. Zhou Dadi, the former director-general of the Energy and Research Institute of the National Development and Reform Commission, says that overcapacity is partly the result of a regime that bases the main indicators of economic growth upon general domestic growth and capital increments. This result is, according to Zhou Dadi, local governments "striving to expand their interests by adding production capacity. Overcapacity is therefore inevitable" (Moody, Andrew, and Lan Lan, "Overcapacity Exacerbated by Recession." *China Daily*, April 12, 2010. http://www.chinadaily.com.cn/bizchina/2010-04/12/content_9714677.htm – accessed April 12, 2010).
18 Letter-24. 因为从来得不到老师和父母的认可和同学的帮助 – 随便贴标签。例如，因学习成绩不好就会遭到父母的变向体罚和老师的漫骂。再比如，我脑子反应稍慢就会受到同学和老师的侮辱，从此我遭受着精神和肉体的折磨。所以，非常自卑总也自信不起来而且性格就内向起来。希望，您能在百忙之中和我交流思想，和我交流心得，使我在心灵上得到净化和教育.
19 Letter-33. 我干麻屡战屡败，我只有在玩电脑和看碟片时才能找到成就感，我要主宰世界，我要让全世界的人都得听我的.
20 See the section "Engulfment" for details. Basically, I use ontological insecurity to mean someone who possesses a partial absence of a secure sense of an autonomous self, which in turn allows anxieties and danger to arise in relation to their own selfhood and the attempts to deal with such dangers and anxieties.
21 Fromm, Erich, *The Fear of Freedom*, 1942, 158.
22 Ibid.
23 在家里老虎，在外面老鼠.
24 *Laoda* 老大 refers to big brother, but can connote the leader/boss of the group. It implies a position of authority and power (and responsibility).
25 Kutner, Lawrence and Cheryl K. Olson, *Grand Theft Childhood: The Surprising Truth About Violent Video Games and What Parents Can Do* (New York: Simon & Schuster, 2008).
26 "Boy, 9, Can Recite 100 Wuhan Bus Routes," *China Daily*, June 27, 2009, 3.
27 Jing Feng, Ian Spence, and Jay Pratt, "Playing an Action video Game Reduces Gender Differences in Spatial Cognition," *Psychological Science*, Vol. 18, (10), 2007, 850–855.
28 Bertman, Stephen, *Hyperculture: The Human Cost of Speed*, 1998, 75–76.
29 Chappell *et al.* also point to excessive gamers of *EverQuest* using the addiction lexicon in a functionally attributive way so as to partly eliminate self-blame. See, Chappell, Darren, Virginia Eatough, Mark N. O. Davies and Mark Griffiths, "*EverQuest*—It's Just a Computer Game Right? An Interpretative Phenomenological Analysis of Online Gaming Addiction," *International Journal of Mental Health and Addiction*, Volume 4, (3), 2006, 205–216
30 Booth Davies, John, *The Myth of Addiction* (Australia: Harwood Academic Publishers, 1997, 37).
31 Chuang Tzu, *Musings of a Chinese Mystic: Selections from the Philosophy of Chuang Tzu*. With Introduction by Lionel Giles (London: John Murray, 1906, 68).
32 Letter-26. 我不愿回家就愿意在外边玩多自由.
33 Mathiesen, Thomas, *Prison on Trial: A Critical Assessment* (London: Sage Publications, 1990, 45).
34 Fromm, Erich, *The Fear of Freedom*, 1942, 16.
35 Ibid.

36 Ibid, 17.
37 Chappell, Darren, Virginia Eatough, Mark N. O. Davies and Mark Griffiths, *"EverQuest*—It's Just a Computer Game Right? An Interpretative Phenomenological Analysis of Online Gaming Addiction," *International Journal of Mental Health and Addiction*, Volume 4, (3), 2006, 205–216.
38 See, O'Connor, S. C., and L.K. Rosenblood, "Affiliation Motivation in Everyday Experience: A Theoretical Comparison," *Journal of Personality and Social Psychology*, Vol. 70, (3), 1996, 513–522.
39 Cha, Ariana Eunjung, "In China, Stern Treatment for Young Internet 'Addicts'," *Washington Post* (http://www.washingtonpost.com/wp-dyn/content/article/2007/02/21/AR2007022102094_3.html – accessed November 13th, 2008).
40 内心向孤岛. I attended a seminar Fu Xueyu gave to parents at Tao Hongkai's four-day course in Beijing.
41 沟通是一剂良药，家庭是孩子的港.
42 Cheng Yingqi, "Psychological Issues Rising Among Students," China Daily, March 10, 2010 (http://www.chinadaily.com.cn/china/2010-03/10/content_9563769.htm – accessed March 10, 2010).
43 Ibid.
44 From the album "Into the Wild" (J-Records, 2007).
45 However, later I argue that the primary ties are, themselves, *suffocating* and so excessive internet use must be partly understood as a *hurried response* to this engulfing condition.
46 Fromm, Erich, *The Fear of Freedom*, 1942, 20.
47 This is why for sociologists like Ferdinard Tönnies modern individualism rests on independence and isolation as opposed to interdependence. Cancian, F. "The History of Love: Theories and Debates." In: Skolnick S. Arlene, and Jerome H. Skolnick, (eds.), *The Family in Transition: Rethinking Marriage, Sexuality, Child Rearing, and Family Organization, 7th Edition* (New York: HarperCollins Publishers, 1992).
48 Chappell, Darren, Virginia Eatough, Mark N. O. Davies and Mark Griffiths, *"EverQuest*–It's Just a Computer Game Right? An Interpretative Phenomenological Analysis of Online Gaming Addiction," *International Journal of Mental Health and Addiction*, Volume 4, (3), 2006, 205–216.
49 Tao Ran, *et al. Analysis and Intervention of Internet Addiction* (Shanghai: Shanghai People's Publishers, 2007). Tao Ran, Ying Li, Yue Shaodong, and Hao Xianghong. *Wang Luo Cheng Yin Tan Xi Yu Gan Yu Zhu* (Shanghai Shi: Shanghai Ren Min Chu Ban she). 陶然等，网络成瘾探析与干预（上海市：上海人民出版社, 2007, 165).
50 Ibid.
51 Cha, Ariana Eunjung, "In China, Stern Treatment for Young Internet 'Addicts'," *Washington Post* (http://www. washingtonpost.com/wp-dyn/content/article/2007/02/21/AR2007022102094_3.html – accessed November 13th, 2008).
52 Hewett, Duncan, *Getting Rich First: Life in a Changing China*, 2007, 181.
53 Ibid.
54 Leary, Timothy, *The Politics of Ecstasy*, 1998, 7.
55 Fromm, Erich, *The Fear of Freedom*, 1942, 206.
56 Li Xiaoshu, "Double Trouble or Twice the Fun?," *Global Times*, April 22, 2010 (http://special.globaltimes.cn/2010-04/525046_2.html – accessed April 24, 2010).
57 In: Talbot, David, "China's Internet Paradox," *Technology Review*, May/June 2010 (http://www.technologyreview.com/web/25032/ – accessed April 24, 2010). Italics added for emphasis.
58 Leary, Timothy, *The Politics of Ecstasy*, 1998.
59 Letter written by concerned psychology student.
60 Žižek, Slovaj, *Violence: Six Sideways Reflections* (New York: Picador, 2008, 70).
61 Virilio, Paul, *Virilio Live: Selected Interviews*. Edited by John Armitage (London: Sage, 2001).

62 Bertman, Stephen, *Hyperculture: The Human Cost of Speed*, 1998, 123.

63 "Sales of China's Online Gaming Industry to Hit 27.5 bln yuan in 2009," *China View* (http://news.xinhuanet.com/english/2009-12/05/content_12594834.htm – accessed March 1, 2010).

64 Perhaps the most important measure of imbalance in contemporary China is income disparity. For example, official figures published during the annual meeting of the National People's Congress in Beijing in 2010 claim that the income disparity between the richest and the poorest 10 percent of the population rose from 7.3-fold in 1988 to 23-fold in 2007. A situation that is causing increasing numbers of people to feel intense anger toward exploitative senior managers of State-owned firms and corrupt officials who use power to create wealth (O'Neill, Mark, "Anger Grows Over Wealth Inequality: Gap Between Haves and Have-nots Fuels Resentment," *South China Morning Post*, March 30, 2010, 8).

65 See, Mao Zedong, *On Guerrilla Warfare*. Translated with introduction by Samuel B. Griffith II (New York: Praeger Publishers, 1961, 12).

66 McNeal, James, and Kara Chan, *Advertising to Children in China*, 2004.

67 One study they cite says that Chinese children influence 68 percent of household purchases.

68 McNeal, James, and Kara Chan, *Advertising to Children in China*, 2004, 4.

69 Fromm, Erich, *The Sane Society*, 1955, 80. Italics in the original.

70 McNeal, James, and Kara Chan, *Advertising to Children in China*, 2004, 8.

71 Nan Du, "Tweeny Bit Spoilt,' *China Daily*, June 8, 2009 (http://www.chinadaily.com. cn/cndy/200906/08/ content_8257628.htm – accessed May 13, 2010).

72 Shao, Alan. T., and Paul Herbig, "Marketing Implications of China's 'Little emperors'," *Review of Business*, Summer/Fall 1994, Vol. 16, Iss. 1, 16–20.

73 Ibid, 17.

74 Nan Du, "Tweeny Bit Spoilt,' *China Daily*, June 8, 2009 (http://www.chinadaily.com. cn/cndy/200906/08/ content_8257628.htm – accessed May 13, 2010). Italics added for emphasis.

75 Said by the son in Letter-25 to his mother while his absent, neglectful, and violent father was away on business. In the original: 家里不给上网，就不上学.

76 Booth Davies, John, *The Myth of Addiction*, 1997.

77 Wu Zengqiang and Zhang Jianguo, *Prevention and Intervention of Adolescent Internet Addiction* (Shanghai: Shanghai Education Publishers, 2008, 14). 吴增强,张建国, "青少年网络成瘾:预防与干预" (上海: 上海教育出版社, 2007, 20).

78 Ibid.

79 Tao Ran, *et al. Analysis and Intervention of Internet Addiction* (Shanghai: Shanghai People's Publishers, 2007). Tao Ran, Ying Li, Yue Shaodong, and Hao Xianghong. *Wang Luo Cheng Yin Tan Xi Yu Gan Yu Zhu* (Shanghai Shi: Shanghai Ren Min Chu Ban she). 陶然等，网络成瘾探析与干预 （上海市: 上海人民出版社, 2007, 165）.

80 Tao Ran, *et al. Analysis and Intervention of Internet Addiction* (Shanghai: Shanghai People's Publishers, 2007).

81 Ibid, 165.

82 叫他吃这个他不吃，叫他不要生气不要动怒，他却动不动就生气还摔东西.

83 See Gershoff, Elizabeth T. "Corporal Punishment by Parents and Associated Child Behaviors and Experiences: A Meta-Analytic and Theoretical Review," *Psychological Bulletin.* (Vol. 128, (4), 2002, 539 –579).

84 Taylor, Catherine, Jennifer A. Manganello, Shawna J. Lee and Janet C. Rice, "Mothers' Spanking of 3-Year-Old Children and Subsequent Risk of Children's Aggressive Behavior," *Pediatrics*, (Vol. 125, (5), May, 2010, 1056–1065).

85 One major flaw of the study is the fact that it only focused upon mothers and so did not account for the father's, or in fact, any other person's use of corporal punishment. The letters here indicate it was the fathers more than the mothers who were using corporal punishment upon their children. Nevertheless, the general finding still seems applicable.

86 In this way we are not dealing simply with a "correlation" but rather an "interpersonal" relation.

87 Park Alice, "Study: Spanking Kids Leads to More Aggressive Behaviour," *Time*, April 12, 2010 (http://www.time.com/time/health/article/0,8599,1981019,00.html – accessed April 12, 2010).

6 Push and pull factors

1 Fromm, Erich, *Man for Himself: An Inquiry Into the Psychology of Ethics*, 1947, 56.
2 Ibid, 109.
3 Ibid, 29.
4 As the letter (after translation) is 3,000 words long, I have cut sections out. However, I have retained as best as possible the mother's own line of argument.
5 Letter-13.
6 *San hao xuesheng* 三好学生. Good in 1) study, 2) attitude, and 3) health.
7 Laing, R.D. *The Divided Self: An Existential Study of Sanity and Madness*, 1965, 44.
8 Significantly, the Chinese term for "spoil" is *ni ai*, with the character *ni* denoting the verb "to drown" or "to be submerged."
9 Laing, R.D. *The Divided Self: An Existential Study of Sanity and Madness*, 1965, 44.
10 我回家不是听你唠叨的, 再唠叨我就走.
11 Laing, R.D. *The Divided Self: An Existential Study of Sanity and Madness*, 1965, 42. Italics in the original.
12 Elias, Norbert, and Eric Dunning, *Quest for Excitement: Sport and Leisure in the Civilizing Process*, 1986.
13 Beck, Ulrich, and Elisabeth Beck-Gernsheim, *Individualization: Institutionalized Individualism and Its Social and Political Consequences*, 2002, xxii.
14 The survey was conducted by World History Institute at the Chinese Academy of Social Sciences. Rosen, Stanley, "Contemporary Chinese Youth and the State," *The Journal of Asian Studies*, Vol. 68, (2), 2009, 359–369.
15 The survey was conducted in Chongqing by the Chongqing University of Posts and Telecommunications "Students Born After 1990 Worship Themselves," *China Daily*, Dec 19, 2008.
16 Called "*Women yuehui ba*" 我们约会吧. Viewed in Hunan TV on June 9, 2010.
17 In understanding the important function the internet plays in China in the *search for happiness*, famous blogger "Hecaitou" said the following: "I like the internet, and I'm willing to throw all of my energy into it and toil for it. Doing something [well] on the internet, whether it's a big or small thing, is what makes me happiest" ("Hecaitou: 'Happiness'," translated by Charlie Custer, *China Geeks*, April 3, 2010).
18 Laing, R.D. *The Divided Self: An Existential Study of Sanity and Madness*, 1965, 53.
19 Ibid, 77.
20 Funk, McKenzie, "I Was a Chinese Internet Addict," *Harper's Magazine*, March 2007, Vol. 314 (1882), 65.
21 由于我过分关注他的学习成绩, 教育方法不当, 更加重了他的逆反心理.
22 我最烦人跟踪.
23 Laing, R.D. *The Divided Self: An Existential Study of Sanity and Madness*, 1965, 186.
24 Bakken, Børge, *The Exemplary Society: Human Improvement, Social Control, and the Dangers of Modernity in China* (Oxford: Oxford University Press, 2000).
25 Fromm, Erich, *The Fear of Freedom*, 1942, 20.
26 现在的教育体制如何不好, 老师家长只知道分数等等.
27 *Bu guan, bu ji, bu pa* 不管, 不急, 不怕.
28 For example, he uses the following sentence: Rational human nature = intelligence, self control, balance. *Heli de renxing = dongshi, zikong, pingheng* 合理的人性 = 董事, 自控, 平衡.
29 Bauman, Zygmunt, *Consuming Life*, 2007.
30 妈妈, 我也想学好, 可我就是管不住自己. It is not clear whether he "really" means it or whether he is just saying that in order to placate his mother, for almost all

the sons would make promises they then promptly broke. Such a strategy was important within the son's art-of-war as placating his mother's anger, fears, and anxiety gave him time. Nevertheless, the example is more theoretical than actual.

31 *Zisi de ai*自私的爱.
32 Cha, Ariana Eunjung, "In China, Stern Treatment for Young Internet 'Addicts'," *Washington Post* (http://www.washingtonpost.com/wp-dyn/content/article/2007/02/21/AR2007022102094_3.html – accessed November 13th, 2008).
33 他完全插入了疯狂状态，足不出户地在家玩电脑游戏. It is not clear whether this is a brother or a cousin as the same form of address is used interchangeably.
34 他要走他自己的路，自己选择未来.
35 *Wang zi cheng long* (望子成龙). The literal meaning of this idiom "hoping the child turns into a dragon" nicely captures the tiger/mouse dichotomy, engulfment, depersonalization, and filiarchy. The parents desire so desperately to see their child become a dragon (a success) that they attempt to do everything they feel is required in order to produce a dragon, but the more he becomes a tiger at home the likelihood of him becoming a mouse outside the home potentially increases.
36 Laing, R.D. *The Divided Self: An Existential Study of Sanity and Madness*, 1965, 45.
37 An essential text signaling the importance of the sociological analysis of this consumer revolution is the book (edited by Deborah Davis) *The Consumer Revolution in Urban China* (Berkeley, California: University of California Press, 2000).
38 In the wake of the 2008 Great Recession and the CCP's subsequent 4 trillion yuan stimulus package favoring State-owned industries, and driven by easy loans, overcapacity has become an even more serious problem in China. In September of 2009, the State Council released a statement noting overcapacity as a serious problem within many industries, because many local governments have expanded capacity "blindly" and have made "duplicated" investments without considering the mid- and long-term implications. That is, they are thinking principally on the *here* and *now* (European Union Chamber of Commerce in China and Roland Berger Strategy Consultants, *Overcapacity in China: Causes, Impacts and Recommendations*, November, 2009. http://www.rolandberger.it/media/pdf/Roland_Berger_Overcapacity_in_China_ 20091201.pdf – accessed April 11, 2010).
39 Farquhar, Judith, *Appetites: Food and Sex in Postsocialist China* (Durham & London: Duke University Press, 2002, 28).
40 Fish, Isaac Stone, "Back to the Land: Why China's 'Happy Farmer' took off," *Newsweek*, April 9, 2010 (http://www.newsweek.com/id/236150 – accessed April 19, 2010).
41 Nan Du, "Tweeny Bit Spoilt," *China Daily*, June 8, 2009 (http://www.chinadaily.com.cn/cndy/200906/08/content_82 57628.htm – accessed May 13, 2010).
42 Bauman, Zygmunt, *Consuming Life*, 2007.
43 *Chengzhen* 城镇.
44 "第 25 次中国互联网络发展状况统计报告," 中国互联网络信息中心 (CNNIC), January, 2010 (available at: www.cnnic.net.cn/en/index/index.htm).
45 379 million is derived from data from The National Bureau of Statistics of the People's Republic of China, but this is just a general guideline (http://www.allcountries.org/china_statistics/4_6_population_by_age_and_sex.html – accessed April 10, 2010).
46 "24th China Internet Development Situation Statistical Report," *China Internet Network Information Center* (CNNIC), July, 2009 (available at: www.cnnic.net.cn/en/index/index.htm).
47 Bauman, Zygmunt, *Consuming Life*, 2007, 6.
48 Brockes, Emma, "I Want to Be Famous!," *The Guardian*, April 17, 2010 (http://www.guardian.co.uk/lifeand style/2010/apr/17/i-want-to-be-famous – accessed April 17, 2010).
49 Kiefer, Anna, "Chinese Youth: Down to Earth People Reaching for the Stars," *Kairos Future*, December, 2007 (http://www.kairosfuture.com/en/system/files/Chinese+Youth+Survey+GW+10+200 7_0.pdf – accessed March 4, 2009).
50 Bauman, Zygmunt, *Consuming Life*, 2007, 13.

51 "War With the Internet Demon." 战网魔 (http://v.youku.com/v_show/id_ XODk3MTkwMDQ=.html – accessed Oct 3, 2009).
52 Ng Tze-wei, "Beijing Says Policy Stability is Its Top Priority for the Rest of the Year," *South China Morning Post*, July 23, 2010, A6.
53 Deleuze, Gilles and Felix Guattari, *Anti-Oedipus: Capitalism and Schizophrenia* (Translated from the French by Robert Hurley, Mark Seem, and Helen R. Lane; preface by Michel Foucault. London: Athlone Press, 1984).
54 *xiaokang shehui* 小康社会.
55 Bauman, Zygmunt, *Consuming Life*, 2007, 31.
56 Ibid, 32.
57 Layard, Richard, *Happiness: Lessons From a New Science* (London: Allen Lane, 2005).
58 The US military-industrial machinery in the film was, in the end, forced to leave Pandora defeated.
59 "Why Are Chinese People So Anxious?" *China Daily*, April 9, 2010 (http://www. chinadaily.com.cn/opinion/2010-04/09/content_9708996.htm – accessed April 10, 2010).
60 Ibid.
61 Bauman, Zygmunt, *Consuming Life*, 2007, 46–47.
62 "Shopaholism" is conceptualized as "compulsive shopping" that apparently "affects" 20 million Americans. "Tanorexia" is described as an "unhealthy dependence" on tanning with "withdrawal symptoms" that are described as being "similar" to those ceasing heavy alcohol and drug use. "Nomophobia" is understood as the fear or anxiety experienced when one is without their mobile phone. See Macartney, Jane, "Glued to the Screen China's Young Fall Victim to Sickness of Internet Addiction," *The Times*, November 11, 2008, 33.
63 Bauman, Zygmunt, *Consuming Life*, 2007, 46.
64 Fromm, Erich, *The Sane Society*, 1955, 127.
65 Deleuze, Gilles and Felix Guattari, *Anti-Oedipus: Capitalism and Schizophrenia*, 1984.
66 Fromm, Erich, *The Sane Society*, 1955, 131.
67 On Anhui TV's *Focus Point* program (*Jiao dian* 焦点). Disc given to me by Tao Hongkai.
68 Fromm, Erich, *The Sane Society*, 1955, 132.
69 Tun Shidai 吞时代. Nan Du, "Tweeny Bit Spoilt,' *China Daily*, June 8, 2009 (http://www. chinadaily.com.cn/ cndy/2009-06/08/content_8257628.htm – accessed May 13, 2010).
70 Nan Du, "Tweeny Bit Spoilt,' *China Daily*, June 8, 2009 (http://www.chinadaily.com. cn/cndy/200906/08/ content_8257628.htm – accessed May 13, 2010).
71 Laing, R.D. *The Divided Self: An Existential Study of Sanity and Madness*, 1965, 34.
72 Ibid, 34.
73 The complementary theoretical frameworks of both Fromm and Laing stem from the following epistemological assumption: The key problem of psychology is not that of the satisfaction or frustration of this or that instinctual need *per se* (re: Freud), but rather that of the specific kind of relatedness of the individual toward the world.
74 Fromm, Erich, *The Fear of Freedom*, 1942, 98–99.
75 Ibid.
76 Ibid, 126.
77 Fromm, Erich, *Man for Himself: An Inquiry Into the Psychology of Ethics*, 1947, 104–107.
78 This datum comes from attending her seminar to parents at the four-day course in Beijing.
79 Such as the need for relatedness; separatedness; transcendence; rootedness; a sense of identity; and a framework of orientation and devotion.
80 *Zhishi* 知识.

81 Presented at the Shandong Healthy Internet Training Base, April 17, 2009.

82 Branigan, Tania, "The Chinese Toddler Chained Through Love and Fear," *The Guardian*, February 4, 2010 (http://www.guardian.co.uk/world/2010/feb/04/chinese-child-chained-picture – accessed February 5, 2010).

83 The father claimed the wife had "learning disabilities" and so was unable to care for the children, while they had no relatives in Beijing. The truth or falsity of the story is unimportant, rather its truth-value resides in its symbolic function.

84 Ibid.

85 Cited at: http://apps.who.int/classifications/apps/icd10online/ – accessed Oct 13, 2009).

86 Laing, R.D. *The Divided Self: An Existential Study of Sanity and Madness*, 1965, 47.

87 现在好人不能活. This critique of society is very similar with the father in Letter-19, who thinks that in a society of "wolves" one must become a wolf themselves in order to survive. There is a strong social Darwinist stance to these perspectives in that only the strongest animal can prevail. This is why the father criticized the mother for teaching the child to be "honest." To the father, a more important survival "trait" is dishonesty, and so parents should be teaching their children to be mistrustful, and not trustful, of the others because public culture is itself based upon mistrust and deception. This offers us a good example of pathology of normalcy.

88 哪知道现在想跟他说，他也不跟你说，这就是惩罚.

89 Laing's theory is not simply a description of the "psychotic." On the contrary, Laing shows how the experiences of the person called psychotic is found in all of us. It is just that what becomes to be seen as psychotic is maybe just an elevated form of what is considered "normal," and so many may get near to the threshold of madness and that each and every one of us is "mad" to some degree. To use Laing's terms is not to imply that excessive gamers are psychotic, but rather that it is an issue of dimension or continuum and not category.

90 Laing, R.D. *The Divided Self: An Existential Study of Sanity and Madness*, 1965, 47.

91 指责老师的教育的方法不当或教育体制不合理.

92 Laing, R.D. *The Divided Self: An Existential Study of Sanity and Madness*, 1965, 52.

93 Bauman, Zygmunt, *Consuming Life*, 2007, 6.

94 Fromm, Erich, *The Sane Society*, 1955, 137–138; Bauman, Zygmunt, *Consuming Life*, 2007, 6.

95 Fromm, Erich, *The Sane Society*, 1955, 137–138.

96 Ibid, 103.

97 Platt, Kevin, "With a Click, Chinese Vault Cultural Walls," *The Christian Science Monitor*, June 1, 2000 (http://www.csmonitor.com/2000/0601/p1s4.html – accessed February 5, 2009).

98 "Beijing Perfect World Signs Agreement with Nestle," *Entrepreneur*, August 1, 2007 (http://www. entrepreneur.com/tradejournals/article/166647698.html – accessed July 8, 2009). Italics added.

99 The translated letter is originally about 5,000 words long, and so I have only included content which helps us contextualize why he was so "enthralled" by online games. The explanation itself analyzes the letter in its entirety.

100 我想也许问题就是全社会给我的压力太大了。比如说，来自家里和学校的压力，我父母和老师总对我"分分!". 我和同学们都没有兄弟姐妹，我本希望我们能成为朋友但我们的关系就跟竞争者似的。这样就这有一个地方可以来逃避这些问题，交朋友哪个地方就是网络. The reference has been lost.

101 Laing, R.D. *Self and Others*, 1969, 82.

102 See, O'Connor, S. C., and L.K. Rosenblood, "Affiliation Motivation in Everyday Experience: A Theoretical Comparison," *Journal of Personality and Social Psychology*, Vol. 70, (3), 1996, 513–522.

103 Reuters, "Game Over for China's Net Addicts,' *China Daily*, December 3, 2007 (http://www.chinadaily.com.cn/china/2007-03/12/content_825231.htm – accessed December 16, 2008). Italics added.

104 Derrida, Jacques, "The Rhetoric of Drugs," *High Culture: reflections on addiction and modernity*, 2003, 19–43.
105 This is why the rapid rise in religious and drug-induced experiences are closely connected to 'internet addiction,' for they stem from the same needs; e.g., the need for spiritual nourishment.
106 Bakken, Børge, *The Exemplary Society: Human Improvement, Social Control, and the Dangers of Modernity in China*, 2000.
107 I myself experienced this firsthand when playing *CS* in internet bars with Renfei and his first cousin Gaorui, for cooperating as a team in the game solidified our real-world friendship. That is, online gaming brought us closer together.
108 Gee, James, *What Video Games Have to Teach Us About Learning and Literacy* (New York: Palgrave Macmillan, 2003).
109 Foucault, Michel, *Discipline and Punish: The Birth of the Prison* (London: Allen Lane, 1977).
110 Derrida, Jacques, "The Rhetoric of Drugs," *High Culture: Reflections on Addiction and Modernity*, 2003, 19–43.
111 Reuters, "Game Over for China's Net Addicts," *China Daily* (http://www.chinadaily.com.cn/china /2007-03/12/content_825231.htm – accessed December 16, 2008).
112 Fromm, Erich, *The Fear of Freedom*, 1942, 16.
113 Fromm, Erich, *Man for Himself: An Inquiry Into the Psychology of Ethics*, 1947, 198.

7 *DSM-IV* – Internet Addiction Disorder

1 Or by a "disobedient personality spreading unchecked"; "no longer being afraid of anyone"; "failing to link up their education?"
2 Laing, R.D. *Self and Others*, 1969, 82.
3 Horwitz, Allan V., *Creating Mental Illness*, 2002, 20.
4 Kong, Linmeng, "Expert: Internet Addiction, Is It a Kind of Mental Illness?" [专家：网络成瘾，是不是一种精神疾病] *Ifengwo.com*, November 17, 2008. (http://www.ifengwo.com/xinwenzhongxin/hulian wang/200811/17-19362.html#digg1 – accessed January 12, 2009).
5 Adams, Jonathan, "In an Increasingly Wired China, Rehab for Internet Addicts," *The Christian Science Monitor*, January 6, 2009 (http://www.csmonitor.com/2009/0106/p01s03-woap.html – accessed January 7, 2009).
6 Wu Zengqiang and Zhang Jianguo, *Prevention and Intervention of Adolescent Internet Addiction* (Shanghai: Shanghai Education Publishers, 2008, 14). 吴增强,张建国, "青少年网络成瘾:预防与干预" (上海: 上海教育出版社, 2007, 20).
7 Horwitz, Allan V., *Creating Mental Illness*, 2002, 11.
8 American Psychiatric Association, *Diagnostic and Statistical Manual of Mental Disorders: DSM-IV* (Washington, DC : American Psychiatric Association, 1994, xxi–xxii) (italics added) .
9 Horwitz, Allan V., *Creating Mental Illness*, 2002, 24.
10 Adams, Jonathan, "In an Increasingly Wired China, Rehab for Internet Addicts," *The Christian Science Monitor*, January 6, 2009 (http://www.csmonitor.com/2009/0106/p01s03-woap.html – accessed January 7, 2009).
11 "Internet Addiction, Should it be Regarded as a Mental Disorder?" *Focus Point* (Anhui TV).
12 Zan Jiefang, "Hooked on Cyberspace. Chinese Psychologists Outline Criteria for Internet Addiction," *Beijing Review*, December 16, 2008 (http://www.bjreview.com.cn/health/txt/200812/16/content_1701 81.htm – accessed December 22, 2008).
13 Ibid.
14 Ibid.
15 Laing, R.D. *Self and Others*, 1969, 22.

16 Significantly, he uses the term "disease" not "mental disorder." This demonstrates a mis-understanding of the very important differences between a "disease" and a "disorder."
17 Anhui TV's *Focus Point* (*Jiao Dian* 焦点).
18 Laing, R.D. *Self and Others*, 1969, 22.
19 Ibid, 25.
20 Fromm, Erich, *The Fear of Freedom*, 1942, 155.
21 Tao Ran, *et al. Analysis and Intervention of Internet Addiction* (Shanghai: Shanghai People's Publishers, 2007).
22 Ibid.
23 Ibid.
24 Adams, Jonathan, "In an Increasingly Wired China, Rehab for Internet Addicts," *The Christian Science Monitor*, January 6, 2009 (http://www.csmonitor.com/2009/0106/p01s03-woap.html – accessed January 7, 2009).
25 *Ibid.*
26 Horwitz, Allan V., *Creating Mental Illness*, 2002, 14.
27 Ng Tze-wei and Fiona Tam, "Blank Faces Return to School Amid the Prayers," *South China Morning Post*, April 20, 2010, 1.
28 American Psychiatric Association, *Diagnostic and Statistical Manual of Mental Disorders: DSM-IV* (Washington, DC : American Psychiatric Association, 1994, xxi-xxii) (italics added).
29 Horwitz, Allan V., *Creating Mental Illness*, 2002, 11.
30 Ibid, 24.
31 Horwitz, Allan V., *Creating Mental Illness*, 2002, 22.
32 Ibid, 35.
33 Laing, R.D. *The Divided Self: An Existential Study of Sanity and Madness*, 1965, 27.
34 Horwitz, Allan V. *Creating Mental Illness*, 2002, 24. Italics added.
35 A professional gamer told me at the China finals of the 2009 World Cyber Games in Shanghai that prior to a competition he and his teammates practice around eight hours per day.
36 Booth Davies, John, *The Myth of Addiction*, 1997, 34.
37 Also known as an "operant conditioning chamber."
38 Internet use cannot be said to have a more measurable pharmacological effect than, say, driving a car.
39 Booth Davies, John, *The Myth of Addiction*, 1997, 31–32.
40 Cha, Ariana Eunjung, "In China, Stern Treatment for Young Internet 'Addicts'," *Washington Post* (http://www.washingtonpost.com/wp-dyn/content/article/2007/02/21/AR2007022102094_3.html – accessed November 13th, 2008).
41 Booth Davies, John, *The Myth of Addiction*, 1997, 31–32.
42 Tao Ran, *et al. Analysis and Intervention of Internet Addiction* (Shanghai: Shanghai People's Publishers, 2007).
43 Ibid. Italics added.
44 Zhang Jin and Zuo Likun, "Quake Victims 'Psychologically Very Weak'," *China Daily*, April 17, 2010 (http://www.chinadaily.com.cn/china/qinghai/2010-04/17/content_9742729.htm – accessed April 17, 2010).
45 Ibid.
46 Booth Davies, John, *The Myth of Addiction*, 1997, 37.
47 Ibid, 36.
48 Ibid, 22.
49 See, Corrigan, Paul, *Schooling the Smash Street Kids* (Basingstake: Macmillan, 1979).
50 Deleuze, Gilles and Felix Guattari, *Anti-Oedipus: Capitalism and Schizophrenia*, 1984, 126.
51 Scheff, Thomas. J. *Being Mentally Ill: A Sociological Theory* (Chicago: Aldine Publishing Company, 1966).
52 Horwitz, Allan V., *Creating Mental Illness*, 2002, 21.

Conclusion: log off

1 Ai Yang, "Grow Up Lonely as the One-and-Only," *China Daily*, July 30, 2010 (http:// www.chinadaily.com.cn/opinion/2010-07/30/content_11074499_2.htm – accessed August 1, 2010).

2 Horwitz, Allan V., *Creating Mental Illness*, 2002, 18.

3 Fromm, Erich, *The Sane Society*, 1955.

4 Ibid, 24.

5 Zhe Zhe, "Internet Addiction Not Just 'Bad Habit'," *China Daily*, November 10, 2008 (http://www.chinadaily.com.cn/china/2008-11/10/content_7188303.htm – accessed November 13, 2008).

6 Hewett, Duncan, *Getting Rich First: Life in a Changing China*, 2007, 166.

7 Fromm, Erich, *The Sane Society*, 1955, 27.

8 Wang Shanshan, "Internet Addicts a Virtual Nightmare for Parents," *China Daily*, December 9, 2006, 3.

9 Wu Meng, "Economic Strength Rising, but We Are Strangers," *Global Times*, September 16, 2009 (http://opinion.globaltimes.cn/observer/2009-09/468186.html – accessed September 17, 2009).

10 Zhang Wen, "*Bo Xilai and Mao Zedong*," (Bo Xilai he Mao Zedong 薄熙来和毛泽东). (http://zhangwen.blshe.com/post/214/527742 – accessed May 2, 2010). The English translation translates "spiritual nourishment" as "nourishment for their minds" (jingshen shiliang 精神食粮). Custer, Charlie, "Zhang Wen: Bo Xilai and Mao Zedong," *ChinaGeeks*, April 19, 2010 (http://chinageeks.org/2010/04 /zhang-wen-bo-xilai-and-mao-zedong/ – accessed May 2, 2010).

11 Funk, McKenzie, "I Was a Chinese Internet Addict," *Harper's Magazine*, March 2007, Vol. 314 (1882), 65.

12 Ibid.

13 The documentary is called "*Young and Restless in China.*" Go to http://www.pbs.org/ wgbh/pages/frontline/ youngchina/

14 Ibid.

15 Reuters, "Students Suffering From Internet Addiction – Study," *stuff.co.nz* (http:// www.stuff.co.nz/technology/ digital-living/3619610/Students-suffering-from-Internet-addiction-study – accessed April 25, 2010).

16 Ibid.

17 Adams, Jonathan, "In an Increasingly Wired China, Rehab for Internet Addicts," *The Christian Science Monitor*, January 6, 2009 (http://www.csmonitor.com/2009/0106/ p01s03-woap.html – accessed January 7, 2009).

18 Associated Press, "Copycat Rampage: Victims as Young as 3," *Sydney Morning Herald*, May 13, 2010 (http://www.smh.com.au/world/copycat-rampage-victims-as-young-as-3-20100513-v0mz.html – accessed May 13, 2010).

19 Ma, Josephine, "Chilling Parallels as Children Again Fall Prey to Crazed Killer," *South China Morning Post*, May 13, 2010, 1.

20 Wang, Xiangwei, "Attacks on Children Signal Deeper Social Ills," *South China Morning Post,* May 10, 2010, 5.

21 Schiller, Bill, "Is China's Boom the Cause of Kindergarten Stabbings?" *thestar.com*, May 12, 2010 (http://www.thestar.com/news/world/article/808191–china-reeling-after-fifth-bizarre-deadly-school-attack – accessed May 13, 2010).

22 Hearne, Chris, "Zhang Wen: China Is Sick"," *ChinaGeeks*, April 28, 2010 (http:// chinageeks.org/2010 /04/zhang-wen-china-is-sick/ – accessed May 2, 2010). Original article: Zhang Wen, "Zhongguo Bing le," *Zhang Wen de Boke* (章文, 中 国病了, 章文的博客), March 31, 2010 (http://zhangwen.blshe.com/post /214/525047 – accessed May 2, 2010).

References

Academic works

American Psychiatric Association. 1994. *Diagnostic and Statistical Manual of Mental Disorders: DSM-IV*. Washington, DC: American Psychiatric Association.

Bakken, Børge. 2000. *The Exemplary Society: Human Improvement, Social Control, and the Dangers of Modernity in China*. Oxford: Oxford University Press.

Bauman, Zygmunt. 2002. "Forward: Individually, Together," In: Beck, Ulrich, and Elisabeth Beck-Gernsheim, *Individualization: Institutionalized Individualism and Its Social and Political* Consequences. London: Sage.

———. 2007. *Consuming Life*. Cambridge; Malden, Massachusetts: Polity Press.

Beck, Ulrich, and Elisabeth Beck-Gernsheim. 2002. *Individualization: Institutionalized Individualism and Its Social and Political Consequences*. London: Sage.

Becker, Howard S. 1973. *Outsiders: Studies in the Sociology of Deviance*. New York: The Free Press of Glencoe, Inc.

Bertman, Stephen. 1998. *Hyperculture: The Human Cost of Speed*. Westport, Connecticut: Praeger Publishers.

Blaszczynski, Alex. 2008. "Commentary: A Response to 'Problems with the Concept of Video Game *Addiction*: Some Case Study Examples'," *International Journal of Mental Health and Addiction*, Vol. 6, (2), 179–181.

Booth Davies, John. 1997. *The Myth of Addiction*. Australia: Harwood Academic Publishers.

Bremmer, Jan N. 1983. "Scapegoat Rituals in Ancient Greece," *Harvard Studies in Classical Philology*, Vol. 87, 299–320.

Burawoy, Michael. 1985. *The Politics of Production: Factory Regimes Under Capitalism and Socialism*. London: Verso.

Callinicos, Alex. 1983. *The Revolutionary Ideas of Karl Marx*. London: Bookmarks.

Cancian, F. 1992. "The History of Love: Theories and Debates." In: Skolnick S. Arlene, and Jerome H. Skolnick, (eds.), *The Family in Transition: Rethinking Marriage, Sexuality, Child Rearing, and Family Organization, 7th Edition*. New York: HarperCollins Publishers.

Canguilhem, Georges. 1989. *The Normal and the Pathological*. Translated by Carolyn R. Fawcett in collaboration with Robert S. Cohen, with an introduction by Michel Foucault. New York: Zone Books.

Castells, Manuel, *The Information Age: Economy, Society and Culture. Volume II. The Power of Identity* (Oxford: Blackwell Publishers, 1997, 125).

Chan, Anita. 1985. *Children of Mao: Personality Development and Political Activism in the Red Guard Generation*. London: Macmillan.

———. 2002. "The Culture of Survival: Lives of Migrant Workers Through the Prism of Private Letters." In: Perry Link, Richard P. Madsen, and Paul G. Pickowicz, (eds.), *Popular China: Unofficial Culture in a Globalizing Society*. Lanham: Rowman and Littlefield Publishers.

Chappell, Darren, Virginia Eatough, Mark N. O. Davies, and Mark Griffiths. 2006. "*EverQuest*—It's Just a Computer Game Right? An Interpretative Phenomenological Analysis of Online Gaming Addiction," *International Journal of Mental Health and Addiction*, Vol. 4, (3), 205–216.

Charlton, John P. 2002. "A Factor-Analytic Investigation of Computer 'Addiction' and Engagement," *British Journal of Psychology*, Vol. 93, (3), 329–344.

Charlton, John P., and Danforth, Ian D. W. 2007. "Distinguishing Addiction and High Engagement in the Context of Online Game Playing," *Computers in Human Behavior*, Vol. 23, (3), 1531–1548.

China Internet Network Information Center. 2009. "24th China Internet Development Situation Statistical Report, July, 2009." (available at: www.cnnic. net.cn/en/index/index. htm).

Chuang Tzu, 1906. *Musings of a Chinese Mystic: Selections From the Philosophy of Chuang Tzu*. With Introduction by Lionel Giles. London: John Murray.

Cochrane, Johanne, Hanhui Chen, Katherine M. Conigrave, and Wei Hao. 2003. "Alcohol Use in China," *Alcohol & Alcoholism*, Vol. 38, (6), 537–542.

Cohen, Stanley. 1987. *Folk Devils and Moral Panics: The Creation of the Mods and Rockers*. Oxford: Blackwell Publishers.

Cole, Helena, and Mark D. Griffiths. 2007. "Social Interactions in Massively Multiplayer Online Role-Playing Gamers," *CyberPsychology & Behavior*, Vol. 10, (4), 575–583.

Colebrook, Claire. 2002. *Gilles Deleuze*. London; New York: Routledge.

Coltrane, Scott and Randall Collins. 2001. *Sociology of Marriage and the Family*. Belmont, California: Wadsworth/Thomson Learning.

Connell, Robert W. 1995. *Masculinities*. Berkely, Los Angeles: University of California Press.

Conrad, Peter and Joseph W. Schneider. 1992. *Deviance and Medicalization: From Badness to Sickness*. Philadelphia: Temple University Press.

Corrigan, Paul. 1979. *Schooling the Smash Street Kids*. Basingstake: Macmillan.

Cover, Rob. 2006. "Gaming (Ad)diction: Discourse, Identity, Time and Play in the Production of The Gamer Addiction Myth," *Game Studies*, Vol. 6, (1). (http://gamestudies. org/0601/articles/ cover – accessed February 25, 2008).

Davis, Deborah. 2000. *The Consumer Revolution in Urban China*. Berkeley, California: University of California Press.

Deleuze, Gilles and Felix Guattari. 1984. *Anti-Oedipus: Capitalism and Schizophrenia*. Translated from French by Robert Hurley, Mark Seem, and Helen R. Lane. Preface by Michel Foucault. London: Athlone Press.

Derrida, Jacques. 1981. *Dissemination*. Translated and Introduction by Barbara Johnson. London: Athlone Press.

———. 2003. "The Rhetoric of Drugs." In: Anna Alexander and Mark S. Roberts, (eds.), *High Culture: Reflections on Addiction and Modernity*. Albany: State University of New York Press.

Elias, Norbert. 1986. "Introduction." In: Elias, Norbert, and Eric Dunning, *Quest for Excitement: Sport and Leisure in the Civilizing Process*. Oxford: Blackwell.

Elias, Norbert, and Eric Dunning. 1986. "The Quest for Excitement in Leisure." In: Elias, Norbert, and Eric Dunning, *Quest for Excitement: Sport and Leisure in the Civilizing Process*. Oxford: Blackwell.

Farquhar, Judith. 2002. *Appetites: Food and Sex in Postsocialist China*. Durham and London: Duke University Press.

Fornäs, Johan, Kajsa Klein, Martina Ladendorf, Jenny Sundén, and Malin Sveningsson. 2002. "Into Digital Borderlands." In: Fornäs, Johan, Kajsa Klein, Martina Ladendorf, Jenny Sundén and Malin Sveningsson, (eds.), *Digital Borderlands: Cultural Studies of Identity and Interactivity on the Internet*. New York: Peter Lang Publishers.

Foucault, Michel. 1977. *Discipline and Punish: The Birth of the Prison*. London: Allen Lane.

Fromm, Erich. 1942. *The Fear of Freedom*. London: Routledge & Kegan Paul.

———. 1947. *Man for Himself: An Inquiry Into the Psychology of Ethics*. Greenwich, Connecticut: Fawcett Publications.

———. 1955. *The Sane Society*. New York: Holt, Rinehart and Winston.

Gee, James. 2003. *What Video Games Have to Teach Us about Learning and Literacy*. New York: Palgrave Macmillan.

Gershoff, Elizabeth T. 2002. "Corporal Punishment by Parents and Associated Child Behaviors and Experiences: A Meta-Analytic and Theoretical Review," *Psychological Bulletin*, Vol. 128, (4), 539 –579.

Golub, Alex, and Kate Lingley. 2008. "'Just Like in the Qing Empire': Internet Addiction, MMOGs, and Moral Crisis in Contemporary China," *Games and Culture*, Vol. 3, (1), 59–74.

Griffiths, Mark D. 1995. *Adolescent Gambling*. London: Routledge.

———. 2005. "Video Games and Health: Video Gaming is Safe for Most Players and Can Be Useful in Health Care," *British Medical Journal*, Vol. 331, (7509), 122–123.

———. 2007. "Videogame Addiction: Fact or fiction?" In: Willoughby, Teena, and Eileen Wood, (eds.), *Children's Learning in a Digital World*. Oxford: Blackwell Publishing.

———. 2008. "Videogame Addiction: Further Thoughts and Observations," *International Journal of Mental Health and Addiction*, Vol. 6, (2), 179–181.

Grüsser, Sabine M., Ralk Thalemann, and Mark D. Griffiths. 2007. "Excessive Computer Game Playing: Evidence for Addiction and Aggression?" *CyberPsychology & Behavior*, Vol. 10, (2), 290–292.

Grusser, S.M., R. Thalemann, U. Albrecht, and C.N. Thalemann. 2005. "Excessive Computer Usage in Adolescents—A Psychometric Evaluation," *Wiener Klinische Wochenschrift*, 117, (5–6), 188–195.

Hewett, Duncan. 2007. *Getting Rich First: Life in a Changing China*. London: Chatto & Windus.

Hofmann, Albert. 1983. *LSD: My Problem Child: Reflections on Sacred Drugs*. Los Angeles: J.P. Tarcher.

Horwitz, Allan V. 2002. *Creating Mental Illness*. Chicago; London: University of Chicago Press.

Huhtamo, Erkki. 2005. "Slots of Fun, Slots of Trouble: An Archaeology of Arcade Gaming." In: Joost Raessens, and Jeffery Goldstein, (eds.), *Handbook of Computer Game Studies*. Cambridge, Massachusetts: MIT Press.

Huizhinga, Johan. 1955. *Homo Ludens: A Study of the Play-Element in Culture*. Boston: Beacon Press.

Jenks, Chris, *Transgression* (London: Routledge, 2003, 25).

Jia, Zhangke. 2005. "The World of Jia Zhangke. An Interview by Patrica R.S. Batto." In: *China Perspectives*, No 60, (July–August), 46–50.

Jiang He, Gu Dongfeng, Chen Jing, and Wu Kigui. 2009. "Premature Deaths Attributable to Blood Pressure in China: A Prospective Cohort Study," *The Lancet*, November 21–27, Vol. 374, (9703), 1765–1772.

Jing Feng, Ian Spence, and Jay Pratt. 2007. "Playing an Action video Game Reduces Gender Differences in Spatial Cognition," *Psychological Science*, Vol. 18, (10), 850–855.

Jones, Steve. 2002. "Postscript: Academia and Internet Research." In: Fornäs, Johan, Kajsa Klein, Martina Ladendorf, Jenny Sundén, and Malin Sveningsson (eds.), *Digital Borderlands: Cultural Studies of Identity and Interactivity on the Internet.* New York: Peter Lang Publishers.

Jordan, Tim. 1999. *Cyberpower: The Culture and Politics of Cyberspace and the Internet.* London; New York: Routledge.

Kipnis, Andrew B. 2011. *Governing Educational Desire: Culture, Politics and Schooling in China.* Chicago: University of Chicago Press.

Kirkland, Russell. 2004. *Taoism: The Enduring Tradition.* New York: Routledge.

Kleinman, Arthur. 1988. *The Illness Narrative: Suffering, Healing, & the Human Condition.* New York: Basic Books.

Kohn, Livia. 2004. *Daoism Handbook.* Boston; Leiden: Brill.

Kutner, Lawrence, and Cherly K. Olsen. 2008. *Grand Theft Childhood: The Surprising Truth About Video Games and What Parents Can Do.* New York: Simon & Schuster.

Laing, R.D. 1965. *The Divided Self: An Existential Study of Sanity and Madness.* Harmondsworth: Penguin Books.

———. 1967. *The Politics of Experience, and, The Bird of Paradise.* Harmondsworth: Penguin.

———. 1969. *Self and Others.* London: Tavistock Publications.

Layard, Richard. 2005. *Happiness: Lessons From a New Science.* London: Allen Lane.

Leary, Timothy. 1998. *The Politics of Ecstasy.* Berkeley: Ronin Publishing.

Mander, Toine (Rapporteur). 2009. "Report: On the Protection of Consumers, in Particular Minors, in Respect of the Use of Video Games," *European Parliament*, February 16, 2009 (http://www.europarl.europa.eu/sides/getDoc.do?langu age=EN&reference=A6-0051/2009 – accessed April 9, 2009).

Mao Zedong, *On Guerrilla Warfare.* Translated with introduction by Samuel B. Griffith II (New York: Praeger Publishers, 1961, 12)

———. 1967. *Quotations from Mao Tse-Tung.* Peking: Foreign Languages Press.

Maté, Gabor. 2000. *Scattered: How Attention Deficit Disorder Originates and What You Can Do About It.* New York: Plume Publishing.

Mathiesen, Thomas. 1990. *Prison on Trial: A Critical Assessment.* London: Sage Publications.

Matthew D. Shane, Barbara J. Pettitt, Craig B. Morgenthal, and C. Daniel Smith. 2008."Should Surgical Novices Trade Their Retractors for Joysticks? Videogame Experience Decreases the Time Needed to Acquire Surgical Skills," *Sugrical Endoscopy*, Vol. 22, (5), 1294–1297.

McNeal, James, and Kara Chan. 2004. *Advertising to Children in China.* Hong Kong: The Chinese University Press.

Munro, Robin. 2002. *Dangerous Minds: Political Psychiatry Today and Its Origin in the Mao Era.* New York: Human Rights Watch; Hilversum, The Netherlands: Geneva Initiative on Psychiatry.

Ng, Brian D., and Peter Wiemer-Hastings. 2005. "Addiction to the Internet and Online Gaming," *CyberPsychology & Behavior*, 8, (2), 110–113.

O'Connor, S. C., and L.K. Rosenblood. 1996. "Affiliation Motivation in Everyday Experience: A Theoretical Comparison," *Journal of Personality and Social Psychology*, Vol. 70, (3), 513–522.

Rofel, Lisa. 2007. *Desiring China*. Durham: Duke University Press.

Rosen, Stanley. 2009. "Contemporary Chinese Youth and the State," *The Journal of Asian Studies*, Vol. 68, (2), 359–369.

Scheff, Thomas J. 1966. *Being Mentally Ill: A Sociological Theory*. Chicago: Aldine Publishing Company.

Shao, Alan T., and Paul Herbig. 1994. "Marketing Implications of China's 'Little emperors'," *Review of Business*, Summer/Fall 1994, Vol. 16, (10), 16–20.

Skinner, Burrhus F. 1953. *Science and Human Behaviour*. New York: Free Press.

Small, Gary W., Teena D Moody, Prabba Siddarth, and Susan Y Bookheimer. 2009. "Your Brain on Google: Patterns of Cerebral Activation During Internet Searching," *The American Journal of Geriatric Psychiatry*, Vol. 17, (2), 116–127.

Steinkuehler, Constance, and Sean Duncan. 2008. "Scientific Habit of Minds in Virtual Worlds," *Journal of Science Education and Technology*, Vol. 17, (6), 530–543.

Sun, Hualin. 2004. Internet Policy and Use: A Field Study of Internet Cafes in China. PhD Thesis, The Florida State University.

Sun Zi. 2007. *The Art of War*. Beijing: Foreign Languages Press.

Sveningsson, Malin. 2002. "Cyberlove: Creating Romantic Relationships on the Net," In: Fornäs, Johan, Kajsa Klein, Martina Ladendorf, Jenny Sundén, and Malin Sveningsson, (eds.), *Digital Borderlands: Cultural Studies of Identity and Interactivity on the Internet*. New York: Peter Lang Publishers.

Tai Zixue. 2006. *The Internet in China: Cyberspace and Civil Society*. New York: Routledge.

Tao Ran, Huang Xiu-qin, Yao Sumin, *et al.* 2007. "Analysis on the Epidemiology of 607 Inpatients With Internet Addiction Disorder," *China Journal of Epidemiology*, May, Vol. 28, (5), 519.

Tao Ran, Ying Li, Yue Shaodong, and Hao Xianghong. 2007. *Analysis and Intervention of Internet Addiction*. Shanghai: Shanghai People's Publishers.

———. 2007. *Wang Luo Cheng Yin Tan Xi Yu Gan Yu Zhu*. Shanghai Shi: Shanghai Ren Min Chu Ban She. 陶然等. 网络成瘾探析与干预. 上海市: 上海人民出版社.

Tao Ran, Huang Xiuqin, Wang Jinan, Zhang Huimin, Zhang Ying, and Li Mengchen. 2010. "Proposed Diagnostic Criteria for Internet Addiction," *Addiction*, Vol. 105, (3), 556–564.

Taylor, Catherine, Jennifer A. Manganello, Shawna J. Lee, and Janet C. Rice. 2010. "Mothers' Spanking of 3-Year-Old Children and Subsequent Risk of Children's Aggressive Behavior," *Pediatrics*, Vol. 125, (5), 1056–1065.

Turkle, Sherry. 1996. *Life on the Screen: Identity in the Age of the Internet*. London: Weidenfeld & Nicolson.

Turner, Nigel E. 2008. "A Comment on "Problems with the Concept of Video Game "Addiction": Some Case Study Examples"," *International Journal of Mental Health and Addiction*, Vol. 6, (2), 186–190.

Virilio, Paul, and Sylvère Lotringer. 1983. *Pure War*. Translated by Mark Poizzotti. New York: Semiotext(e).

———. 1991. *The Lost Dimension*. Translated by Daniel Moshenberg. New York: Semiotext(e).

———. 2001. *Virilio Live: Selected Interviews*. Edited by John Armitage. London: Sage.

Wakefield, Jerome C. 1992. "Disorder as Harmful Dysfunction: A Conceptual Critique of DSM-III-R's Definition of Mental Disorder," *Psychological Review*, Vol. 99, (2), 232–247.

Wallace, Patricia. 1999. *The Psychology of the Internet*. Cambridge: Cambridge University Press.

Walter, Glenn D. 1999. *The Addiction Concept: Working Hypothesis or Self-fulfilling Prophesy?* Boston: Allyn & Bacon.

Weber, Max. 1949. *The Methodology of the Social Sciences*. Translated and edited by Edward A. Shils, and Henry A. Finch. New York: Free Press.

Wood, Richard T. A. 2008. "Problems with the Concept of Video Game "Addiction": Some Case Study Examples," *International Journal of Mental Health and Addiction*, Vol. 6, (2), 169–78.

——. 2008. "A Response to Blaszczynski, Griffiths and Turners' Comments on the Paper "Problems with the Concept of Video Game "Addiction": Some Case Study Examples"," *International Journal of Mental Health and Addiction*, Vol. 6, (2), 179–181.

Wood, Richard T. A., and Griffiths, Mark D. 2007. "A Qualitative Investigation of Problem Gambling as an Escape-Based Coping Strategy." *Psychology and Psychotherapy: Theory, Research and Practise*, Vol. 80, (1), 107–125.

Wood, Richard T. A., Griffiths, Mark D., and Parke, Adrian. 2007. "Experiences of Time Loss Among Videogame Players: An Empirical Study," *Cyberpsychology and Behavior*, 10, (1), 38–44.

Wu Zengqiang, and Zhang Jianguo. 2008. *Prevention and Intervention of Adolescent Internet Addiction*. Shanghai: Shanghai Education Publishers.

——. 2008. *Qing shao nian wangluo chengyin yufang yu ganyu*. Shanghai: Shanghai jiaoyu chu ban she. 吴增强,张建国. 青少年网络成瘾:预防与干预. 上海: 上海教育出版社.

Yang Guobin. 2009. *The Power of the Internet in China: Citizen Activism Online*. New York: Columbia University Press.

Yang Wenying, Lu Juming, Weng Jianping, Jia Weiping, Linong Ji, Jianzhong Xiao, *et al.* 2010. "Prevalence of Diabetes Among Men and Women in China," *The New England Journal of Medicine*, Vol. 362, (12), March 25, 1090–1101.

Young, Kimberly S. 1998. *Caught in the Net: How to Recognize the Signs of Internet Addiction – And a Winning Strategy for Recovery*. New York: John Wiley & Sons, Inc.

Zimmerman, Eric. 2005. "Game Design and Meaningful Play." In: Joost, Raessens, Jeffery Goldstein, (eds.), *Handbook of Computer Game Studies*. Cambridge, Massachusetts: MIT Press.

Žižek, Slovaj. 2008. *Violence: Six Sideways Reflections*. New York: Picador.

Works in the popular press

Adams, Jonathan. 2009. "In an Increasingly Wired China, Rehab for Internet Addicts," *The Christian Science Monitor*, January 6, 2009 (http://www.csmonitor.com/2009/0106/p01s03-woap.html – accessed January 7, 2009).

Ai Yang. 2010. "Grow Up Lonely as the One-and-Only," *China Daily*, July 30 (http://www.chinadaily.com.cn/opinion/2010-07/30/content_11074499_2.htm – accessed August 1, 2010).

"As China Transitions, Beware Suicide Risk," *Global Times*, September 10, 2009, 8.

Associated Press. 2010. "Copycat Rampage: Victims as Young as 3," *Sydney Morning Herald*, May 13 (http://www.smh.com.au/world/copycat-rampage-victims-as-young-as-320100513 v0mz.html – accessed May 13, 2010).

Associated Press, 2009. "Good Times Blamed for Resurgence of Syphilis," *South China Morning Post*, November 5, 7.

Associated Press. 2009. "Is No 3 Lama Prepared to Take the Reins?" *South China Morning Post*, March 13, A4.

"Beijing Perfect World Signs Agreement with Nestle," *Entrepreneur*, August 1, 2007 (http://www.entrepreneur.com/tradejournals/article/166647698.html – accessed July 8, 2009).

Branigan, Tania. 2010. "The Chinese Toddler Chained Through Love and Fear," *The Guardian*, February 4 (http://www.guardian.co.uk/world/2010/feb/04/chinese-child-chained-picture – accessed February 5, 2010).

Brockes, Emma. 2010. "I Want to Be Famous!," *The Guardian*, April 17 (http://www.guardian.co.uk/lifeandstyle/2010/apr/17/i-want-to-be-famous – accessed April 17, 2010).

"Boy, 10, Chained at Home," *South China Morning Post*, July 20, 2010, A6.

Cha, Ariana Eunjung. 2007. "In China, Stern Treatment for Young Internet 'Addicts'," *Washington Post*, February 21 (http://www.washingtonpost.com/wp-dyn/content/article/2007/02/21/AR2007022102094_3.html – accessed November 13th, 2008).

Cheng Yingqi. 2010. "Psychological Issues Rising Among Students," *China Daily*, March 10 (http://www.chinadaily.com.cn/china/2010-03/10/content_9563769.htm – accessed March 10, 2010).

"China Statistics and Related Data Information Links," *China Today* (http://www.chinatoday.com/data/data.htm – accessed November 4, 2009).

"China's Hu Vows to 'Purify' Internet," *OpenNet Initiative* (http://opennet.net/blog/2007/02/chinas-hu-vows-purify-internet-reuters – accessed January 29, 2010).

"Clinic Expert Defends His Internet-Addiction Claim in Face of Criticism," *China Economic Net*, November 26, 2008 (http://en.ce.cn/National/Local/200811/26/t20081126_17506423.shtml – accessed December 23, 2008).

Curley, Fia. 2006. "Detox Clinic Opening for Video Addicts," June 8 (http://www.breitbart.com/article.php?id=D8I489R80&show_article=1 – accessed on June 3, 2008).

Custer, Charlie. 2010. "Zhang Wen: Bo Xilai and Mao Zedong," *ChinaGeeks*, April 19 (http://chinageeks.org/2010/04/zhang-wen-bo-xilai-and-mao-zedong/ – accessed May 2, 2010).

Davis, Rowenna. 2009. "Game Overload," *South China Morning Post*, March 11, C1.

Dan Chongshan. 2009. "The Death of the Internet Addict Youth Deng Senshen, *Southern Metropolis Weekly*, August 14. English translation by *EastSouthWestNorth* (http://www.zonaeuropa.com/20090826_1.htm – accessed August 26, 2009).

Ding Gang. 2009. "Lost Souls Falling Through Fast Social Change," *Global Times*, September 10, 9.

European Union Chamber of Commerce in China and Roland Berger Strategy Consultants. 2009. *Overcapacity in China: Causes, Impacts and Recommendations*, (http://www.rolandberger.it/media/pdf/Roland_Berger_Overcapacity_in_China20091201.pdf – accessed April 11, 2010).

Fish, Isaac Stone. 2010. "Back to the Land: Why China's 'Happy Farmer' took off," *Newsweek*, April 9 (http://www.newsweek.com/id/236150 – accessed April 19, 2010).

Funk, McKenzie. 2007. "I Was a Chinese Internet Addict," *Harper's Magazine*, March, Vol. 314, (1882), 65.

Hearne, Chris. 2010. "Zhang Wen: 'China Is Sick'," *ChinaGeeks*, April 28 (http://chinageeks.org/2010/04/zhang-wen-china-is-sick/ – accessed May 2, 2010). Original article: Zhang Wen, "Zhongguo Bing le," *Zhang Wen de Boke* (章文, 中 国病了, 章文的博客), March 31, 2010 (http://zhangwen.blshe.com/post/214/525047 – accessed May 2, 2010).

"Hecaitou: 'Happiness'," translated by Charlie Custer, *China Geeks*, April 3, 2010.

Jiang, Jessie. 2009. "Inside China's Fight Against Internet Addiction," *Time*, January 8, (http://www.time.com/time/world/article/0,8599,1874380,00.html – accessed January 18, 2009).

Ji Beibei. 2009. "'High-pressure' Huawei Sets Up In-house Health Center," *Global Times*, June 19, 5.

"Juvenile Crime on Rise in China," *The Sunday Times*, December 6, 2007 (http://www. asiaone. com/News/AsiaOne+News/Asia/Story/A1Story20071206-39928.html – accessed May 21, 2009).

Kiefer, Anna. 2007. "Chinese Youth: Down to Earth People Reaching for the Stars," *Kairos Future*, December (http://www.kairosfuture.com/en/system/files/Chinese+Youth +Survey+GW+10+2007_0.pdf – accessed March 4, 2009).

Kong, Linmeng. 2008. "Expert: Internet Addiction, Is It a Kind of Mental Illness?" (专家：网络成瘾，是不是一种精神疾病) *Ifengwo.com*, November 17 (http://www.ifengwo. com/xinwenzhongxin/hulianwang/200811/119362.html#digg1 – accessed January 12, 2009).

LaFraniere, Sharon. 2009. "China College Entry Test Is an Obsession," *The New York Times*, June 12 (http://www.nytimes.com/2009/06/13/world/asia/13exam.html?ref=global-home – accessed June 13, 2009).

Lai Chloe. 2010. "Foxconn Deaths Spur Boycott of New iPhone," *South China Morning Post*, May 25, 2.

Lau Mimi. 2009. "Infertility Levels Raise Alarm on the Mainland," *South China Morning Post*, October 7, 4.

Lin-Liu, Jennifer. 2006. "China's e-Junkies Head for Rehab," *IEEE Spectrum*, February, (http:// ieeexplore.ieee.org/stamp/stamp.jsp?arnumber=1584358&isnumber=33435 – accessed June 12, 2008).

Liu, Irene Jay, and Fox Yi Hui. 2010. "At Foxconn, Success and Tragedy Linked," *South China Morning Post*, June 1, 1.

Liu Xin, Alice. 2009. "Internet Addict Swallows Steel Saw Blade," *Danwei.org*, January 9 (http://www.danwei.org/ – accessed January 9, 2009). Original article, 郝涛, 贾儒, "网瘾男子吞下钢锯条 术后仍念叨网游词语," 北京晨报, January 9, 2009 (http://news.xin-huanet.com/internet/2009-01/06/content_10607845.htm – accessed Jan 9, 2009).

Li Xiaoshu. 2010. "Double Trouble or Twice the Fun?," *Global Times*, April 22 (http:// special.globaltimes.cn/2010-04/525046_2.html – accessed April 24, 2010).

Lott, Tim. 2009. "My Virtual Support Network," *The Guardian*, May 12 (http://www. guardian.co.uk/lifeandstyle/2009/may/12/cbt-nhs-beating-blues-computer – accessed May 12, 2009).

Macartney, Jane. 2008. "Glued to the Screen China's Young Fall Victim to Sickness of Internet Addiction," *The Times*, November 11, 33.

——. 2009. "In God They Trust," *Post Magazine*, [date unknown], 14–17.

Maguire, Paddy. 2008. "Compulsive Gamers not 'Addicts'," BBC News, November 25 (http://news.bbc.co.uk/1/hi/technology/7746471.stm – accessed November 26, 2008).

Ma, Josephine. 2010. "Chilling Parallels as Children Again Fall Prey to Crazed Killer," *South China Morning Post*, May 13, 1.

"Man Poisons His Family Over Game Addiction," *BBGSITE@com*, November 17, 2008 (http://news.bbgsite.com/content/2008-11-16/20081116082600795.shtml – accessed December 23, 2008).

Moody, Andrew, and Lan Lan. 2010 "Overcapacity Exacerbated by Recession," *China Daily*, April 12 (http://www.chinadaily.com.cn/bizchina/2010-04/12/content_9714677. htm – accessed April 12, 2010).

Musgrove, Mike. 2008. "Video Game Technology Gives Veterans New Lease on Life," *The Washington Post*, November 21 (http://www.washingtonpost.com/wpdyn/content/ article/2008/11/20/AR2008 11200 3731.html – accessed November 23, 2008).

Nan Du. 2009. "Tweeny Bit Spoilt," *China Daily*, June 8 (http://www.chinadaily.com.cn/cndy/2 009-06/08/content_8257628.htm – accessed May 13, 2010).

Ng Tze-wei and Fiona Tam. 2010. "Blank Faces Return to School Amid the Prayers," *South China Morning Post*, April 20, 1.

Ng Tze-wei. 2010. "Beijing Says Policy Stability Is Its Top Priority for the Rest of the Year," *South China Morning Post*, July 23, A6.

O'Neill, Mark. 2010. "Anger Grows Over Wealth Inequality: Gap Between Haves and Have-Nots Fuels Resentment," *South China Morning Post*, March 30, 8.

Park Alice. 2010. "Study: Spanking Kids Leads to More Aggressive Behaviour," *Time*, April 12 (http://www.time.com/time/health/article/0,8599,1981019,00.html – accessed April 12, 2010).

Platt, Kevin. 2000. "With a Click, Chinese Vault Cultural Walls," *The Christian Science Monitor*, June 1 (http://www.csmonitor.com/2000/0601/p1s4.html – accessed February 5, 2009).

Reuters. 2007. "Game Over for China's Net Addicts," *China Daily*, December 3 (http://www.chinadaily.com.cn/china/2007-03/12/content_825231.htm – accessed December 16, 2008).

Reuters. 2007. "Online Addict Dies After Marathon Session," *Reuters*, February 28 (http://www.reuters.com/article/idUSPEK26772020070228 – accessed March 4, 2008).

Reuters. 2010. "Students Suffering From Internet Addiction – Study," *stuff.co.nz* (http://www.stuff.co.nz/technology/digital-living/3619610/Students-suffering-from-Internet-addiction-study – accessed April 25.

"Sales of China's Online Gaming Industry to Hit 27.5 bln yuan in 2009," *China View* (http://news.xinhuanet.com/english/2009-12/05/content_12594834.htm – accessed March 1, 2010).

Schiller, Bill. 2010. "Is China's Boom the Cause of Kindergarten Stabbings?," *thestar.com*, May 12 (http://www.thestar.com/news/world/article/808191–china-reeling-after-fifth-bizarre-deadly-school-attack – accessed May 13, 2010).

Stewart, Christopher S. 2010. "Obsessed With the Internet: A Tale From China," *Wired*, January 13 (http://www.wired.com/magazine/2010/01/ff_internetaddiction/all/1 – accessed May 31, 2010).

"Students Born After 1990 Worship Themselves," *China Daily*, December 19, 2008.

Sun Uking. 2010 "Chinese Society Mobilized for Gaokao Battle," *China Daily*, June 4 (http://www.chinadaily.com.cn/china/2010-06/04/content_9935778.htm – accessed June 5, 2010).

Talbot, David. 2010. "China's Internet Paradox," *Technology Review*, May/June (http://www.technologyreview.com/web/25032/ – accessed April 24, 2010).

"Teenager Sells Family Car to Fuel Internet Addiction," *China Daily*, January 12, 2009, 5.

"The Diary of Tobacco Bureau Chief," *EastSouthWestNorth* (http://www.zonaeuropa.com/20100302_1.htm – accessed March 5, 2010).

Thompson, Clive. 2009. "How Video Games Blind Us With Science," *Wired*, August 8, 2009 (http://www.wired.com/gaming/gamingreviews/commentary/games/2008/09/gamesfrontiers 0908 – accessed August 12, 2009).

Tian Bingxin. 2005. "Zhang Chunliang: Damned Internet Games," *Southcn.com*, January 2 (http://www.southcn.com/nfsq/ywhc/tbxst/shentan/200510260380.htm – accessed June 4, 2010).

"Troubled Teen Survives Jump to Expose Boot Camp," *YNET.com*, June 7, 2008 (http://bjtoday.ynet.com/article.jsp?oid=21243835&pageno=4 – accessed April 28, 2009).

Vause, John. 2010 "Inside China Factory Hit by Suicides," *CNN*, June 1 (http://edition.cnn.com/2010/WORLD/asiapcf/06/01/china.foxconn.inside.factory/index.html?hpt=C2 – accessed June 2, 2010).

Wang, Xiangwei. 2010. "Attacks on Children Signal Deeper Social Ills," *South China Morning Post,* May 10, 5.

Wang Shanshan. 2006. "Internet Addicts a Virtual Nightmare for Parents," *China Daily*, December 9, 3. "War With the Internet Demon." 战网魔 (http://v.youku.com/v_show/id XODk3MTkwMDQ=.html – accessed October 3, 2009).

"War: Retreat of the 20,000," *Time*, December 18, 1950 (http://www.time.com/time/magazine/article/0,9171,858986,00.html – accessed February 22, 2010).

Watts, Jonathan. 2010. "China's 'Cancer Villages' Reveal Dark Side of Economic Boom," *The Guardian*, June 7 (http://www.guardian.co.uk/environment/2010/jun/07/china-cancer-villages-industrial-pollution – accessed June 7, 2010).

"Why are Chinese People So Anxious?" *China Daily*, April 9, 2010 (http://www.chinadaily.com.cn/opinion/2010-04/09/content_9708996.htm – accessed April 10, 2010).

Wu Meng. 2009. "Economic Strength Rising, but We Are Strangers," *Global Times*, September 16, (http://opinion.globaltimes.cn/observer/2009-09/468186.html – accessed September 17 2009).

Xinhua. 2009. "Road Accidents Kill Over 15,000 in the First Quarter," *China Daily*, May 4 (http://www.chinadaily.com.cn/china/2009-04/05/content_7650094.htm – accessed November 4, 2009).

Xinhua. 2010. "China's First Law on Online Games Takes Effect, *China Daily*, August 1 (http://www.chinadaily.com.cn/china/2010-08/01/content_11077080.htm – accessed August 1, 2010).

Xu Shenglan. 2009. "Bonus Inspires Independence," *Global Times*, September 10, 6.

Zan Jiefang. 2008. "Hooked on Cyberspace. Chinese Psychologists Outline Criteria for Internet Addiction," *Beijing Review*, December 16 (http://www.bjreview.com.cn/health/txt/20 08-12/16/content_170181.htm – accessed December 22, 2008).

Zhang Jiawei. 2010. "China's Middle Class Under Great Pressure," *China Daily*, April 22 (http://www.chinadaily.com.cn/china/2010-04/22/content_9762269.htm – accessed April 22, 2010).

Zhang Jin and Zuo Likun. 2010. "Quake Victims 'Psychologically Very Weak'," *China Daily*, April 17 (http://www.chinadaily.com.cn/china/qinghai/2010-04/17/content_9742729.htm – accessed April 17, 2010).

Zhe Zhe. 2008. "Internet Addiction Not Just 'Bad Habit'," *China Daily*, November 10 (http://www.chinadaily.com.cn/china/2008-11/10/content_7188303.htm – accessed November 13, 2008).

Index

abnormal 15, 18, 26, 32, 33, 34, 110, 165, 166; life 37, 84; looks 69, 72; situation 124, 127, 132; symptoms 29; thoughts 19
Age of excess 84
alcohol 54, 57, 83, 121, 144, 176, 198n, 205n
alcoholic 25, 35, 42, 45, 61, 174
alcoholism 26, 44, 174, 176
American Psychiatric Association 5, 10, 11, 33, 41, 46, 172, 196n, 207n, 208n
anxiety 40, 85, 87, 142, 165, 168, 169; consumerism and 141–2; depression and 68; drugs and 118; parents and 96–7, 133, 170, 204n; to relieve 44, 61, 73, 118; withdrawal and 41, 55
Aristotle 6, 77, 78
attribution 26, 103, 111, 116, 120, 121, 130, 173
authoritarian 8, 70, 72, 75, 80, 87, 92, 94
autonomy 91, 94, 150, 154; freedom and 131, 136; individuality and 89, 123, 130; sacrifice of 89; saving one's 129; to preserve one's 90

bad 52, 92, 118; behaviour 31, 120, 174; choices 174; education system 133; friends 70, 120, 177, 179; influence 60; people 14; sick and 31, 33, 34, 42, 57, 67
badness 33, 47, 64, 91, 152
Bakken, Børge 132, 160
Bakker, Keith 16–17
Bauman, Zygmunt 88, 91, 140–2, 182, 193n, 198n, 199n
behaviour: rectify 2, 19, 30, 34, 63, 148
being in the world 8, 53, 186n
Berners-Lee, Tim 37
biographical solutions (to social problems) 8, 81, 85, 94, 106, 129, 130, 180–1, 183–4

biomedical model 2, 5, 6, 9, 10, 16, 20, 46, 123, 165, 168
biopsychosocial 11, 52, 71, 193n
Blaszczynski, Alex 46, 53–4, 55, 60, 62

Cai Peng 117–18
canary in the coal mine 112
cancer 83–4, 198n
Castells, Manual 36
children of Mao 89, 93, 114, 137, 199n
children of the market 89, 91, 93, 94, 130–1, 137, 154
China Internet Network Information Center 137, 204n
Chinese Classification of Mental Disorders 32, 46
Chinese Communist Party (CCP) see also Party-State 30, 75, 137, 144, 182, 184, 200n, 204n; Cultural Revolution and 112; ideology of 76, 168; political strategy of 183; propaganda 142; socialism and 112; well-off society and 84, 140, 141
Chinese youth 84–5, 92–3, 143, 171, 180, 190n; as scape-goats 79; as vulnerable 29; as grade-making machines 82; individuation process and 130; internet and 27, 28, 61, 85, 111, 137, 181, 193n; middle-class 138; online gaming and 73, 89; personal power and 53, 109, 130, 132; search for freedom and 53; weak self control and 29
Christianity 18, 82, 163, 182
chronic stressors 20–1, 119, 167–8, 180, 188n
civil society 8, 183
classmates 100, 150, 160, 172, 182; as rivals 80, 153, 156; competing with 132; internet bar and 23, 27; relations with 118, 128, 155–6, 157, 159, 171

commodification: of the subject 86, 91, 134, 138–9, 140, 147–8, 151–2, 153
communication 16, 41, 59–60; breakdown of 21, 50, 87, 97, 104, 108, 148; lack of 180; reduced 39; skills 47; technology 37, 43, 187n; with parents 104, 106, 125, 148
competition 4, 103, 154, 175, 208n; as ethic 7, 75, 112, 132; between education system and gaming industry 108; mathematics 99, 102, 135; online gaming and 40, 75, 126, 132, 162–3; with classmates 132, 155, 156
conform i, 17, 33, 113
conformity 166, 174, 178, 199n; with outside directives 131; with peers 132
Conrad & Schneider 33
consumer 4, 51, 84, 113, 140–5, 195n, 199n; fashions 154; goods 114, 140; life 137, 138; love 137; revolutionaries 93; transformed into commodity 151
consumerism 17, 84, 140–5, 150, 193n, 199n
consumer-driven society 11, 84,138, 141, 163, 181
consumer revolution 84, 91–4, 137, 145, 204n
consuming love 135, 137, 145
Counter Strike 14, 73, 126, 132, 135
coping mechanism 61, 71, 77, 87, 171
Cover, Rob 54
Cultural Revolution 89, 93, 112, 114
culture of excess 6, 9, 80–6, 94, 100, 137, 181, 200n; intensification of life and 11, 111, 147; world out of balance and 94
cyberspace 43, 60, 69, 86, 124, 164, 168, 187n; as black hole 44; as space of equality 70; being a *laoda* in 153; internet bar and 13; migration to 71, 94, 112, 138, 154; search for freedom and 14, 111

Dalian 13, 73, 187n
danwei 87, 198n
Daoism 49, 134
death 123, 136, 165, 172, 180, 189n; as chronic stressor 20, 119; at military-style boot camp 50–2; attributed to internet addiction 82; cancer and 83; of a father 95, 119, 120; of a loved one 67, 167; premature 83; social 137; suicide and 82; thinking about 68, 70, 97, 119; workplace 28

Deng Fei 50–1, 52
Deng Senshan 50–2, 57
Deng Xiaoping 84, 141, 197n
deregulation 88, 129
dehumanization i, 7, 9, 38, 49, 73, 82, 94
depersonalization 147–53, 159, 168–9, 180, 204n; engulfment and 90, 95, 118, 123, 165
Derrrida, Jacques 79
desire: as a revolutionary force 178; for freedom 70, 109, 178; for power and domination 99, 101, 139, 154, 162; for the internet 41, 54; to avoid aloneness 53, 81, 108; to be part of a world outside oneself 8, 53, 72, 171; to be someone 7, 53, 138–9, 158; to become a *laoda* 153, 154; to blow off steam 6, 73; to excel others 99; to express one's individuality 53; to feel in control 57, 73, 153; to feel like a winner 53, 132, 139, 158; to inflate the ego 54, 101, 154, 158; to play online games 87, 96, 111, 178, 183
destruction 101–2, 106, 121, 135, 183
deviance 67, 100, 119, 131, 148, 166, 172, 174–5; internet use and 122; levels of 63, 65; space of 48
deviant youth 30, 42, 50, 79; social control and 30
devotion 31–2, 81, 123, 162, 184, 185, 197–8n, 205n; to online games /the internet 4, 12, 81, 85, 87, 102, 163, 185; to school work 4, 27, 85, 89, 115, 122, 137
diabetes 83
diagnosis 16, 30, 58, 65, 127
diagnostic model 34–9, 4; and time 34–7; and value judgment 34, 36
disobedient personality 119, 173, 207n
disorientation 82, 87
discipline 36, 85, 92, 127; control and 36, 39, 52, 74, 94, 103, 109; measures 5, 50, 78, 87, 103, 109, 124, 127, 131, 133, 170; military-style 18, 19, 34, 65, 68, 78, 178; punishment and 39, 50, 152, 87, 116, 152
domination 101–2, 108, 123, 136, 145, 183; over others 8, 135, 154, 162; power and 99
DSM-III (American Psychiatric Association's Diagnostic and Statistical Manual, Third Edition) 65–6
DSM-IV (American Psychiatric Association's Diagnostic and Statistical Manual, Fourth Edition) v, 5, 11, 22, 52, 65–8, 95, 100, 165–79, 180, 188n

DSM-V (American Psychiatric Association's Diagnostic and Statistical Manual, Fifth Edition) 5, 41, 65
Durkheim, Emile 36

economic development 8, 37, 39, 84, 112, 184
education system 16, 73, 74, 76, 103, 144, 150, 162, 172; competitive 7, 17, 60, 113, 148, 154; gaming industry and 4, 34, 108, 158, 162; online gaming and 77; rejection of 93; school grades and 100, 125, 133
ego 54, 64, 77
electric-shock treatment/electroshock therapy 1, 2, 31, 50, 137, 139, 181, 186n
electronic opium i, 3, 24, 44, 49, 79, 129, 188n
Elias, Norbert 71, 72–4, 77, 93–4
Elias & Dunning 39, 74, 154–5
escaping reality 7, 76, 93, 160, 161, 182–3
estrangement 153, 156–7, 159, 182
ethics 8, 56, 75, 129, 135, 185; capitalist 75, 87, 92; dominant 7, 123; work 92, 112
EverQuest 35, 53, 72, 105, 108, 200n
exam *see also gaokao* 3, 151, 155, 159, 174; grade 2, 115, 125, 150, 152, 159; preparing for 73, 103, 150; pressure of 40, 95, 165
exchange value 39–40, 60, 90, 134, 150, 177; internet use and 50; school grades and 7; use value and 8, 39, 91, 112, 147, 151–2
excitement 73–4, 77–8, 129; gambling and 55; of the internet 24, 43, 64; online gaming and 4, 93, 106, 162, 163, 164; quest for 154–5
existential needs 11, 53, 61, 84–6, 105, 146, 181–4; economic development and 8; online gaming and 6
existential trophies 7, 139
expectable response 68, 100, 139, 177, 179; or unexpectable response 28; to a stress condition 67, 100, 167–8, 171, 172–3, 175, 188n

facelessness 15, 70, 72, 138, 171
family war-machine 91, 93, 116, 121–2, 141, 145, 147; beginning of 111; ideal type and 97; over internet use 108, 114, 130

fan gan (*see also* rebellious psychology) 5, 94, 105, 122, 130, 133, 155, 159; as oppositional defiant disorde117; confinement and 104; depersonalization and 147; engulfment and 90, 124, 131, 133; internet bar and 21; strategies 114, 120; violence and 121
fantasy 8, 43, 54, 60, 62, 74, 158
fa xie 6, 73, 76, 106, 131, 133, 148, 160, 170, 184
fear 137, 147, 148, 150, 164, 177, 180, 204n, 205n; of authority 119; of internet gaming 150; of love 146; of the real world 80; of the stranger 14; parental 4, 48, 50, 51, 52, 86, 91, 133, 134, 151
filiarchy 7, 89, 113–16, 119, 139, 153, 186n, 204n
Foxconn 28, 38, 58
freedom 70, 87, 107–10, 122, 131, 145, 146, 153; from authority and control 8, 87, 92, 94, 108, 109, 112, 115, 157; from discrimination 72; from engulfment 133; from primary ties 87, 107–8, 122, 132; from school 116; individual/personal 4, 54, 86, 87, 89, 104, 107, 109, 130; of the internet 90, 123 satisfaction and 69, 70, 79–80, 91; search for 4, 14, 53, 87, 92, 95, 113, 122, 129, 178; struggle for 101, 130, 154; suppression of 87, 108, 110, 111
Freudian psychoanalysis 66
Fromm, Erich 9, 81–91, 101–2, 121, 132–3, 142–3, 161; existential needs 183–5; domination and destruction 135, 183; filiarchy 113; frame for orientation and devotion 123; individuation process 107, 128; loneliness 105; love 145–6; marketing orientation 151; pathology of normalcy 6, 180–1; receptive orientation 144; sane society 184; thwarted life 8, 154, 183–4
Funk, McKenzie 68
future 3, 113, 134, 155, 156, 174, 184; child's successful 4, 134, 136, 147; development 39; exchange value 152; in gaming 126, 134

gaming industry 4, 34, 79, 92, 112, 143, 202n, 218n
gambling addiction 26, 42, 46, 52–3, 55, 64, 144

gaokao (college entrance examination) 40, 108, 136, 152, 153, 155, 156, 174
gold farmer 40, 164, 175, 192n
grade-making machine 7, 82, 90, 100, 118, 136, 153, 172, 174, 180; depersonalization and 124, 133, 147, 149, 150
gratification 137, 140, 141,158, 193n
Griffiths, Mark 32, 46, 53–6, 57–8, 59, 60, 61–3, 71, 77

happiness 52, 84–6, 89, 114, 130, 140–3, 182, 203n; extreme 2, 4; freedom and 70; gaming and 106, 130, 134, 158, 160, 161; genuine 51; love and 145; medication and 135; reduced feelings of 38, 39, 79, 166, 167; self-realization and 7, 8, 94; with life 90, 149
harmonious society 94
hearts and minds 4, 34, 89, 144, 154
Hewett, Duncan 8
Horwitz, Allan 65–7
Huang He 1–2, 50, 80, 137, 139, 162, 171
Huawei 27
Huizinga, Johan 98–9
Hu Jintao 30
hurried existence 103, 111, 132, 151, 185
hyperculture 109–12, 132, 174
hypertension 83

ideal type 10, 97, 119, 120, 124, 135, 154, 170
individual pathology 9, 48, 79, 112, 122, 142; DSM and 66; internet addiction as 3, 16, 95; pathology of normalcy and 81
individualization 87–8, 110, 129–30, 198n, 199n
individuation 113; process 86–7, 107–9, 111, 122, 128, 129–30, 132, 138
information pollution 6, 29, 30, 76, 96
intensive internet use 11, 37, 63, 101–2, 123, 130, 154, 179, 193n; loneliness and 105; model 2, 5, 10, 69; ontological insecurity and 122; time and 39; underlying mechanisms of 180
intensive gaming 11, 93, 101, 165, 168; as critique of *status quo* 92; producing interpersonal problems 61; push factors of 90, 154; the family and 95
internal dysfunction 34, 67, 68, 72, 100, 139, 158, 172–5, 178–9
internet: as a monastery/sanctuary 70, 105, 131; attraction towards 14, 91, 153, 160, 162, 171, 188n; penetration rate and 137–8; preoccupation towards 5, 41, 54–5

internet bar 13–15, 18, 24, 108, 126, 174, 178, 187n; as a kind of monastery/ sanctuary 49, 90, 101, 123, 130; as a poison/toxin 49, 116; as social conduit 143; as a space of deviance 48–9, 116; attraction of 12, 70; autonomy and 130; hangout out at 12, 23, 27, 120, 121; happiness and 134; physical structure of 13; sneaking off to 97, 135, 136, 145, 148, 171; thinking about 34; time and 13, 125, 167; time spent at 26, 87, 108, 133
'internet addict': as product of reform- period 11, 40, 82, 84, 91, 93, 142, 144, 160, 180–1; as scapegoat 79; bullying and 16; death of parent and 95, 104, 119, 120, 123–4, 165, 166, 167, 172; hospitalization of 30, 169, 173, 176; isolation of 16, 105; mental illness and 29, 33, 58, 118, 166, 169, 170, 173; parent's occupation and 117–18; social transformation and 18–19, 61, 111–12; troubled social existence of 16, 18, 63, 69–70, 119–20, 165, 167–8, 172, 180; weak self control and 43, 44, 103, 117, 171, 177, 178; visualization of 28–9, 33–4, 43, 168–9, 173, 176
'internet addiction': abuse and 50, 52, 60, 65, 66; agency and 17; aggression and 7, 29, 32, 109, 112, 120–1, 133; alcohol use and 57; alcoholism and 26, 44 176; alcoholic and 25, 35, 42, 45, 61; alleviation of negative emotions and 41, 61–3; attribution and 103, 120, 173, 177, 200n; Christianity and 18, 82, 182; compulsivity and 37, 44, 71, 142; crime and 26, 32; criteria of 34–45, 46, 52–3, 58, 64, 66–7, 68, 167, 179; deception and 23, 33, 41, 63–4, 65, 169, 170, 173; dependence and 43, 44, 60, 62, 64–5, 134, 135; diagnostic model and 34–5, 67, 68, 167–8, 170, 173, 175, 178; drug use and 54, 64; drug addiction and 26, drug addict and 6, 26, 42, 45, 55, 144; gambling and 16, 30, 41, 44, 45, 46, 53, 55, 57, 64; gambling addiction/ addict and 6, 26, 42, 52, 64, 144; habit and 26, 53, 56, 64, 138; harmful consequences and 41, 42, 49–50, 57–8, 64, 76, 92, 166; harming social

functioning and 10, 37–42, 47, 59, 85;
high levels of engagement and 52, 54,
64; impaired control and 55; loss of
social communications and interests
and 41, 59; medication and 30, 168,
181; mining and 26; misuse of 60, 65;
negative reinforcement and 62; normal
functioning of society and 6, 8, 11,
28–9, 34, 40, 68, 171, 178; positive
reinforcement and 62; preoccupation
and 5, 41, 44, 52, 54–5, 79; reliability
and 10, 37, 41, 45, 57, 64–5, 66–7;
social characteristics and 36, 105,
118; stigmatization and 18, 86; suicide
and 27, 82; time and 8, 26, 29, 34–7,
39–40, 43, 52, 59–60, 64, 112, 158,
175, 176; tolerance and 41, 55–6, 64;
value judgment and 34, 36, 40, 59, 60,
64, 158, 175; withdrawal and 24–5,
34, 41, 55, 58, 64, 118, 169–70, 177,
182, 194n, 205n; as epidemic 2, 44; as
escape from reality 11, 61, 70, 71, 80,
168, 182–3; as impulse-control 41–2,
47, 56–7, 62; as mental disorder 5, 11,
21, 22, 26, 28–9, 30, 32, 34, 46, 65–8,
118, 165–79, 180, 188n; as mental
illness 11, 18, 19, 28, 47, 96, 102,
150; effects of 25, 26, 58, 65; signs of
5, 10, 24, 42–3, 45, 61, 62, 170, 182;
symptoms of 5, 10, 38, 44–5, 53, 63,
64, 65, 68, 166–71, 179
internet addiction narrative 21, 96
internet addiction disorder *see also*
    Young-Tao model 20, 40, 41, 45, 60,
    63, 65, 67, 68, 167, 179; accepting
    48; as individual pathology 3, 166;
    as social tool 178; biomedical-based
    2, 42–3; catching 36; dehumanistic
    9; medication and 168; misuse of 50;
    value judgment and 71
internet addiction phenomenon 2, 4, 7, 8,
    28, 36, 63, 79, 154; as moral panic 48,
    92; parental fear and 50; underlying
    mechanisms of 81, 86, 88, 115
internet information addiction 56
internet trading addiction 56
internet use *see also* online gaming:
    autonomy and 90, 91, 94, 123, 129,
    130, 136, 154; belonging and 15,
    17, 18, 157, 158, 163; expression of
    feelings and 15, 69–70, 77–8, 80, 106,
    152; facelessness and 15, 171; freedom
    and 69, 70, 89, 90, 92, 108, 109–11,
    115, 116, 153, 157; friendship and 14,

59–60, 69, 70, 72, 137, 160–1, 163;
loneliness and 68, 73, 103, 105, 157,
159, 162–4; positive effects and 58, 59,
80; relatedness and 15, 18, 123, 157–8,
160–1, 163, 181; role of government
and 27, 112, 141; role of marketplace
and 27, 142, 144; satisfaction and 41,
44, 52, 54, 55–6, 60, 64, 70, 79–80,
158; security and 106, 112, 136;
venting pressure and 52; as detrimental
to schoolwork 50, 59, 60, 172; as
remedy 42, 73, 106, 169, 171, 182;
controlling 3, 35, 57, 71, 103, 116, 171;
socially problematic 2, 3, 6, 9, 10, 11,
19, 33, 74, 82, 88, 119
interpersonal relations 21, 51, 91, 100,
148, 150, 15; depersonalization and
149; parent–child 60, 89, 108, 128;
with parents 17; with peers 10; within
the family 2, 7, 49, 90, 94
intrapersonal 42, 50, 71, 129, 148, 164;
lifeworld 2; factors 11, 176;
changes 87
introverted personality 24, 25, 27, 29,
100, 149, 173–4, 177

Jiang Zemin 75, 76

karaoke 14, 73, 74
Kleinman, Arthur 21

label: attaching 20; rejection of 18
labeled: addicted to online games 61; an
    addict 35; an internet addict 2, 8, 9, 11,
    12, 13, 18, 52, 68, 95, 112; as mentally
    disordered 88, 170, 171; randomly 100
labeling 26, 68, 93, 102, 110, 166, 169,
    179; behaviour an addiction 60
Laing, R.D. 7, 9, 30, 89–90, 101, 123,
    128–9, 145, 148, 150, 156, 168, 205n
laoda 80, 139, 153, 158, 162, 200n;
    becoming a 101, 154; effect 7, 161
leisure 4, 19, 37, 89, 146; activity 39, 77,
    136, 139, 148, 155, 162; internet use
    for 35, 36, 50; life of 85; pursuits 4, 77,
    113, 139, 144, 172; time 113; use value
    and 8, 60; work and 4, 71, 72–4, 93,
    116, 134, 175
letters 20–2; letter-6 97–8; letter-13
    124–6; manager Chen's 95–6; Xiao
    Chuan's 2–3; Xiao Kang's 154–64;
    Xiao Wang's 23–4, 69–70
living out of balance 6, 83, 85, 112,
    153, 171

loneliness 73, 105, 106, 164; experiencing 155, 156; feelings of 157, 162–3; overcoming 159; within the child 96
love 108, 120, 165; as behavioural addiction 41; chained 4–5, 90, 130, 147, 153, 206n; deathly 90, 130–1, 137, 145, 153; dominating 146; engulfing 7, 89, 95, 124, 128, 131, 136, 147; excessive 134–5, 146, 147; for the child 89, 100, 119, 146, 147; lack of 16, 20, 63, 168; misdirected 150; of consumption 136–7, 138, 144, 145; oneself 17, 130, 139; parents 31; productive 145, 146; selfish 134
LSD 54, 92

maladjustment 6, 81, 166, 167
Maoism 87, 89, 93, 160, 182
Maoist-era 87, 111
Mao Zedong 19, 112
market orientation 90, 147, 151, 184
Marx, Karl 19
massively multiplayer online role-playing games (MMORPGs) 55, 72, 74, 76
materialism 11, 17, 85, 88, 136, 140–1, 182, 183
McNeal, James 113
me generation 109–10, 154
medical crusader 28, 33, 48, 82, 139, 178
medicalization 30–1, 33, 65, 68, 78, 93, 135, 165, 168–9, 170, 190n
medicine/medication 30, 65, 68, 135, 168, 169, 170, 190n
mental/mentally diseased 3, 28, 30, 33,42, 179, 189n
mental disorder 21, 28–9, 47–8, 65–8, 93, 165–79, 189n, 208n; classification of a 32, 67, 188n; definition of a 5, 11, 22, 64, 65, 95; legitimate 26, 46; suffering from a 34, 118; valid 67, 68, 180
mental illness 18, 47–8, 57, 72, 96, 150, 183; *DSM-III* and 65–6; internet addiction and 11,19, 28
methodology 9, 12–13
military-style boot camp 18, 19, 21, 23, 30–31, 84, 105, 170; abuse and 50–2; as a panacea 51, 57; parents and 18, 50–1, 97, 115, 130; punishment and 44
mimic/mimetic 73, 74, 75, 77, 78, 103
Ministry of Culture 18, 76
Ministry of Health 50, 63
moral crisis 79, 184

moral entrepreneur 28, 33, 48, 82, 139, 178, 191n
moral panic 28, 44, 48, 50, 54, 57, 92, 112
motivation 5, 7, 34, 41, 42, 43, 54, 55, 71, 93, 109, 173

netizen 13, 15, 112, 153
normal functioning of society 4, 29, 34, 37, 76, 85, 87, 109, 127, 162, 180–1, 182; adhering to the 89; adjusting to the 171; as bringing suffering 40, 94; cutting oneself off from the 8, 130, 134; dealing with the 47, 106; existential needs and 11; going against the 68, 99; internet addiction and 6; isolated from 12; online games and 74; pressure from the 135; questioning the 112; submit to the 94; rejecting the 178; removed from the 26

obedience 5, 18, 51, 57, 75, 120, 135, 152, 170
obsessive-compulsive disorder 68
one-child policy 17, 88
online gaming *see also* internet use: as poison 3; as remedy 31, 77–8, 79, 82, 94, 129, 153, 160, 164; as competitive skill-based activity 54, 75, 132, 162; being enthralled in 96, 149, 155, 156, 157–8; being infatuated with 96, 111, 124, 125, 126, 127, 134; being intoxicated with 159; capitalist ethics and 112, 123, 132, 139, 144, 158; cathartic effect and 77–8; creation of tension and 77; economic development and 37, 112, 132, 141–2; exchange value and 40, 50, 60; feelings of superiority and 70, 80, 101, 123, 139, 154, 155, 160, 161, 162–3; friendship and 14, 60, 63, 70, 105, 120, 121, 157, 158, 159, 160–3, gaining respect and 157, 158, 159; happiness and 134, 158, 160, 161; morality and 76–7; personalized meanings and 54, 77, 80; prior negative emotions and 17, 73, 77–8; satisfaction 108, 123, 130, 136, 157–61; sense of achievement and 101, 103, 108, 130, 136, 158, 161, 177; science and 74, 76, 159, 161–2; self-esteem and 72, 139, 157, 158, 160, 161, 162; spirituality and 73; team play and 14, 72, 105, 160–1, 162; time loss and 59, 64; violence and 32

online pornography addiction 56
ontological insecurity 101, 122, 134, 148, 153, 154, 200n
opening up and reform 82, 83, 87–8, 90, 91, 112, 142, 160
opium: addict 2, 24, 25; den 3, 48–9, 149, 163
oppositional defiant disorder 117, 118
orientation and devotion 81, 123, 184, 185, 197n, 205n

parents: absent 20, 95, 115, 116, 117, 119, 121, 150, 165, 180; chained love 4–5, 90, 147, 153; deathly love 90, 130, 131, 134–5, 137, 145–7, 153; depersonalization and 90, 95, 118, 133, 147–53, 159, 165, 180; distress and 170-1; divorce 95, 148–9, 180; engulfing love 124, 128, 131, 136, 147; engulfment 7, 17, 89, 90, 95, 117, 127–32, 133, 134, 136, 146, 165, 180; expectations 57, 100, 132, 135, 151, 155, 164, 174; fear 48, 50, 51, 52, 86, 91, 134, 147, 150, 151; material rewards and 4, 88, 89, 115, 127, 135–6, 141, 142, 152, 153; neglect 5, 20, 116, 117, 120–1, 131, 148–9, 159, 165, 168, 180; over-investment 90, 95, 115, 124, 128, 165; pressure to conform 17, 113, 115, 135, 139, 152; problematic educational methods 17, 63, 111, 116–20, 131, 133; problematic socialization methods (17, 91, 103, 111, 116–20, 137, 145,156; school grades and 7, 17, 89, 90, 96–7, 100, 127–8, 131, 133, 146, 149, 150; violence 4, 20, 32, 63, 87, 91, 95, 96, 104–5, 116, 117, 127, 133, 168, 171, 180
Party-State *see also* CCP 11, 75, 76, 84, 87, 93, 111–12, 188n; capitalist reforms and 81; economic development and 8; internet and 70, 72; media and 48
pathology of normalcy 6–7, 8–84, 103, 141, 178, 184, 185, 206n; as the normal functioning of society 94, 127, 180; culture of excess and 9; detaching from 90; freedom from 86; resisting 86; saving oneself from 154
People's Liberation Army (PLA) 18, 19, 25, 30
Perfect World 14, 146, 153, 181, 187n; as a metaphor 14
pharmakon 6, 78–9, 94

pleasure 134; consumerism and 19, 137, 143; online gaming and 6, 40, 77, 154, 160, 161, 162, 164; the internet and 6, 7, 78, 91, 151, 193n
poison 40, 96, 136; internet bar as 49; online games as 6, 7, 31, 92; remedy and 73, 78–80, 94, 106, 129
post-1980s generation 88, 89, 93, 109, 111, 112, 137
pride 80, 104, 115, 121, 156
primary ties 86–7, 107–8, 113, 122, 132, 201n
privatization 88, 129
professional gamer 40, 99, 134, 136, 164, 175, 192n, 208n
psychological needs 183–4
pull factors 5, 7, 17, 52, 57, 70, 91, 108, 91, 108, 123, 154, 161
push factors 7, 70, 90, 91, 123, 130, 150, 154

QQ 15, 72, 78, 143, 146, 171, 181, 187n
quick-fix 51, 193n
quest for excitement 74, 154–5

rebel 79, 90, 129, 130, 159, 164; cultural 69; going against social norms 67, 68; with a cause 42, 86
rebellion 21 92, 93, 94, 128, 150
rebellious 29, 79, 88, 117, 165, 177; journey 92; psychology 90, 126, 131, 135, 170; youth 89
Red Guards 89, 93
reliability 64, 65, 66–7
remedy 77, 78–9, 109; internet as 42, 73, 80, 106, 169, 177, 182; online gaming as 6, 31, 94, 129, 153, 160; poison and 6
Renfei 12–15, 73, 76, 106, 137, 150, 187n, 207n
resistance: and rebellion 92, 94, 104, 116, 117, 121; engulfing love and 128; punishment producing 105
resistant 5, 29, 33, 88, 104 133
revenge 183
road accidents 28
rootedness 81, 107, 163, 184, 185, 205n

sacrifice 4, 79, 89, 114, 130, 136, 145, 153–4
SARS 2, 43
scapegoat 79
school stabbings 183

scientific outlook on development 76, 163, 168
search for happiness 134, 141–2, 203n
self: preserving autonomy of 7, 123, 129, 130, 149, 150, 154; inflation of 6, 54, 77, 80, 101, 139, 154, 157, 158, 163; maintenance of 6, 77, 80, 129; survival of 6, 71, 77, 101, 105, 123, 128, 131, 154, 164
self control 17, 73, 111, 134, 151, 173n; weak 5, 29, 43, 96, 102, 103, 117, 134, 177
self-preservation 123, 129, 156–7
self-realisation 7, 8, 51, 86, 94
sexual revolution 83
Shandong Healthy Internet Training Base 18, 99, 106, 206n
shopaholism 142
sick18, 81, 116, 119, 168; bad and 31, 33–4, 42, 47, 57, 64, 67; pathologically 3; society 80, 81–2, 168, 184–5; youths 30
Skinner, B.F. 62, 175–6, 178, 195n
Skinner-box 175–6, 178
social Darwinism 132, 206n
social existence 2, 3, 9, 10, 28, 69, 156, 181, 184; disordered 7, 16, 79
social expectations 34, 42, 47, 57, 64, 70, 85, 184
social functioning 7, 37–9, 47–8, 50, 59, 72, 79, 8
social transformation 6, 8, 12, 19, 61, 77, 171, 182
socialism with Chinese characteristics 75, 139
socially problematic internet use 2, 3, 6, 10, 19, 33, 74, 88, 119
solitary confinement 51, 57, 104–5, 109
spiritual needs 49, 81, 84–5, 103, 180, 182, 183, 185
spiritual nourishment 81, 182, 185, 209n
spoilt 88, 89, 111, 114, 117, 203n
stranger 14, 15, 80, 181–2; fear of 14
stubborn personality 104, 115–16
suicide 27–8, 38, 81–2
Sun Hualin 49
suzhi (quality) 16

Tai Zixue 8
Tao Hongkai 5, 9, 19, 31, 79, 97, 151, 174, 179; consumerism and 17, 144; education system and 16, 17; letters written to 10, 20, 21, 23, 69, 95; parenting and 16, 17, 99–100, 101–2,

111, 133–5, 136–7, 145, 146, 170; quality education (*suzhi jiaoyu*) and 15, 17, 170; work history and 15, 18
Tao Ran 9, 16, 17, 25, 30, 44, 48, 53, 58, 79, 80, 108–9; as moral crusader 33, 178; as moral entrepreneur 33, 178; confession letters and 31, 99; diagnostic model and 34–42, 59, 68, 166, 167, 170; electric-shock treatment and 31; exchange value and 39–40; ex-patients and 31, 182; force-feeding medication and 31, 68, 168, 170, 173; individual pathology and 16, 118, 166, 173; medicalization and 33–4, 46, 118–19, 131, 165, 168–9; on physiological effects of internet addiction 25, 57–8, 118, 166, 169; patient's troubled social existence 16, 63, 71, 165, 167–8; professional background 25; traditional Chinese medical theory and 30; visualization of internet addict 28–9, 80, 173, 176
tension 55, 73, 77–8, 94, 129; creation of 6, 73, 7; loosening of 6, 76, 77, 118
thwarted life 2, 9, 101, 122, 135, 154, 183
tiger-and-mouse phenomenon 101, 104, 115, 123, 153–4, 155, 157, 180, 204n
time: experience of 13, 36–7; loss of 59, 64; wasting 8, 29, 39, 43, 96, 112, 158
transcendence 81, 123, 163, 184, 185, 205n
treatment centre 19, 23, 25, 30, 44, 50, 60, 79, 86, 170
Turkle, Sherry 13
Turner, Nigel 46, 53, 62
turn on, boot up, log in 92, 94, 103, 137

unobtainium 140–1

valid 5, 10, 32, 41, 45, 54, 67, 68, 165, 167
validity 11, 36, 37, 52, 53, 63, 64, 65, 66
violence 32, 100, 148, 160, 165, 180; as method of conflict resolution 105–6; between parents 120–1; parental 4, 16, 32, 63, 87, 116, 117, 119, 133, 168, 171; Red Guards and 93; symbolic 4, 100, 117, 121, 127, 133; war-machine and 4, 91
Virilio, Paul 36–7
volition 5, 43

wangyin see also internet addiction i, 2, 4, 19
wang zi cheng long 17, 136 204n

well-off society (*xiaokang shehui*) 84, 140, 141, 142
Wen Jiabao 140
Wood, Richard. T.A. 46, 48, 52, 53, 54, 55, 56, 57, 59, 61, 62
World Cyber Games 92, 99, 192n, 208n
World Health Organization (WHO) 46, 47; definition of mental disorders 47–8, 64
World of Warcraft 12, 14, 55, 62, 75, 76, 78, 81, 146, 153
world-out-of-balance 70, 80, 94, 160, 171, 184
Wu Zengqiang 29, 34

use value 7, 8, 39, 60, 91, 112, 147, 152, 177

videogame addiction 45

Xiao Chuan 2–7
Xiao Kang 6, 11, 77, 154–64, 171, 177
Xiao Liang 124–35
Xiao Wang 23–4, 25, 26, 27, 29, 32, 34, 43, 57, 69–70, 71, 72, 79

Yang Xiong 88, 109, 181
Yang Yongxin 1–2, 50, 82, 137, 139, 178
youth: crime and 3; existential trophies and 139; individualising 4, 130; transforming 4, 109–10, 112
Young, Kimberly 42–4, 46, 48, 53, 71
Young-Tao Model 5, 44–5, 52–67, 69, 71, 72, 167; bias toward exchange value 90; *DSM-IV* and 165; harming social functioning and 85; main pillars of 10

Zhang Chunliang 48–9
Zhang Jiangguo 29, 34

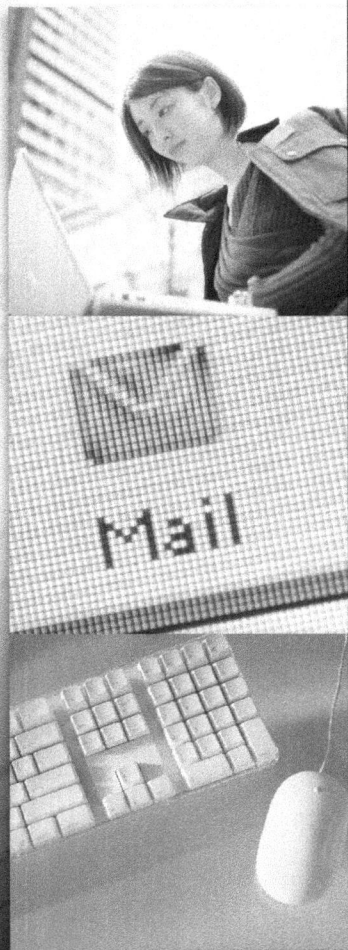

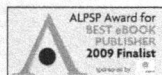

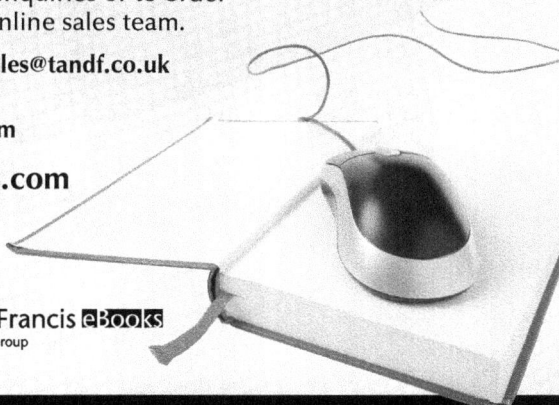

For Product Safety Concerns and Information please contact our EU
representative GPSR@taylorandfrancis.com
Taylor & Francis Verlag GmbH, Kaufingerstraße 24, 80331 München, Germany

www.ingramcontent.com/pod-product-compliance
Lightning Source LLC
Chambersburg PA
CBHW062019270326
41929CB00014B/2260